Pharmacy: Science and Technology

Pharmacy: Science and Technology

Editor: Corey Harrelson

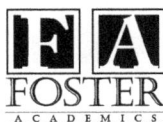

FA FOSTER
A C A D E M I C S

www.fosteracademics.com

www.fosteracademics.com

FA
FOSTER
ACADEMICS

Cataloging-in-Publication Data

Pharmacy : science and technology / edited by Corey Harrelson.
    p. cm.
Includes bibliographical references and index.
ISBN 978-1-63242-830-1
1. Pharmacy. 2. Drugs. 3. Materia medica. 4. Pharmacology. I. Harrelson, Corey.
RS153 .P43 2019
615--dc23

Foster Academics,
118-35 Queens Blvd., Suite 400,
Forest Hills, NY 11375, USA

ISBN 978-1-63242-830-1 (Hardback)

Contents

Preface

The science and technique associated with the preparation and distribution of drugs is known as pharmacy. It acts as a link between health sciences and chemical sciences. Its main goal is to ensure the safety and efficacy of pharmaceutical drugs. The health professionals involved in the practice of pharmacy are called pharmacists or chemists. They are experts in drug therapy. The main sub-disciplines of pharmacy include pharmaceutics, medicinal chemistry, pharmacognosy, pharmacy practice, pharmacology and pharmacoinformatics. Biochemical mechanisms and action of drugs, therapeutic effects, potential drug interactions, etc. are important focus areas of pharmaceutical sciences. This book provides significant information of this discipline to help develop a good understanding of pharmacy and related fields. The various sub-fields of pharmacy along with technological progress that have future implications are glanced at in it. As this field is emerging at a rapid pace, the contents of this book will help the readers understand the modern concepts and applications of the subject.

This book has been the outcome of endless efforts put in by authors and researchers on various issues and topics within the field. The book is a comprehensive collection of significant researches that are addressed in a variety of chapters. It will surely enhance the knowledge of the field among readers across the globe.

It gives us an immense pleasure to thank our researchers and authors for their efforts to submit their piece of writing before the deadlines. Finally in the end, I would like to thank my family and colleagues who have been a great source of inspiration and support.

Editor

Implementation of Competency-Based Pharmacy Education (CBPE)

Andries Koster [1],*, Tom Schalekamp [2] and Irma Meijerman [3]

[1] Department of Pharmaceutical Sciences, Utrecht University, The Netherlands and European Association of Faculties of Pharmacy (EAFP), Utrecht 3508 TB, The Netherlands

[2] Department of Pharmaceutical Sciences, Utrecht University, Utrecht 3508 TB, The Netherlands; T.Schalekamp@uu.nl

[3] Department of Pharmaceutical Sciences, The Netherlands and Centre for Teaching and Learning, Utrecht University, Utrecht 3508 TB, The Netherlands; I.Meijerman@uu.nl

* Correspondence: A.S.Koster@uu.nl

Academic Editor: Jeffrey Atkinson

Abstract: Implementation of competency-based pharmacy education (CBPE) is a time-consuming, complicated process, which requires agreement on the tasks of a pharmacist, commitment, institutional stability, and a goal-directed developmental perspective of all stakeholders involved. In this article the main steps in the development of a fully-developed competency-based pharmacy curriculum (bachelor, master) are described and tips are given for a successful implementation. After the choice for entering into CBPE is made and a competency framework is adopted (step 1), intended learning outcomes are defined (step 2), followed by analyzing the required developmental trajectory (step 3) and the selection of appropriate assessment methods (step 4). Designing the teaching-learning environment involves the selection of learning activities, student experiences, and instructional methods (step 5). Finally, an iterative process of evaluation and adjustment of individual courses, and the curriculum as a whole, is entered (step 6). Successful implementation of CBPE requires a system of effective quality management and continuous professional development as a teacher. In this article suggestions for the organization of CBPE and references to more detailed literature are given, hoping to facilitate the implementation of CBPE.

Keywords: assessment; competence; competency-based education; constructive alignment; curriculum; development; entrustable professional activity; learning outcomes

1. Introduction

If you want to grow a worthwhile plant: a rose, a fruit tree, a vine of paan, then you need effort.

You must water, apply manure, weed it, prune it.

It is not simple.

So it is with the world.

Vikram Seth: A suitable boy

National and international tendencies indicate that competency-based educational models are becoming dominant for the education of heath care professionals, such as nursing [1], dentistry [2], medicine [3], and pharmacy [4,5]. The main driver for adopting competency-based educational designs is the need to prepare pharmacists for their societal role, ultimately leading to improvement of health care and patient safety [6–9]. However, implementation of a competency-base pharmacy curriculum is a formidable task, in particular if an existing curriculum is organized in a disciplinary, content-driven, teacher-centered way, in which students are expected to mainly attend lectures and to perform in well-structured practical exercises reproducing compounding and analytical tasks as described in national formularies of pharmacopoeias. Even though this description of a 'traditional' curriculum can be considered stereotypical, most readers will recognize elements of this description in their local pharmacy curricula. An additional problem in developing a pharmacy curriculum is the recent change in the tasks of the pharmacist, which, during the last decades, has shown a shift from product-orientation to more patient-orientation (FIP 2012, [4]). Transforming a 'traditional' educational practice into competency-based pharmacy education (CBPE), which pays attention to both the science-based and patient-oriented aspects of pharmacy in a balanced way, will involve re-thinking of the roles of teachers, the roles of students, and re-designing of assessment tasks and many educational activities [10,11]. Moreover, a pharmacy department or faculty is usually organized along disciplines ranging from medicinal chemistry, via biopharmacy to pharmacotherapeutics and social pharmacy. It is, therefore, necessary to create a curriculum management structure and a human resources allocation model, which may interfere or conflict with existing hierarchies and research interests.

This paper describes the essential steps in designing a competency-based pharmacy curriculum and gives tips for a successful organization, development, and implementation of such curricula. Suggestions will be based on literature references whenever possible, but will also be 'colored' by the authors' experiences with implementing new curricula in the field of pharmacy and pharmaceutical sciences [12,13]. Readers should be aware that the possibility to make radical changes in existing curricula depend heavily on the local situation, in particular with respect to the experienced need for change, the preparedness to embark on a complicated journey, and the willingness of the formal departmental and/or university structure to support and facilitate the change process. The experiences of the authors are 'colored' by the way a curriculum renewal was handled in a positive and stimulating way by the departmental leadership (cf. [14]). It is, therefore, uncertain whether all aspects, which refer to the authors' own experiences, can be easily implemented in other environments. Nevertheless, we hope that this article can be a guide in starting an interesting journey towards competency-based pharmacy education (CBPE).

2. Competency-Based Pharmacy Education

The attention for competency-based pharmacy education is relatively recent, compared to other health care professional programs. The American Association of Colleges of Pharmacy has pioneered the development of educational outcome-based guidelines since the early 1990s (AACP 2013, [10]) and a global competency framework was published by the International Pharmaceutical Federation more recently (FIP 2012, [4]). Descriptions of the entry-into-practice requirements for professional pharmacists are available for Canada (AFPC 2010), the United Kingdom (GPhC 2011), Australia (NCSF 2010 [15]), and Europe (EPCF 2016, [9]). These descriptions can be based on different models and may have more or less official legal status, but they all intend to function as guiding principles for the evaluation and 're-engineering' of existing curricula and the design and development of new curricula. The requirements for entry-level pharmacists are usually defined in terms of learning outcomes or competencies and are ordered on the basis of Miller's pyramid of clinical competence [16]. The diversity of frameworks (see Appendix A) illustrates that no 'golden standard' for a competency framework exists. As long as the framework is internally consistent and captures all aspects of the required professional competence, it can be used as a tool for the analysis, development, and structuring of a curriculum. Existing frameworks for pharmacy education appear to be similar across jurisdictions [17] and health care competency frameworks in general appear to address the same aspects of professional competence. The use of competency standards for undergraduate pharmacy education was recently reviewed by Nash et al. [5].

Apart from competency frameworks covering the complete initial Pharmacy higher education program, competency profiles have been developed for separate curriculum domains, e.g., advanced pharmacy practice [18], professional development skills [19], or related specialization areas, such as clinical pharmacology [20] or pharmaceutical medicine [21].

3. Terminology and Definitions

The implementation of CBPE is often complicated by concepts and terminology, which is experienced as ill-defined or confusing [22,23]. Medical competence is defined as "The array of abilities across multiple domains or aspects of physician performance in a certain context. Statements about competence require descriptive qualifiers to define the relevant abilities, context, and stage of training. Competence is multi-dimensional and dynamic. It changes with time, experience, and setting" (cited from [3], (p. 641)). We suggest that the same definition can be used for other health care professionals, including pharmacists, by changing the use of 'physician' into any other relevant professional job description.

The definition of competence makes clear that competence of a student or pharmacist can only be observed or assessed in the context of specific well-defined circumstances. Being competent in one professional situation does not necessarily imply competence in another situation (competence is *contextual*), and students need time to become competent in different aspects of their intended profession (competence is *developmental*). Moreover, it is highly unlikely that all students can acquire competence at the same rate and with the same amount of training provided; large inter-individual differences are usually encountered. Finally, competence is only demonstrated when all relevant knowledge, skills, and behavior is used in an integrated way which is relevant in a particular professional situation (competence is *multidimensional*). The contextual, developmental, and multidimensional nature of the competence to be achieved by a curriculum has important consequences for the organization of CBPE, in particular with respect to assessment and progression of students through the curriculum [3,24].

An approach to deal with the complex nature of CBPE is to use *entrustable professional activities* (EPAs) for the operationalization of educational outcomes at the transition of undergraduate education to professional working life. EPAs are carefully described aspects of professional acting, respecting the contextual and developmental aspects of competence, which are used to structure learning, training, and assessment of starting professionals enrolled in medical specialization programs [23]. By proposing the use of EPAs as a way of structuring medical education at an earlier stage, the undergraduate curriculum, medical educators intend to ease the abrupt transition from undergraduate to graduate education [24]. In this conception, undergraduate education, entry into professional life, further specialization, and postgraduate training become a flexible educational continuum where training and assessment is structured by using EPAs as building blocks of competence. In the context of pharmacy education, EPAs are used for structuring the advanced pharmacy practice experience of the University of Minnesota College of Pharmacy, USA [25] and the postgraduate 'advanced community pharmacy' specialization in the Netherlands [26].

Competence can be conceptualized as consisting of various ingredients, or building blocks, which together enables the student to function in a competent way. These building blocks of competence are designated as competencies (singular: *competency*). Competencies are preferably specified as observable abilities of a pharmacist, integrating multiple components such as knowledge, skills, values, and attitudes, and expressed as actual behavior. Since competencies are observable, they can be measured and assessed to ensure that students have acquired them [3]. Moreover, progression of students through the curriculum can be guided and monitored by defining intermediate stages in the acquirement of competencies (see below). These intermediate stages can be used as anchor points to structure the curriculum and/or as critical points for assessing whether students are progressing according to expectations. Competencies are acquired by the students while they progress through the curriculum and must be considered a personal qualities or abilities of the student [23].

In order to guide the development of assessment formats and teaching-learning activities (see below) competencies usually need to be further broken down in their constituent elements.

Most competencies, as defined in existing competency frameworks, each consist of a unique mixture of knowledge in particular disciplines, cognitive skills, non-cognitive skills, and attitudinal aspects, which need to be used or applied in an integrated way. In undergraduate education different fields of knowledge (disciplinary or otherwise) and a variety of skills (technical, cognitive, non-cognitive, etc.) can be taught or trained in several ways, but assessment is largely done with dedicated assessment formats, which are aimed at capturing specific learning objectives. The results of assessments can be considered the observable *learning outcome* of competency-based education and are defined in terms of knowledge, skills, and behavior. Intended learning outcomes are preferably described with action verbs, which indicate the required cognitive level. Furthermore, the conditions under which the concrete behavior is expected to be demonstrated, must be specified in the intended learning outcomes [27,28]. Examples of intended learning outcomes for a content domain and for a generic skill are given below (Section 5). Learning outcomes can be ordered in different domains and different developmental stages to guide curriculum development.

In the previous paragraph the term 'learning outcome' is used in a specific sense to describe the results of assessment of the knowledge and skills elements of individual competencies; a learning outcome in this case is subordinate to a competency. It must be remarked that in the literature the term 'learning outcome' is also used in a more general way to describe the results of an educational program at different levels of integration; acquired competencies and entrusted professional activities can also be described as learning outcomes [15,22].

4. Curriculum Design Process

The design of a competency-based curriculum ideally follows a specific sequence from competencies to learning outcomes, to assessments, to teaching-learning activities. This process can be described in six steps (Figure 1, adapted from [3]). Depending on the local situation, a curriculum change process can be more or less challenging, and success or failure will depend on the felt sense of urgency, the creation of a shared explicit vision on the future, and the willingness of all participants to engage in discussing fundamental issues, related to scientific identity and societal responsibility. Involvement of a diversity of stakeholders, both within and outside academia, and a careful 'orchestration' of the change process is necessary [29,30]. In our experience a combination of strong external pressure (e.g., a critical visitation or a critical attitude of professional organizations), internal dissatisfaction with the existing educational quality (often latent among teachers, students, and alumni), and courage of the institutional leadership to make a fundamental change, will make transformation from a 'traditional' curriculum to a competency-based curriculum possible. Even then, it is advised to monitor the change process carefully and to be aware of the socio-political aspects of the way the change process is organized [29].

Once a decision is made to embark on the journey to CBPE, the first two steps (Figure 1) are mainly strategic and intend to position the curriculum in the local context. The first step can be complex because the pharmacy profession has evolved from a nearly exclusively product-orientation to a more patient-orientation. Within a faculty or department a certain degree of consensus must be reached on the consequences of this shift, which necessitates more attention to softer disciplines such as pharmacotherapeutics and patient counselling, including communication skills. A pitfall in the first curriculum development step can be the introduction of new disciplines and new skills without reducing more traditional ones, resulting in overburdening the curriculum. Moreover, the main driving force for a curriculum rebuilding must be the learning process of the students and the responsibility to educate them to competent professionals, who can function adequately in the context of the local health care system or the local pharmaceutical research environment [16,31]. This means that—even though competency frameworks can be used as guidelines—interpretation and fine-tuning of the required competencies and competence levels is necessary. Another aspect is the need to consider accommodating a certain degree of specialization or profiling within the curriculum. The result of the strategic choices made will be a description of competencies and learning outcomes, which is more detailed than the general framework used as a starting point. Several examples of curriculum implementations in different contexts can be found in the literature (see Table 1).

- **Tip 1: Use a competency framework.** Several competency frameworks are available (see Appendix A). All can be used as a starting point for curriculum development but interpretation and fine-tuning to the local situation is necessary.
- **Tip 2: Consult all your stakeholders.** In designing a new curriculum consultation of the outside world is necessary to align the competences of recent graduates to the local professional and healthcare needs.
- **Tip 3: Think forward (scenarios).** Curriculum changes are usually implemented gradually, starting from the first year of the program. This means, that your newly-educated graduates will enter practice at least five years from now!

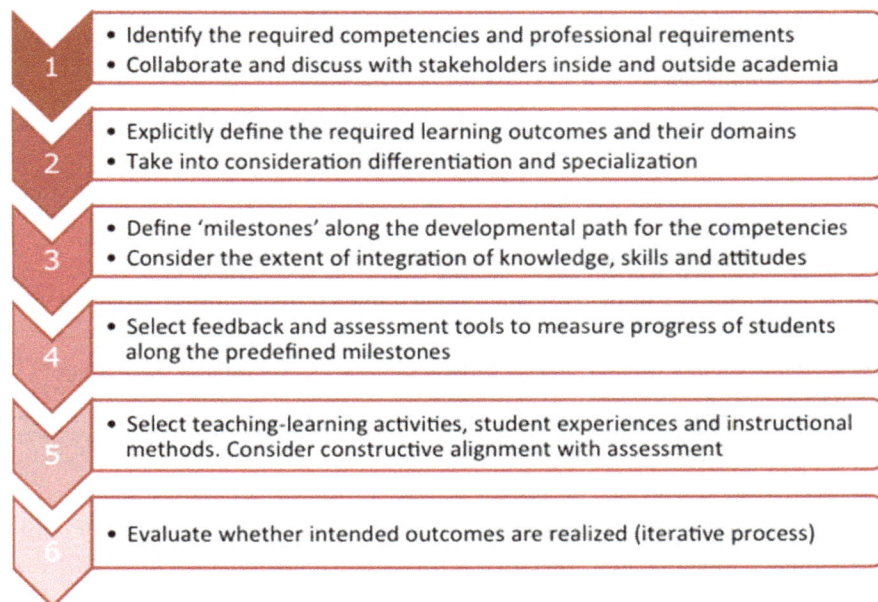

1	• Identify the required competencies and professional requirements • Collaborate and discuss with stakeholders inside and outside academia
2	• Explicitly define the required learning outcomes and their domains • Take into consideration differentiation and specialization
3	• Define 'milestones' along the developmental path for the competencies • Consider the extent of integration of knowledge, skills and attitudes
4	• Select feedback and assessment tools to measure progress of students along the predefined milestones
5	• Select teaching-learning activities, student experiences and instructional methods. Consider constructive alignment with assessment
6	• Evaluate whether intended outcomes are realized (iterative process)

Figure 1. The curriculum design process.

Table 1. Examples of curriculum design and construction.

Curriculum	Description	Reference
B.Sc.	Content and generic skills for a pre-professional curriculum (nationwide, USA)	[32]
B.Pharm.	Design of an outcomes-based Pharmacy curriculum (Hong-Kong, China)	[33]
B.Pharm.Sc.	Undergraduate honours programme for the training of pharmaceutical researchers (Utrecht, the Netherlands)	[12]
Pharm.D.	An integrated professional pharmacy curriculum (Denver, USA)	[34]
B.Sc. + M.Sc.	Design of a complete bachelor and master programme (Helsinki, Finland)	[31]
Ph.D.	Research training for clinical pharmaceutical sciences: assessments and rubrics (Pittsburgh, USA)	[35]
M.D.	Content and skills for the core curriculum of a medical school (Sheffield, United Kingdom)	[36]
M.D.	Teaching, training, and assessment of professional behaviour in medicine (Amsterdam, The Netherlands)	[37]
Physician assistants	Teaching, training and assessment for physician assistants (Utrecht, The Netherlands)	[38]

5. Curriculum Construction

Step 3 of the curriculum implementation process (Figure 1) is a crucial one. A competency-based curriculum is much more than a collection of courses: curricular elements, such as individual courses, (research) projects and pharmacy practice placements need to be organized in a logical sequence and decisions must be made about the obligatory or elective nature of the elements, taking into account possible specializations or profiling of students during the curriculum. It is helpful to explicitly formulate principles for the curriculum construction, which can serve as an internal 'frame of reference' or 'reflection tool' for steering and adjusting the construction process. Sharing these principles with teachers, students, and others involved in the curriculum implementation can ease the development process. In Table 2 an example is given of the principles that we have used during the curriculum design process at Utrecht University in the past.

Table 2. Seven principles for design and construction of a curriculum.

1	The curriculum is designed as a coherent program.
2	The program stimulates active study behaviour, is challenging and varied.
3	Acquisition, application and integration of knowledge and skills take place in a context relevant for the future profession.
4	Within the program systematic and explicit attention is paid to the development of academic and personal skills and values.
5	Direction of the learning process is gradually shifted from teacher to student.
6	The program enables students to follow individual interests by offering elective courses and a patient- or product-oriented profile.
7	A well-balanced system of mentoring and assessment is used, which takes into account the steering effects of testing.

Example of guiding principles used for the design of a new pharmacy curriculum (bachelor, master) at Utrecht University in 2001, cited from [13].

Two aspects of the curriculum design need further attention: integration of content and skills in curricular elements and the longitudinal development of knowledge and skills, also described as horizontal and vertical integration, respectively [11]. The first aspect—integration of knowledge and skills—is a fundamental requirement in CBPE because students are expected to acquire complex competences during their study, where the required knowledge, cognitive and non-cognitive skills are expected to be used in an integrated way (AACP 2013, AFPC 2010, [11]). For the design of a competency-based curriculum this raises the question where, when, and how integration can be realized. In traditional curricula the change from non-integrated to integrated learning can be very abrupt, usually when a student is confronted with pharmacy practice for the first time, either during rotations or entry into professional practice. In less traditional curricula a more gradual approach, where students are moving from learning skills in isolation to application of skills in the context of professionally relevant tasks—with a gradual increase in complexity—is advocated [11,39]. This can be achieved by using problem-based and project-based learning methods of a relatively restricted nature in early phases of the curriculum, and a gradual increase in the complexity of assignments or projects as the curriculum progresses [12]. In later stages of the curriculum, simulations of pharmacy practice (e.g., the pharmacy game Gimmics®, [40]) and organizing the curriculum around EPAs (see above) can train students in real-life pharmacy practice situations under complex, but still safe and supervised, conditions without giving students full responsibility.

A gradual increase in the extent of integration of skills as the curriculum progresses requires that the development of skills and their integration with the content of the curriculum is explicitly analyzed and translated into teaching and learning activities, which confront students with challenging tasks during the whole curriculum. This requires that knowledge about the learning of skills must be present among the teachers and that some overarching description is available of the way development of skills is organized, monitored and assessed. In our situation in Utrecht this is realized by making selected teachers responsible for the development of different skills tracks, such as 'pharmaceutical calculations', 'compounding', 'research methodology', 'oral communication', and 'written communication'. These teachers are stimulated to specialize in these didactic areas and participate in local networks with teachers from other faculties or universities. Within the pharmacy program, they function as consultants to the teachers who are responsible for the different courses of the curriculum. Similar track or stream coordination functions have been described for other curricula [31,41,42].

Analogous to the progression of skills, the development of content knowledge in the curriculum requires an explicit analysis of the way knowledge in different curricular domains is built up during the curriculum. These analyses can be used to explicitly formulate learning outcomes, which students are expected to have reached at intermediate stages of the curriculum. Once these intermediate stages (or 'milestones') are described, they can be used to inspire student assessment formats and guide the definition of actual course content on different levels of the curriculum. Examples of explicit intended learning outcomes at intermediate stages (end of year one, bachelor degree, and master degree) for a content domain and a skills domain of a curriculum are given in Figures 2 and 3. In the example of the content domain 'pharmacokinetics' (Figure 2), the gradual built up of knowledge from basic concepts to practice-oriented applications is illustrated. In the example of the skills domain 'oral communication' (Figure 3), it can be seen that the requirements gradually increase in complexity and that some profiling is specified during the master phase.

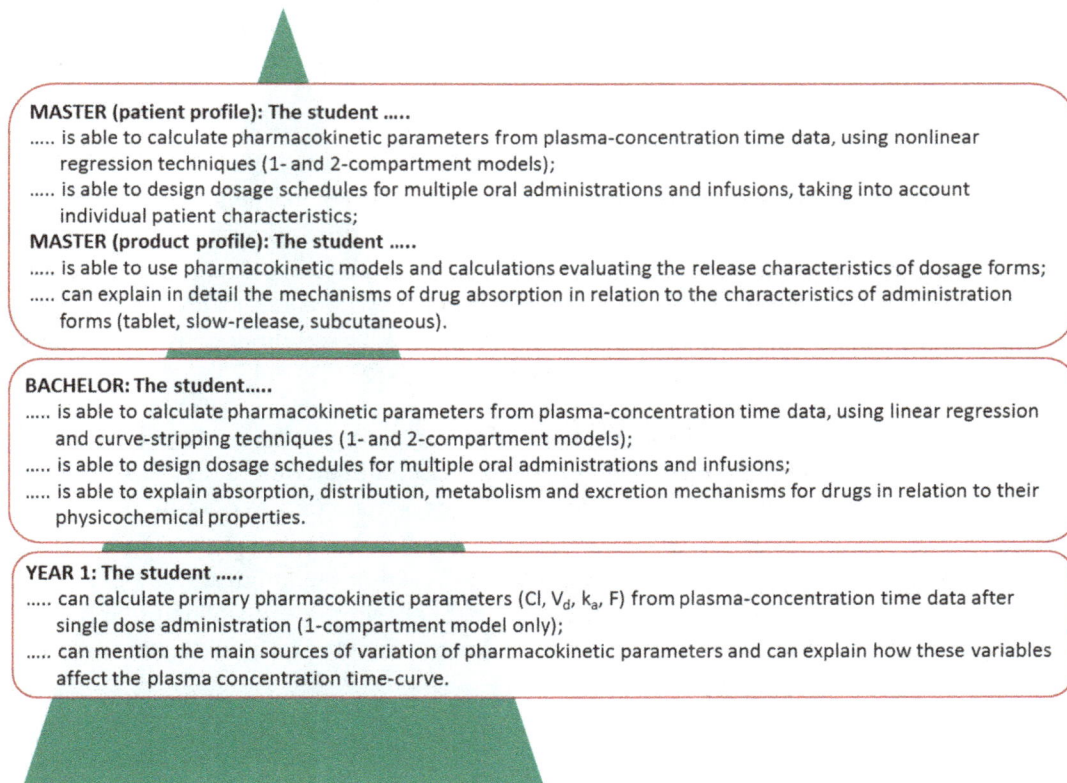

MASTER (patient profile): The student …..
….. is able to calculate pharmacokinetic parameters from plasma-concentration time data, using nonlinear regression techniques (1- and 2-compartment models);
….. is able to design dosage schedules for multiple oral administrations and infusions, taking into account individual patient characteristics;

MASTER (product profile): The student …..
….. is able to use pharmacokinetic models and calculations evaluating the release characteristics of dosage forms;
….. can explain in detail the mechanisms of drug absorption in relation to the characteristics of administration forms (tablet, slow-release, subcutaneous).

BACHELOR: The student…..
….. is able to calculate pharmacokinetic parameters from plasma-concentration time data, using linear regression and curve-stripping techniques (1- and 2-compartment models);
….. is able to design dosage schedules for multiple oral administrations and infusions;
….. is able to explain absorption, distribution, metabolism and excretion mechanisms for drugs in relation to their physicochemical properties.

YEAR 1: The student …..
….. can calculate primary pharmacokinetic parameters (Cl, V_d, k_a, F) from plasma-concentration time data after single dose administration (1-compartment model only);
….. can mention the main sources of variation of pharmacokinetic parameters and can explain how these variables affect the plasma concentration time-curve.

Figure 2. Example of curriculum layers for a content domain. Learning outcomes for the domain 'pharmacokinetics' at intermediate stages of the pharmacy curriculum in Utrecht. In this curriculum nine different content domains are distinguished, and learning outcomes are specified for the end of year one, for the bachelor degree, and for the master degree.

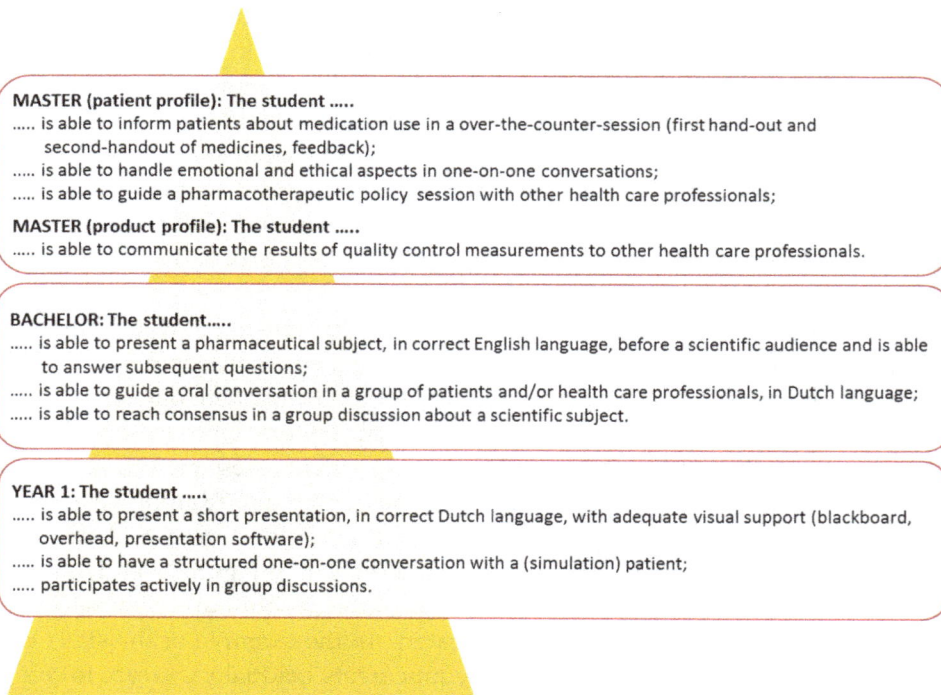

MASTER (patient profile): The student .....
..... is able to inform patients about medication use in a over-the-counter-session (first hand-out and second-handout of medicines, feedback);
..... is able to handle emotional and ethical aspects in one-on-one conversations;
..... is able to guide a pharmacotherapeutic policy session with other health care professionals;

MASTER (product profile): The student .....
..... is able to communicate the results of quality control measurements to other health care professionals.

BACHELOR: The student.....
..... is able to present a pharmaceutical subject, in correct English language, before a scientific audience and is able to answer subsequent questions;
..... is able to guide a oral conversation in a group of patients and/or health care professionals, in Dutch language;
..... is able to reach consensus in a group discussion about a scientific subject.

YEAR 1: The student .....
..... is able to present a short presentation, in correct Dutch language, with adequate visual support (blackboard, overhead, presentation software);
..... is able to have a structured one-on-one conversation with a (simulation) patient;
..... participates actively in group discussions.

Figure 3. Example of curriculum layers for a skills domain. Learning outcomes for the skill 'oral communication' at intermediate stages of the pharmacy curriculum in Utrecht. In this curriculum nine different skills domains are distinguished in total, and learning outcomes are specified for the end of year one, for the bachelor degree, and for the master degree.

Designing a curriculum is essentially a creative process, which requires the contribution of variously-minded individuals, and is best done with a combination of teachers, students, educational specialists, and administrative support personnel. Both creative, bird-like, leaders and meticulous, ant-like, workers are needed in different stages of the process [29]. In our experience, this can be organized as a curriculum committee with a flexible structure where sub-tasks can be allocated to smaller subsets of the committee as the need arises (see also [29]). Descriptions of available curriculum design processes may function as an inspiration for the reader [12,33,34,36].

- **Tip 4: Integrate content and skills as far as possible.** Skills can initially be trained in isolation, but must be integrated with course content as the curriculum advances. Professional activities usually require that knowledge, cognitive skills, and non-cognitive skills are used in an integrated way.
- **Tip 5: Appoint curriculum coordinators.** CBPE requires that the longitudinal development of knowledge and skills progresses gradually from relatively simple and isolated to more complex and integrated. This requires monitoring and readjustment of the curriculum structure by skills consultants and/or stream coordinators.

6. Student Assessment

In the next step of the implementation process (step 4 in Figure 1) formats for the summative and formative assessment of students are designed [43,44]. The goal of summative assessment (or: assessment *of* learning) is to evaluate and grade students at the end of the different curricular elements by comparing it to some standard or benchmark. The overall purpose of summative assessments in a curriculum is to guarantee that each individual student has fulfilled the curricular requirements. In the context of CBPE this means that the total of summative assessments is supposed to be representative for all required competencies. As a consequence, the student can be considered 'competent' at the level specified by the description of the required degree competencies.

The goal of formative assessment is different. Formative assessment (or: assessment *for* learning) is intended to monitor student learning, and to inform teachers and students about progress in the learning process. Formative assessment essentially has a feedback purpose and can help students to identify their strengths and weaknesses and to identify areas that need additional attention. The results of formative assessments can help teachers to identify areas which appear to be problematic for students, and can help them to adapt and improve their teaching.

Designing assessment tasks, which have a clear relation to the required competencies in CBPE, is a challenging task [22,45]. As the focus in CBPE, compared to more traditional educational formats, is strongly emphasizing the development of student abilities [3], authentic assessment tasks are called for. Authentic assessment tasks mimic aspects of the future professional life of the students and can greatly contribute to student motivation. As the curriculum progresses, assessment tasks can increase in complexity to maintain consistency with the gradual evolution of the curriculum in the direction of professional identity (illustrated in Figure 4; see also [16,24,25]). In order to maintain student motivation and to prevent student burnout, overburdening the curriculum with multiple summative assessments should be prevented. In our experience it is better to concentrate on a limited number of well-chosen summative assessments, and invest more in frequent formative assessments. Spreading assessment periods over the study year and making assessment an integral part of curricular elements (courses, projects, rotations) results in a system of 'continuous assessment', which improves study behavior and minimizes test anxiety and student burnout. Investing in the development of formative assessment tasks emphasizes the function of assessment-for-learning (formative), rather than the function of assessment-of-learning (summative) [44,45].

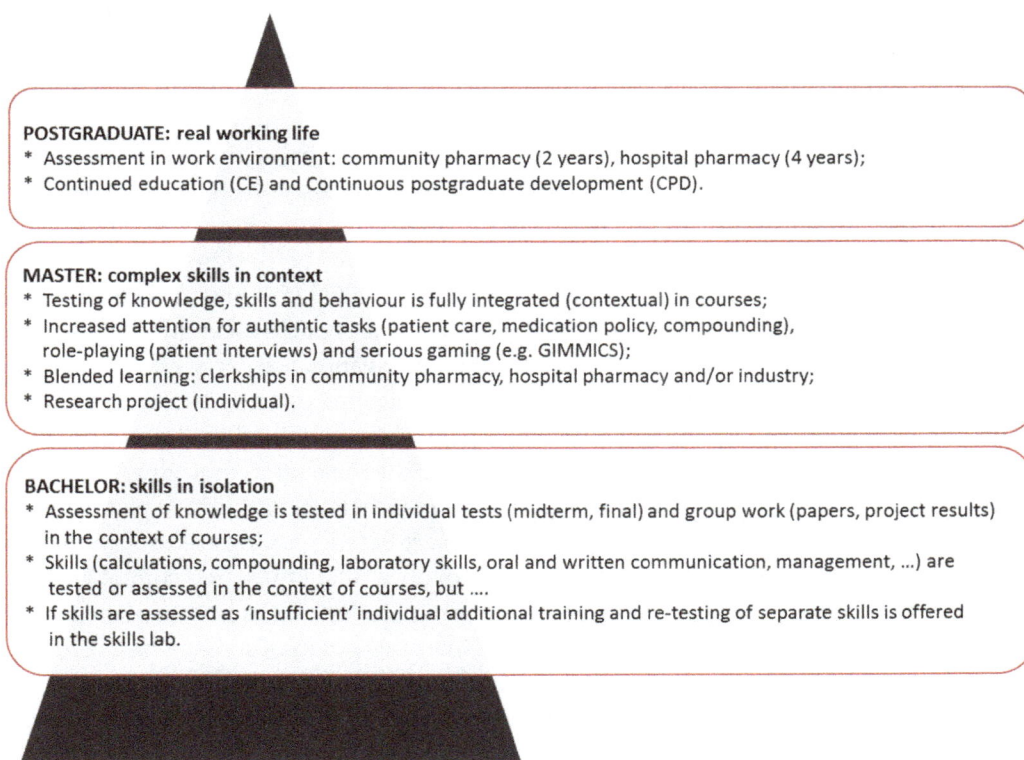

POSTGRADUATE: real working life
* Assessment in work environment: community pharmacy (2 years), hospital pharmacy (4 years);
* Continued education (CE) and Continuous postgraduate development (CPD).

MASTER: complex skills in context
* Testing of knowledge, skills and behaviour is fully integrated (contextual) in courses;
* Increased attention for authentic tasks (patient care, medication policy, compounding), role-playing (patient interviews) and serious gaming (e.g. GIMMICS);
* Blended learning: clerkships in community pharmacy, hospital pharmacy and/or industry;
* Research project (individual).

BACHELOR: skills in isolation
* Assessment of knowledge is tested in individual tests (midterm, final) and group work (papers, project results) in the context of courses;
* Skills (calculations, compounding, laboratory skills, oral and written communication, management, ...) are tested or assessed in the context of courses, but ....
* If skills are assessed as 'insufficient' individual additional training and re-testing of separate skills is offered in the skills lab.

Figure 4. Example of curriculum layers for assessment of skills. Assessment formats in the curriculum ideally should move from simple, isolated assessments to more integrated, complex assessment formats. In this example the assessment principles of the pharmacy curriculum in Utrecht, including subsequent postgraduate education, are given as an example.

Several assessment formats have been developed for formative assessment in competency-based education, such as serious games [40], and tools for self-evaluation and reflection, such as portfolios [46,47]. Objective structured clinical examinations (OSCEs, [48]) and an internet-based assessment tool for the assessment of advanced pharmacy practice experiences [18] can be used for summative assessment. It is beyond the scope of this article to fully evaluate the range of available assessment tools and their use in CBPE (but see [22] for a recent overview of the issues involved).

- **Tip 6: Less is more, in particular for summative assessment.** A pharmacy curriculum is easily overburdened; this can lead to burnout of students and teachers. Restrict contact hours and high-stakes examinations to a well-chosen minimum; concentrate on non-summative feedback.
- **Tip 7: Use authentic assessment tasks.** Authentic learning activities and assessment tasks (cases, OSCE), simulations (serious gaming) and the use of entrustable professional activities (EPAs) can motivate students and can prepare them for their professional life.

7. Effective Learning and Constructive Alignment

Competency-based education heavily relies on constructivist psychological principles, in which educational methods focus on the learning of students [27,49,50], where students construct meaning from what they do during their learning activities. In step 5 of the curriculum design process (Figure 1), the role of the teachers is to design the teaching-learning environment (TLE) in such a way that the student cannot escape from learning. In order to reach this goal all aspects of the TLE needs to be carefully designed. The learning of students is not only influenced by their perception of the assessment tasks (see above), but also by the way teaching is delivered, by the teacher behavior, and by the rules and regulations which pertain to the curriculum. The principles of *constructive alignment* [27,31,51] can be used to align all aspects of the TLE as good as possible. Several examples of carefully designed pharmacy curricula are described in the literature (see Table 1).

It is recommended to use an explicit, evidence-based, educational model to guide the development of learning tasks and design principles for a curriculum (see Table 2 for an example). Once formulated, the model can be used to make argued choices for teaching and learning activities, assessment of students and organizational aspects, whenever discussions arise during the actual implementation of the curriculum. Having an explicit model for the learning process will also protect against taking potentially counterproductive measures (see [27], pp. 309–315).

Effective TLEs with high-quality learning outcomes need to be designed in such a way that students are motivated for deep, self-regulated, learning [31,44,52]. Several aspects of a model for effective learning are summarized in Figure 5. Extensive educational research has shown that—in addition to cognitive capacity—personality characteristics, motivational aspects, and teacher behaviors can contribute to the quality of learning [27,52]. Autonomous motivation, in contrast to controlled motivation, can contribute to high-quality outcomes [52,53]. As explained by the self-determination theory, student motivation is enhanced by giving students *autonomy* in studying and by creating opportunities to develop *relatedness* to fellow students and teachers, in addition to paying attention to the development of *competence* [52]. Problem- and/or project-based learning are educational methods, which are well-aligned with the development of the autonomy, relatedness and competence elements of this educational model [27,31]. Designing challenging student tasks and explicit attention for *reflection on learning* also will enhance the quality of learning outcomes. Case-based learning, for example, can be very effective for studying pharmacotherapy-oriented tasks and for practicing patient- and physician-directed communication. It is beyond the scope of this paper to describe all aspects of designing effective TLEs; excellent literature sources are available [12,27,51,52].

A newly-developed curriculum is seldom ideal from the start [54], and several years may be necessary to improve upon the original design. As a final step of the curriculum design process (Step 6 in Figure 1) a cycle of curriculum evaluation and refinement is needed. Both short-term and long-term feedback loops are necessary. In the short-term feedback loop all curricular elements (e.g., courses) are evaluated on a regular, usually annual, basis. In the long-term feedback loop the curriculum is undergoing review every five to ten years. This review may be synchronized with external evaluations or visitations, but is preferably also done internally.

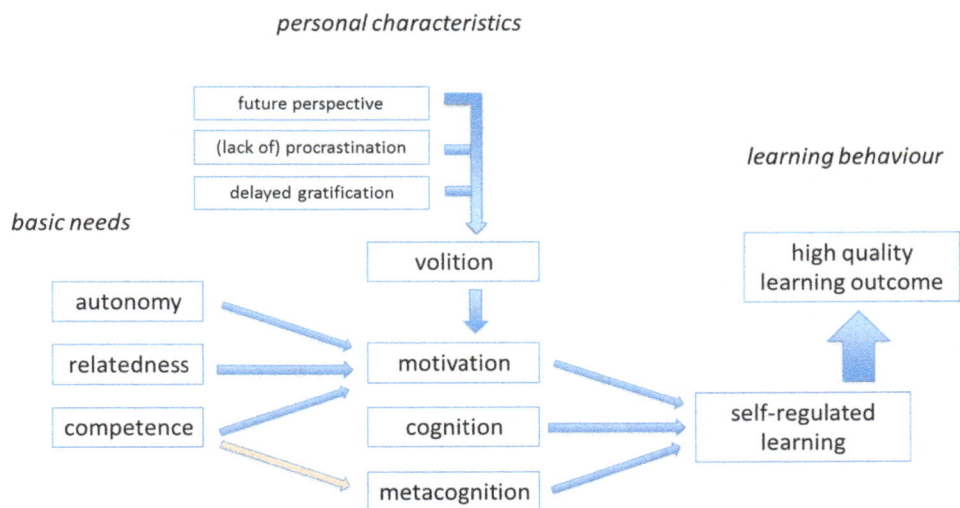

Figure 5. A model for effective learning.

Evaluation of the curriculum *as a whole* is usually done by mapping the curriculum using an existing framework [42,55]. Curriculum mapping can serve different purposes, but in the context of this paper the main purpose will be providing guidance in further improvement of the curriculum, as described by Farris et al. [30] and Zelenitsky et al. [56]. Mapping the *experienced curriculum* (the curriculum as perceived by the students) on the *intended curriculum* (the designed curriculum) can be very useful for identifying gaps, overlaps, and discontinuities in the curriculum construction [55,57].

- **Tip 8: Adopt frameworks for cognitive and skills development.** An explicit, evidence-based, educational model can guide choices for assessments, learning tasks, and can protect against counterproductive measures.
- **Tip 9: Use curriculum mapping for internal quality enhancement.** Mapping the various curricular elements (course, etc.) against existing frameworks can be very helpful in identifying curricular gaps, overlaps, and discontinuities.

8. Management and Quality Enhancement

When a new curriculum is designed, a continuous process of refinement and optimization is started. This is a long-term and laborious process, which may last several years [30,54] and requires an effective quality management system [58]. It is advised that continuity for this process is organized at the highest possible organizational level (faculty, institute) and that the adopted design principles (Section 5) and an explicit educational model (Section 7) are used as an internal 'frame of reference' to guide all discussions with the involved teachers, students, and other stakeholders. Open-minded and frequent communication with everybody involved is necessary to prevent misalignment of curricular elements and to assure that the delivered curriculum (the curriculum as presented to the students) is as close as possible to the designed curriculum. It is advised to use evaluation- and feedback-cycles at both the course level and the curriculum level (see above) to maintain flexibility and adaptability [58].

Integration of curricular disciplinary content, integration of knowledge and skills, and the use of novel assessment formats require that some teachers are given the opportunity to pay attention to these aspects of the curriculum, preferably on a curriculum level (i.e., under direct responsibility of a director of education or a curriculum manager). In this way the consistency of educational approaches in different curricular elements (across courses) can be improved. Appointment of stream coordinators, skills consultants, or specialization of teachers in novel assessment methodology is called for [59]. Another potential new teacher role is the role of a tutor, who can advise students in their personal development. All these non-traditional roles are preferably organized as temporary part-time tasks besides a primary role as teacher, responsible for delivering disciplinary content in the curriculum. By organizing non-traditional roles in this way, the connection with other teachers and flexibility of the organization can be maintained as good as possible. We strongly advise against a strict separation between teachers having traditional and non-traditional roles in the organization of the curriculum.

New roles for teachers require development of new educational expertise and the introduction of a trajectory for continuous professional development *as a teacher* [60]. This can be organized in a more or less structured way, ranging from formal training in teaching methodology [59], to a personal development trajectory for future program leaders [61,62]. Suggestions for the collaborative development of specific expertise can be found in the educational literature [63]. Depending on the local situation (such as size of a faculty or institution, number of teachers involved, existing university policy) educational development programs can range from informal, small-scale initiatives to relatively large-scale formal training and development programs [64]. Engaging in a scholarly approach to teaching and learning (SoTL), involving reflection on teaching experiences, use of educational research literature, and evidence-based development of teaching, can contribute to the quality enhancement of CBPE [65,66]. In our experience, the content and scale of training or development activities should be carefully adapted or 'titrated' to the needs felt by teachers [59,65]. Effective development programs usually involve a combination of individual and collaborative projects, sharing of knowledge and experiences, interaction with other like-minded teachers, and goal-directed development of educational innovations [61,64].

- **Tip 10: Assure management continuity.** Development and optimization of CBPE requires a long-term perspective and continuity in the educational development. This is best achieved by appointing a director of education and/or by forming a curriculum management team.
- **Tip 11: Develop educational expertise and specialization.** A competency-based curriculum requires teachers to develop expertise in the fields of autonomy-supportive teaching and competency assessment.
- **Tip 12: Develop scholarship of teaching and learning (SoTL).** Building a competence-based curriculum requires the development and testing of non-standard teaching-learning activities and novel assessment formats. Teachers and curriculum developers can benefit from a scholarly approach, using educational literature, exchange of good practices and training or coaching in (inter)national networks.

9. Summary and Conclusions

Implementing CBPE is a time-consuming and complicated process, which requires 'translation' of formulated competencies into intended learning outcomes and assessment formats. Conscious choices and decisions on all organizational levels are needed to achieve consistency between learning tasks, feedback to students, teacher roles, and organization of the curriculum. Formulating design principles and adopting an explicit educational model, based on evidence-based educational psychology, can be helpful in guiding curriculum development and optimization. Finally, the institutional management structure should support the required human resources allocation, which involves training of teachers for new roles and the stimulation of teacher professional development.

Acknowledgments: The authors to thank Antonio Sánchez Pozo (University of Granada, Spain), Aukje Mantel-Teeuwisse (Utrecht University, The Netherlands), and Daisy Volmer (Institute for Pharmacy, Tartu, Estonia) for commenting on an early version of this paper.

Author Contributions: Since 2000 the authors have been actively involved in developing competency-based curricula for undergraduate pharmacy (Andries Koster and Tom Schalekamp) and pharmaceutical sciences (Irma Meijerman) degrees. Andries Koster conceived the paper and wrote the first version; Tom Schalekamp and Irma Meijerman commented on several draft versions of the paper.

Appendix A. Competency- or Outcome-Based Frameworks

AACP 2013. CAPE Educational outcomes, American Association of Faculties of Pharmacy (AACP), Chicago 2013. Available online at www.aacp.org/resources/education/cape/Pages/default. aspx (last accessed on 8 February 2017).

AFPC 2010. Educational Outcomes for First Professional Degree Programs in Pharmacy (Entry to Practice Pharmacy Programs) in Canada. Association of Faculties of Pharmacy of Canada (AFPC), Vancouver 2010. Available online at http://www.afpc.info/node/39 (last accessed on 8 February 2017).

EPCF 2016. European Pharmacy Competency Framework, The Phar-QA Quality in Pharmacy Education in Europe consortium and European Association of Faculties of Pharmacy (EAFP), Brussels and Malta 2016. Available online at eec-pet.eu/pharmacy-education/competency-framework/ (last accessed on 8 February 2017).

FIP 2012. A global framework for services provided by Pharmacy workforce. International Pharmaceutical Federation (FIP), The Hague, 2012. Available online at www.fip.org/files/fip/ PharmacyEducation/GbCF_v1.pdf (last accessed on 1 December 2016).

GPhC 2011. Standards for the initial education and training of pharmacists, General Pharmaceutical Council (GPhC), 2011. Available online at www.pharmacyregulation.org/sites/ default/files/GPhC_Future_Pharmacists.pdf (last accessed on 1 December 2016).

NCSF 2010. National Competency Standards Framework for Pharmacists in Australia, Pharmaceutical Society for Australia (PSA), 2010. Available online at www.psa.org.au/downloads/ standards/competency-standards-complete.pdf (last accessed on 1 December 2016).

References

1. Girot, E.A. Assessment of Competence in Clinical Practice—A Review of the Literature. *Nurse Educ. Today* **1993**, *13*, 83–90. [CrossRef]
2. Spielman, A.I.; Fulmer, T.; Eisenberg, E.S.; Alfano, M.C. Dentistry, Nursing, and Medicine: A Comparison of Core Competencies. *J. Dent. Educ.* **2005**, *69*, 1257–1271. [PubMed]
3. Frank, J.R.; Snell, L.S.; Cate, O.T.; Holmboe, E.S.; Carraccio, C.; Swing, S.R.; Harris, P.; Glasgow, N.J.; Campbell, C.; Dath, D.; et al. Competency-Based Medical Education: Theory to Practice. *Med. Teach.* **2010**, *32*, 638–645. [CrossRef] [PubMed]
4. Bruno, A.; Bates, I.; Brock, T.; Anderson, C. Towards a Global Competency Framework. *Am. J. Pharm. Educ.* **2010**, *74*, 56. [CrossRef] [PubMed]
5. Nash, R.E.; Chalmers, L.; Brown, N.; Jackson, S.; Peterson, G. An International Review of the use of Competency Standards in Undergraduate Pharmacy Education. *Pharm. Educ.* **2015**, *15*, 131–141.
6. Hepler, C.D. Clinical Pharmacy, Pharmaceutical Care, and the Quality of Drug Therapy. *Pharmacotherapy* **2004**, *24*, 1491–1498. [CrossRef] [PubMed]
7. Miller, B.M.; Moore, D.E.; Stead, W.W.; Balser, J.R. Beyond Flexner: A New Model for Continuous Learning in the Health Professions. *Acad. Med.* **2010**, *85*, 266–272. [CrossRef] [PubMed]
8. Van Mil, J.W.F.; Schulz, M.; Tromp, T.F.J. Pharmaceutical Care, European Developments in Concepts, Implementation, Teaching, and Research: A Review. *Pharm. World Sci.* **2004**, *26*, 303–311. [PubMed]
9. Atkinson, J.; De Paepe, K.; Sanchez Pozo, A.; Rekkas, D.; Volmer, D.; Hirvonen, J.; Bozic, B.; Skowron, A.; Mirciou, C.; Marcincal, A.; et al. The Second Round of the Phar-QA Survey of Competences for Pharmacy Practice. *Pharmacy* **2016**, *4*, 27. [CrossRef]
10. Medina, M.S.; Plaza, C.M.; Stowe, C.D.; Robinson, E.T.; DeLander, G.; Beck, D.E.; Melchert, R.B.; Supernaw, R.B.; Roche, V.F.; Gleason, B.L.; et al. Center for the Advancement of Pharmacy Education 2013 Educational Outcomes. *Am. J. Pharm. Educ.* **2013**, *77*, 162. [CrossRef] [PubMed]
11. Pearson, M.L.; Hubball, H.T. Curricular Integration in Pharmacy Education. *Am. J. Pharm. Educ.* **2012**, *76*, 204. [CrossRef] [PubMed]
12. Meijerman, I.; Nab, J.; Koster, A.S. Designing and Implementing an Inquiry-Based Undergraduate Curriculum in Pharmaceutical Sciences. *Curr. Pharm. Teach. Learn.* **2016**, *8*, 905–919. [CrossRef]

13. Koster, A.S.; Meijerman, I.; Blom, L.T.G.; Schalekamp, T. Pharmacy Education at Utrecht University: An Educational Continuum. *Dosis Sci. J. Pharm.* **2009**, *25*, 85–93.

14. Gibbs, G.; Knapper, C.; Piccinin, S. Disciplinary and Contextually Appropriate Approaches to Leadership of Teaching in Research-Intensive Academic Departments in Higher Education. *High. Educ. Q.* **2008**, *62*, 416–436. [CrossRef]

15. Stupans, I.; McAllister, S.; Clifford, R.; Hughes, J.; Krass, I.; March, G.; Owen, S.; Woulfe, J. Nationwide Collaborative Development of Learning Outcomes and Exemplar Standards for Australian Pharmacy Programmes. *Int. J. Pharm. Pract.* **2015**, *23*, 283–291. [CrossRef] [PubMed]

16. Miller, G.E. The Assessment of Clinical Skills/Competence/Performance. *Acad. Med.* **1990**, *65*, S63–S67. [CrossRef] [PubMed]

17. Stupans, I.; Atkinson, J.; Mestrovic, A.; Nash, R.; Rouse, M.J. A Shared Focus: Comparing the Australian, Canadian, United Kingdom and United States Pharmacy Learning Outcome Frameworks and the Global Competency Framework. *Pharmacy* **2016**, *4*, 26. [CrossRef]

18. Ried, L.D.; Doty, R.E.; Nemire, R.E. A Psychometric Evaluation of an Advanced Pharmacy Practice Experience Clinical Competency Framework. *Am. J. Pharm. Educ.* **2015**, *79*, 19. [CrossRef] [PubMed]

19. Ramia, E.; Salameh, P.; Btaiche, I.F.; Saad, A.H. Mapping and Assessment of Personal and Professional Development Skills in a Pharmacy Curriculum. *BMC Med. Educ.* **2016**, *16*, 533. [CrossRef] [PubMed]

20. Midlöv, P.; Höglund, P.; Eriksson, T.; Diehl, A.; Edgren, G. Developing a Competency-Based Curriculum in Basic and Clinical Pharmacology—A Delphi Study among Physicians. *Basic Clin. Pharm. Toxicol.* **2015**, *117*, 413–420. [CrossRef] [PubMed]

21. Silva, H.; Stonier, P.; Buhler, F.; Deslypere, J.-P.; Criscuolo, D.; Nell, G.; Massud, J.; Geary, S.; Schenk, J.; Kerpel-Fronius, S.; et al. Core Competencies for Pharmaceutical Physicians and Drug Development Scientists. *Front. Pharm.* **2013**, *4*, 105. [CrossRef] [PubMed]

22. Hawkins, R.E.; Welcher, C.M.; Holmboe, E.S.; Kirk, L.M.; Norcini, J.J.; Simons, K.B.; Skochelak, S.E. Implementation of Competency-Based Medical Education: Are We Addressing the Concerns and Challenges? *Med. Educ.* **2015**, *49*, 1086–1102. [CrossRef] [PubMed]

23. Ten Cate, O.; Scheele, F. Viewpoint: Competency-Based Postgraduate Training: Can We Bridge the Gap between Theory and Clinical Practice? *Acad. Med.* **2007**, *82*, 542–547. [CrossRef] [PubMed]

24. Chen, H.C.; van den Broek, W.E.S.; Ten Cate, O. The Case for use of Entrustable Professional Activities in Undergraduate Medical Education. *Acad. Med.* **2015**, *90*, 431–436. [CrossRef] [PubMed]

25. Pittenger, A.L.; Chapman, S.A.; Frail, C.K.; Moon, J.Y.; Undeberg, M.R.; Orzoff, J.H. Entrustable Professional Activities for Pharmacy Practice. *Am. J. Pharm. Educ.* **2016**, *80*, 57. [CrossRef] [PubMed]

26. Buurma, H.J. *Advanced Community Pharmacist Education Programme*; Royal Dutch Pharmacists Association: The Hague, The Netherlands, 2012.

27. Biggs, J.; Tang, C. *Teaching for Quality Learning at University*, 4th ed.; SRHE and Open University Press, McGraw-Hill: Maidenhead, UK, 2011.

28. Harden, R.M. Learning Outcomes as a Tool to Assess Progression. *Med. Teach.* **2007**, *29*, 678–682. [CrossRef] [PubMed]

29. Al-Eraky, M.M. Curriculum Navigator: Aspiring Towards a Comprehensive Package for Curriculum Planning. *Med. Teach.* **2012**, *34*, 724–732. [CrossRef] [PubMed]

30. Farris, K.B.; Demb, A.; Janke, K.K.; Kelley, K.; Scott, S.A. Assessment to Transform Competency-Based Curricula. *Am. J. Pharm. Educ.* **2009**, *73*, 158. [CrossRef] [PubMed]

31. Katajavuori, N.; Hakkarainen, K.; Kuosa, T.; Airaksinen, M.; Hirvonen, J.; Holm, Y. Curriculum Reform in Finnish Pharmacy Education. *Am. J. Pharm. Educ.* **2009**, *73*, 151. [CrossRef] [PubMed]

32. Boyce, E.G.; Lawson, L.A. Preprofessional Curriculum in Preparation for Doctor of Pharmacy Educational Programs. *Am. J. Pharm. Educ.* **2009**, *73*, 155. [CrossRef] [PubMed]

33. Ho, S.S.S.; Kember, D.; Lau, C.B.S.; Au Yeung, M.Y.M.; Leung, D.Y.P.; Chow, M.S.S. An Outcomes-Based Approach to Curriculum Development in Pharmacy. *Am. J. Pharm. Educ.* **2009**, *73*, 14. [CrossRef] [PubMed]

34. Nelson, M.; Allison, S.D.; McCollum, M.; Luckey, S.W.; Clark, D.R.; Paulsen, S.M.; Malhotra, J.; Brunner, L.J. The Regis Model for Pharmacy Education: A Highly Integrated Curriculum Delivered by Team-Based Learning™ (TBL). *Curr. Pharm. Teach. Learn.* **2013**, *5*, 555–563. [CrossRef]

35. Poloyac, S.M.; Empey, K.M.; Rohan, L.C.; Skledar, S.J.; Empey, P.E.; Nolin, T.D.; Bies, R.R.; Gibbs, R.B.; Folan, M.; Kroboth, P.D. Core Competencies for Research Training in the Clinical Pharmaceutical Sciences. *Am. J. Pharm. Educ.* **2011**, *75*, 27. [CrossRef] [PubMed]

36. Newble, D.; Stark, P.; Bax, N.; Lawson, M. Developing an Outcome-Focused Core Curriculum. *Med. Educ.* **2005**, *39*, 680–687. [CrossRef] [PubMed]

37. Mak-Van Der Vossen, M.; Peerdeman, S.; Kleinveld, J.; Kusurkar, R. How We Designed and Implemented Teaching, Training, and Assessment of Professional Behaviour at VUmc School of Medical Sciences Amsterdam. *Med. Teach.* **2013**, *35*, 709–714. [CrossRef] [PubMed]

38. Mulder, H.; Cate, O.T.; Daalder, R.; Berkvens, J. Building a Competency-Based Workplace Curriculum around Entrustable Professional Activities: The Case of Physician Assistant Training. *Med. Teach.* **2010**, *32*, e453–e459. [CrossRef] [PubMed]

39. Husband, A.K.; Todd, A.; Fulton, J. Integrating Science and Practice in Pharmacy Curricula. *Am. J. Pharm. Educ.* **2014**, *78*, 63. [CrossRef] [PubMed]

40. Van der Werf, J.J.; Dekens-Konter, J.; Brouwers, J.R.B.J. A New Model for Teaching Pharmaceutical Care Services Management. *Pharm. Educ.* **2004**, *4*, 165–169. [CrossRef]

41. Conway, S.E.; Medina, M.S.; Letassy, N.A.; Britton, M.L. Assessment of Streams of Knowledge, Skill, and Attitude Development across the Doctor of Pharmacy Curriculum. *Am. J. Pharm. Educ.* **2011**, *75*, 83. [CrossRef] [PubMed]

42. Malone, D.T.; Short, J.L.; Naidu, S.; White, P.J.; Kirkpatrick, C.M. Mapping of the Australian Qualifications Framework Standards Onto an Undergraduate Bachelor of Pharmacy Course. *Pharm. Educ.* **2015**, *15*, 261–269.

43. Van Der Vleuten, C.P.M.; Schuwirth, L.W.T.; Driessen, E.W.; Dijkstra, J.; Tigelaar, D.; Baartman, L.K.J.; van Tartwijk, J. A Model for Programmatic Assessment Fit for Purpose. *Med. Teach.* **2012**, *34*, 205–214. [CrossRef] [PubMed]

44. Nicol, D.; MacFarlane-Dick, D. Formative Assessment and Selfregulated Learning: A Model and Seven Principles of Good Feedback Practice. *Stud. High. Educ.* **2006**, *31*, 199–218. [CrossRef]

45. Schuwirth, L.W.T.; Van der Vleuten, C.P.M. Programmatic Assessment: From Assessment of Learning to Assessment for Learning. *Med. Teach.* **2011**, *33*, 478–485. [CrossRef] [PubMed]

46. Stupans, I.; March, G.; Owen, S.M. Enhancing Learning in Clinical Placements: Reflective Practice, Self-Assessment, Rubrics and Scaffolding. *Assess. Eval. High. Educ.* **2013**, *38*, 507–519. [CrossRef]

47. Allen, S.; Waterfield, J.; Rivers, P. An Investigation of Pharmacy Student Perception of Competence-Based Learning using the Individual Skills Evaluation and Development Program, iSED®. *Pharm. Educ.* **2016**, *16*, 72–80.

48. Branch, C. An Assessment of Students' Performance and Satisfaction with an OSCE Early in an Undergraduate Pharmacy Curriculum. *Curr. Pharm. Teach. Learn.* **2014**, *6*, 22–31. [CrossRef]

49. Ten Cate, O.; Snell, L.; Mann, K.; Vermunt, J. Orienting Teaching toward the Learning Process. *Acad. Med.* **2004**, *79*, 219–228. [CrossRef] [PubMed]

50. Blumberg, P. Maximizing Learning through Course Alignment and Experience with Different Types of Knowledge. *Innov. High. Educ.* **2009**, *34*, 93–103. [CrossRef]

51. Kaartinen-Koutaniemi, M.; Katajavuori, N. Enhancing the Development of Pharmacy Education by Changing Pharmacy Teaching. *Pharm. Educ.* **2006**, *6*, 197–208. [CrossRef]

52. Ten Cate, T.J.; Kusurkar, R.A.; Williams, G.C. How Self-Determination Theory can Assist our Understanding of the Teaching and Learning Processes in Medical Education. *AMEE Guide No. 59. Med. Teach.* **2011**, *33*, 961–973. [PubMed]

53. Niemiec, C.P.; Ryan, R.M. Autonomy, Competence, and Relatedness in the Classroom: Applying Self-Determination Theory to Educational Practice. *Theor. Res. Educ.* **2009**, *7*, 133–144. [CrossRef]

54. Remington, T.L.; Hershock, C.; Klein, K.C.; Niemer, R.K.; Bleske, B.E. Lessons from the Trenches: Implementing Team-Based Learning Across several Courses. *Curr. Pharm. Teach. Learn.* **2015**, *7*, 121–130. [CrossRef]

55. Plaza, C.M.; Draugalis, J.R.; Slack, M.K.; Skrepnek, G.H.; Sauer, K.A. Curriculum Mapping in Program Assessment and Evaluation. *Am. J. Pharm. Educ.* **2007**, *71*, 20. [CrossRef] [PubMed]

56. Zelenitsky, S.; Vercaigne, L.; Davies, N.M.; Davis, C.; Renaud, R.; Kristjanson, C. Using Curriculum Mapping to Engage Faculty Members in the Analysis of a Pharmacy Program. *Am. J. Pharm. Educ.* **2014**, *78*, 139. [CrossRef] [PubMed]

57. Kirkpatrick, M.A.F.; Pugh, C.B. Assessment of Curricular Competency Outcomes. *Am. J. Pharm. Educ.* **2001**, *65*, 217–224.

58. Kleijnen, J.; Dolmans, D.; Willems, J.; van Hout, H. Effective Quality Management Requires a Systematic Approach and a Flexible Organisational Culture: A Qualitative Study among Academic Staff. *Q. High Educ.* **2014**, *20*, 103–126. [CrossRef]

59. Andurkar, S.; Fjortoft, N.; Sincak, C.; Todd, T. Development of a Center for Teaching Excellence. *Am. J. Pharm. Educ.* **2010**, *74*, 123. [CrossRef] [PubMed]

60. Al-Eraky, M.M.; Donkers, J.; Wajid, G.; Van Merrienboer, J.J.G. Faculty Development for Learning and Teaching of Medical Professionalism. *Med. Teach.* **2015**, *37*, S40–S46. [CrossRef] [PubMed]

61. Tofade, T.; Abate, M.; Fu, Y. Perceptions of a Continuing Professional Development Portfolio Model to Enhance the Scholarship of Teaching and Learning. *J. Pharm. Pract.* **2014**, *27*, 131–137. [CrossRef] [PubMed]

62. Grunefeld, H.; van Tartwijk, J.; Jongen, H.; Wubbels, T. Design and Effects of an Academic Development Programme on Leadership for Educational Change. *Int. J. Acad. Dev.* **2015**, *20*, 306–318. [CrossRef]

63. Vos, S.S.; Trewet, C.B. A Comprehensive Approach to Preceptor Development. *Am. J. Pharm. Educ.* **2012**, *76*, 47. [CrossRef] [PubMed]

64. Mårtensson, K.; Roxå, T.; Olsson, T. Developing a Quality Culture through the Scholarship of Teaching and Learning. *High. Educ. Res. Dev.* **2011**, *30*, 51–62. [CrossRef]

65. Medina, M.; Hammer, D.; Rose, R.; Scott, S.; Creekmore, F.M.; Pittenger, A.; Soltis, R.; Bouldin, A.; Schwarz, L.; Piascik, P. Demonstrating Excellence in Pharmacy Teaching through Scholarship. *Curr. Pharm. Teach. Learn.* **2011**, *3*, 255–259. [CrossRef]

66. Dolmans, D.H.J.M.; Tigelaar, D. Building Bridges between Theory and Practice in Medical Education using a Design-Based Research Approach: AMEE Guide No. 60. *Med. Teach.* **2012**, *34*, 1–10. [CrossRef] [PubMed]

2

Evaluation of a Tool to Measure Pharmacists' Readiness to Manage Intimate Partner Violence

Marie Barnard * [iD], Donna West-Strum [iD], Yi Yang and Erin Holmes

Department of Pharmacy Administration, School of Pharmacy, University of Mississippi, 223 Faser Hall, University, MS 38677, USA; dswest@olemiss.edu (D.W.-S.); yiyang@olemiss.edu (Y.Y.); erholmes@olemiss.edu (E.H.)
* Correspondence: mbarnard@olemiss.edu

Abstract: Intimate partner violence (IPV) is a public health problem that demands a comprehensive health care response. Provider education and training is needed for the entire health care team, including pharmacists, to competently care for IPV-impacted patients. Standardized assessments are needed to determine need for training and to evaluate the effectiveness of IPV training initiatives. The Physician Readiness to Manage Intimate Partner Violence Survey (PREMIS) has previously been validated for physicians. This study adapted and evaluated the PREMIS instrument for use with pharmacists to assess knowledge, attitudes, behaviors, and intentions related to IPV and IPV screening. A total of 144 surveys from community pharmacists were analyzed. Pharmacists had low levels of IPV knowledge. Exploratory factor analysis revealed a five-factor structure: workplace and self-efficacy, preparation, legal requirements, alcohol and drugs, and constraints. This instrument can be utilized to guide the development and implementation of IPV-related training initiatives for pharmacists.

Keywords: community pharmacy; intimate partner violence; advanced pharmacy services; assessment; continuing professional education; pharmacy education

1. Introduction

Intimate partner violence (IPV) is a public health problem of epidemic proportion in the United States, impacting more than 11 million people each year [1]. IPV has negative health impacts that include physical injuries, exacerbation of chronic medical conditions, harmful mental health impacts, and poor health behaviors, including poor medication adherence [2–7]. The health care system has recognized the seriousness of IPV and has been actively recommending screening for over two decades [8–10]. While the guidance and standards of care for most health care providers call for routine screening, and universal screening is widely promoted, most investigations have found that screening is poorly adopted and implemented in practice [4,11–16]. Clearly, there is a need to expand the health care response to IPV.

One health care field, pharmacy, has not been included in the effort to address IPV. This is unfortunate because for many patients, pharmacists are the health care professional with whom they have the most accessible and frequent contact. Engaging community pharmacists in this public health effort could provide an additional opportunity to improve the care of IPV-impacted patients. Pharmacists are actively involved in public health initiatives, from counseling patients on smoking cessation and diabetes management, to health screenings and provision of vaccinations [17–21]. Patients report that pharmacists are one of the most trusted members of the health care team and utilization of the expanding pharmacy services continues to increase, including engagement in partnerships in public health [22–26]. Patients exposed to IPV are more likely to utilize prescription medications, including mental health and antihypertensive drugs [27–29]. Patients exposed to IPV are at greater risk for cost-related medication nonadherence and are less likely to utilize contraception [30,31]. Given that IPV negatively impacts health behaviors, including medication compliance, increased knowledge and awareness of IPV and its impact on patients can improve pharmacy care and provide an additional prevention and intervention opportunity within the health care system to address IPV [6,32,33].

The development of education and training programs to prepare pharmacists to care for IPV-impacted patients requires assessment tools to evaluate training outcomes. Currently, no such instrument exists for use with pharmacists. It is difficult to develop successful educational and training programs to build skills and improve confidence in treating these patients without a tool to better understand health care providers' educational needs and to assess training program outcomes. One such instrument has been developed for measuring physicians' readiness to manage IPV. The instrument, developed and validated by Short et al. in 2006, is the PREMIS (Physician Readiness to Manage Intimate Partner Violence Survey) [34]. PREMIS is a 67-item comprehensive survey that measures a physician's preparedness to manage IPV patients. The tool examines knowledge, attitudes, beliefs, and self-reported practice behaviors related to IPV. The survey items were developed by a review of existing survey tools in the literature. A content analysis was conducted through review by an outside group of IPV educators. The characteristics of the instrument were evaluated in two separate populations of physicians. PREMIS was shown to be reliable and valid, sensitive to change, and capable of discriminating trained from untrained providers [34]. Construct validity checks included evaluation of the Rand coefficient for the relationship between the empirically derived scales and the objective values assigned to the original theoretical constructs developed by the expert panel. The Rand coefficient was 0.89, indicating a high degree of association between the original theoretical constructs and the empirically derived scales. Construct validity was also assessed by examining the correlations between related instrument scales and the extent to which self-evaluated knowledge, attitudes, and beliefs predicted self-reported behaviors. These analyses found significant correlation between scores on practice issues, all background scales, actual knowledge, and six of the eight opinion scales (alcohol/drugs and victim autonomy were not significantly associated with practice issues). An external validity study conducted site visits to physicians' offices and compared observed practice activities to reported practice activities related to IPV and found a high correlation between the two.

Two other studies have examined the PREMIS instrument. The first adapted it for use in a population of students in medicine, nursing, social work, and dentistry [35]. A factor analysis of the adapted student PREMIS instrument identified six of the eight factors identified in the original PREMIS instrument (see Table 1). The Workplace Issues and the Constraints scales were not identified, which was expected as this was a student population. The adapted instrument found a new scale, IPV screening, that had good reliability ($\alpha = 0.74$). The Connor et al. study demonstrated that the PREMIS scale can successfully be modified for use in other provider groups in addition to physicians. The second study translated the PREMIS instrument into another language (Greek) and tested it in a sample of primary care physicians in Greece [36]. The translated measure found all of the scales found in the original PREMIS study and the IPV screening scale found in the student study (see Table 1). The PREMIS instrument has demonstrated that it can be adapted for other health care provider groups and settings, making it an ideal scale for adapting to the pharmacist population. The development of a pharmacy-specific measure could guide the development of education and training for this unique provider group.

Table 1. PREMIS Scales in Prior Studies.

Scales	Short et al. Physicians n = 67			Connor et al. Health Professions Students n = 286			Papadaki et al. Greek Physicians n = 80		
	Alpha	Total Items	Mean (SD)[1]	Alpha	Total Items	Mean (SD)[1]	Alpha	Total Items	Mean (SD)[1]
BACKGROUND									
Perceived Preparation	0.96	12	3.67 (1.05)	0.97	12	3.80 (1.52)	0.93	9	4.08 (1.17)
Perceived Knowledge	0.96	16	3.55 (0.97)	0.97	16	3.83 (1.42)	0.96	16	3.36 (1.22)
Actual Knowledge	n/a	18	26.0 (5.18)	n/a	18	23.9 (5.68)	n/a	18	18.52 (4.58)
OPINIONS									
Preparation	0.85	5	4.20 (1.11)	0.89	4	NR[2]	0.78	4	3.70 (1.24)
Legal Requirements	0.82	4	3.92 (1.15)	0.91	3	NR	–	–	–
Workplace Issues	0.79	6	4.18 (1.05)	–	–	–	0.78	5	3.09 (1.13)
Self-efficacy	0.69	6	3.68 (1.26)	0.80	7	NR	0.75	3	4.78 (1.22)
Alcohol & Drugs	0.70	3	4.46 (0.61)	0.48	2	NR	0.50	2	4.05 (0.80)
Victim Understanding	0.69	7	5.06 (0.78)	0.46	3	NR	0.63	4	4.10 (1.24)
Constraints	0.47	2	4.65 (1.26)	–	–	–	0.61	3	4.33 (1.38)
Victim Autonomy	0.37	3	4.32 (0.83)	0.36	3	NR	–	–	–
IPV Screening	–	–	–	0.74	2	NR	0.58	2	34.45 (1.40)

[1] On a scale from 1 (strongly disagree) to 7 (strongly agree); [2] NR = not reported.

2. Purpose

The main purpose of this study is to evaluate an instrument for use with community pharmacists that assesses knowledge, attitudes, behaviors, and intentions related to IPV and IPV screening. An instrument such as this is necessary for two reasons. First, it allows a standardized evaluation of pharmacists' knowledge, attitudes, behaviors, and intentions related to IPV and IPV screening that can be compared to other health care providers. Secondly, the data collected with this instrument can guide the development of future educational initiatives, policy recommendations, and potentially the future development of screening programs in the community pharmacy setting. Any differences between the pharmacist version and other versions are important to understand as these potential differences have implications for the design, implementation, and evaluation of interventions to prepare pharmacists to provide high quality care to patients exposed to intimate partner violence.

3. Materials and Methods

3.1. Study Design

This study utilized a cross-sectional online survey. The study was approved by the University of Mississippi Institutional Review Board (protocol #12-235).

3.2. Instrument

This study was designed to adapt and evaluate the PREMIS instrument in pharmacists. Modifications to develop a PREMIS for Pharmacists instrument occurred in several steps. First, the original PREMIS items were adapted for use with pharmacists to address the unique practice characteristics, activities, and concerns of a pharmacy practitioner. Additionally, the opinions section was adapted to reword clinical examination terms and items to assess intention to screen were added as it is anticipated that few pharmacists have conducted screening to date, so assessing screening behavior only is less optimal for this population. Finally, the demographic and IPV history items were adapted as the PREMIS instrument did not use standardized demographic or IPV history items. The demographic and IPV history items were replaced with those utilized in the national Behavioral Risk Factor Surveillance System (BRFSS) surveys. Next, we conducted an expert review of the measure by researchers with expertise in IPV screening, community pharmacy practice, and health behavior theory. Suggested revisions were incorporated and a pilot instrument was finalized. Before the instrument was pilot tested, cognitive interviews were conducted. Cognitive interviews, a recommended step prior to administering a pilot survey, can detect any challenges in understanding navigation, wording of directions and questions, visual layout, etc. [37]. Three cognitive interviews were conducted with a convenience sample of practicing community pharmacists. Revisions based on the cognitive interviews were made and the revised instrument was then pilot tested with a convenience sample of faculty in a school of pharmacy and local practicing community pharmacists. The final survey instrument was then programmed into Qualtrics, an online survey system, for administration with the study sample (see Supplementary Material 1 for the complete survey).

3.3. Survey Administration

The adapted measure, PREMIS for Pharmacists, was distributed via email in March 2012 to a national sample of 6000 community pharmacists enrolled in a panel with Integrated Medical Data, a data services company. Multiple email prompts, following the tailored design method, and a $10 gift card incentive were utilized to encourage participation with the survey remaining open for 8 weeks [38]. A total of 189 pharmacists responded. After a review of the data, 45 responses were not included in the analyses as they had not completed 90% of the survey, resulting in a final analytic sample of 144 participants. Once the final analytic sample was prepared, coding was completed, including reverse scoring relevant items.

3.4. Psychometric Studies

Maximum likelihood exploratory factor analysis was utilized to evaluate the psychometric properties of the adapted PREMIS for Pharmacists instrument. Results were compared to the original results by Short et al. and to the results of the instrument adapted for use in two additional populations, health care students and Greek physicians [34–36]. Exploratory factor analysis was appropriate for this study as the measure being tested has only been utilized in three studies, two of which utilized an adaptation of the original instrument and found slightly different factor structures compared to the original study. The current study adapted the measure for use with practicing community pharmacists and this adapted measure has never been tested before. Because the training and practice of community pharmacists are considerably different from physicians, a different factor structure was possible. All analyses were conducted utilizing SPSS 20.0. Three steps were taken prior to analysis to examine the factorability of the data. First, the variable-to-case ratio was calculated to determine if the study met the recommendation of a 1:5–10 ratio for factor analysis [39]. Second, Bartlett's test for sphericity was estimated to test for the presence of correlations among the variables. Finally, the Kaiser–Meyer–Olkin measure of sampling adequacy (KMO MSA) was calculated.

Maximum likelihood exploratory factor analysis with an oblique rotation based on eigenvalues greater than one was used to replicate the analysis approach that was used in all three of the studies of this instrument [34–36]. This iterative method of factor analysis is a preferred extraction method because it employs a statistical test to determine the number of factors to be extracted. The procedure begins with one factor and adds one factor in each iteration until the model achieves goodness of fit as demonstrated by the X^2 test. Once the appropriate number of factors has been determined, the extracted factors will be subjected to oblique rotation to foster interpretability. Oblique rotation was selected because it is anticipated that the factors may be intercorrelated and oblique rotation allows this, whereas orthogonal rotation does not. Following the recommendation of Thompson, the promax method of oblique rotation was utilized with a pivot power of 4 [40]. Factors were examined for both statistical and theoretical soundness. Items were considered for deletion if a factor loading was lower than 0.32 or if an item cross-loaded on multiple factors. Only factor loadings greater than 0.20 were displayed in the analysis. Reliability and validity were then evaluated.

Validity was examined in several ways, including following Schaffer, DeGeest, and Li's 2016 guidelines to assess discriminant validity [41]. Construct validity assessment followed Flake, Pek, and Hehman's 2017 guidance to examine substantive, structural, and external evidence [42]. Substantive evidence included expert review and cognitive interviews; structural evidence included item analysis, factor analysis, and reliability assessments, including Cronbach's alpha to examine internal consistency within identified scales. Further, correlation between the scales was used in the assessment. Correlations were considered weak if $r < 0.30$, moderate if r is between 0.30 and 0.70, and strong if $r > 0.70$. External evidence in the form of comparison with previous administrations of PREMIS in other populations was also conducted. Statistical significance for all tests was set at $\alpha < 0.05$.

4. Results

4.1. Study Participants

The mean age of the pharmacists in this study was 47.9 years ($\pm$11.8 years), with a range of 28 to 80 years of age. Table 2 reports the sex and race of the study participants. In order to characterize the training characteristics, participants were asked to report their most advanced pharmacy training and to indicate any postgraduate training they may have had. The majority of participants had either a B.S. in Pharmacy or a Pharm.D. Participants also reported completion of training in areas such as anticoagulation therapy, diabetes education, nuclear pharmacy, health care management, and geriatric care. Participants reported that they have been practicing an average of 23.3 years ($\pm$12.5) (range 0 to 60), including their residency. Most of the participants had no IPV-related training (67.4%). For those that had any training, they reported their training included reading their institution's protocol (13.2%), watching a video (11.1%), or attending a lecture on IPV (9.0%). Additional participant characteristics are included in Supplementary Material 2.

Table 2. Participant Demographics.

	Percent	n
Sex		
Female	52.8%	76
Male	47.2%	68
Race		
White	84.7%	122
Black/African American	3.5%	5
Asian	7.6%	11
Native Hawaiian/Pacific Islander	0.7%	1
American Indian/Alaskan Native	0.7%	1
Other	2.8%	4
Hispanic		
Yes	5.6%	8
No	93.8%	135
Don't know/Not sure	0.7%	1
Most advanced pharmacy training		
B.S. in Pharmacy	59.7%	86
Pharm.D.	37.5%	54
M.S. in Pharmacy	2.1%	3
Other	0.7%	1

4.2. Measurement Model Exploration

4.2.1. Background Scales

The original PREMIS instrument had three background scales assessing Perceived Knowledge, Perceived Preparation, and Actual Knowledge and these scales were adapted and utilized in the PREMIS for Pharmacists. The Perceived Preparation scale included 12 items that assessed how prepared pharmacists felt to work with IPV victims and responses ranged from 1 (not prepared) to 7 (quite well prepared). The mean composite score on this 12-item scale was 27.76 ($\pm$17.28). The internal consistency of this scale was high ($\alpha = 0.970$). The Perceived Knowledge scale contained 16 items that assessed respondents' perceived knowledge about IPV. Responses on these items ranged from

1 (nothing) to 7 (very much) and the mean composite scale score was 35.36 ($\pm$23.06). The internal consistency of this scale was also high (α = 0.978). The IPV Actual Knowledge scale included 18 items, with a possible range from 6 to 32, and the mean composite score on this scale was 20.83 ($\pm$6.04).

4.2.2. Opinion Scales

Exploratory factor analysis was employed with the 32 opinion items of the PREMIS for Pharmacists instrument to explore and refine the underlying structure of the items in this population. In order to determine the factorability of the data in this sample, the variable-to-case ratio was examined. A total number of 32 variables was considered in this analysis, making the variable-to-case ratio 32 to 144. The Kaiser–Meyer–Olkin (KMO) measure of sampling adequacy was 0.731, indicating the suitability of the data for factor analysis. Bartlett's test of sphericity was significant (X^2 = 2370.63; df = 465; $p < 0.001$), indicating sufficient correlation between the items and thus the appropriateness of factor analysis for these data. Maximum Likelihood Factor (MLF) analysis with oblique rotation of the 32 opinion items identified a 9-factor solution that was statistically sound (X^2 = 277.57; df = 222; $p < 0.007$) that explained 54.65% of the variance; however, 23 of the items had similar loadings in at least two factors, indicating complex loadings. Although this solution was statistically sound, the solution lacked a good theoretical basis. Variables with low communalities or loading scores below 0.32 were removed from analysis. The final MLF factor solution had five factors utilizing 18 items and accounted for 64.16% of the variance. Only loadings greater than 0.20 were shown; all of the items loaded exclusively on one factor in the final solution. Four of the five identified scales had Cronbach's $\alpha > 0.70$ and were thus considered to have acceptable reliability. The fifth scale demonstrated moderate reliability (α = 0.676). The identified scales, with reliability coefficients and sample items, are included in Table 3.

Table 3. PREMIS for Pharmacists Scales.

Scales	Alpha	Total Items	Item Mean (SD) [1]	Sample Item
BACKGROUND				
Perceived Preparation	0.97	12	2.31 (0.003)	How prepared do you feel to appropriately respond to disclosure?
Perceived Knowledge	0.98	16	2.21 (0.004)	How much do you feel you know about what questions to ask to identify IPV?
Actual Knowledge	n/a	18	20.83 (6.04)	What is the strongest single risk factor for being a victim of IPV?
Practice Issues	n/a	21	9.44 (6.95)	For every IPV victim you have identified in the past 6 months, how often have you documented patient's statements about IPV in record?
OPINIONS				
Efficacy-workplace/self	0.86	7	2.68 (0.013)	I feel comfortable discussing IPV with my patients. My practice setting allows me adequate time to respond to victims of IPV.
Preparation	0.96	3	3.01 (0.0001)	I don't have the necessary skills to discuss abuse with an IPV victim who is female.
Legal Requirements	0.95	3	2.93 (0.007)	I am aware of the legal requirements in this state regarding reporting of suspected case of IPV.
Alcohol & Drugs	0.80	2	4.63 (0.01)	Use of alcohol or drugs is related to IPV victimization.
Constraints	0.68	3	4.31 (0.031)	Pharmacists do not have the time to assist patients in addressing IPV.

[1] On a scale from 1 (strongly disagree) to 7 (strongly agree).

4.2.3. Assessing Validity

Utilizing the guidance of Shaffer, DeGeest, and Li (2016) and Flake, Pek, and Hehman (2017), validity was assessed in multiple steps starting with a literature review to look for any similar measures in the field of pharmacy [41]. As none were found, the next step was to evaluate construct validity utilizing a multitrait, multimethod matrix. This was assessed by estimating the correlation between the instrument's scales. Similar to both Short et al. and Connor et al., in the PREMIS for Pharmacists, the Perceived Knowledge score was strongly correlated with the Perceived Preparation score ($r = 0.889$; $p = 0.01$) and moderately correlated with the amount of previous training ($r = 0.402$; $p = 0.01$); a moderate correlation between Perceived Preparation and hours of previous IPV training was also found ($r = 0.402$; $p = 0.01$). Similar to Connor et al., we found no significant correlation between Actual Knowledge of IPV and Perceived Knowledge, Perceived Preparation, and hours of previous IPV training (Table 4).

Table 4. Correlation between Preparation and Knowledge Items/Scales in PREMIS for Pharmacists.

	Perceived Preparation	Perceived Knowledge	Actual Knowledge	Practice Issues	Hours IPV Training
Perceived Preparation	1				
Perceived Knowledge	0.889 **	1			
Actual Knowledge	0.119	0.106	1		
Practice Issues	0.126	0.086	−0.041	1	
Hours IPV Training	0.409 **	0.402 **	0.213	0.126	1

** $p < 0.01$ (all two-tailed).

In contrast, Short et al. did find a correlation between Actual Knowledge and Perceived Knowledge ($r = 0.201$). Perceived Preparation and Perceived Knowledge were significantly correlated with all of the Opinion scales, although none of the correlations were strong (Table 5). These findings are also similar to Short et al. and Connor et al. Finally, the Opinion scales were examined and a moderate correlation between Workplace and Self-Efficacy and Legal Requirements was found ($r = 0.526$; $p < 0.01$). Weak but significant correlations were found among several of the other Opinion scales (Table 6).

Table 5. Correlation between Opinion and Background Scale Items/Scales in PREMIS for Pharmacists.

	Perceived Preparation	Perceived Knowledge	Actual Knowledge	Hours IPV Training
Workplace/Self-Efficacy	0.606 **	0.623 **	0.129	0.323 *
Staff Preparation	0.262 **	0.243 **	0.009	0.268
Legal Requirements	0.531 **	0.636 **	0.240 **	0.084
Alcohol/Drugs	0.277 **	0.245 **	−0.110	0.174
Constraints	−0.022	−0.052	0.175	0.309 *

* $p < 0.05$; ** $p < 0.01$ (all two-tailed).

Table 6. Correlation between Opinion Scales in PREMIS for Pharmacists.

	Work/Self-Efficacy	Staff Preparation	Legal Requirements	Alcohol/Drugs	Constraints
Work/Self-Efficacy	1				
Staff Preparation	0.217 **	1			
Legal Requirements	0.526 **	0.155	1		
Alcohol/Drugs	0.241 **	−0.074	0.168 *	1	
Constraints	0.125	0.174 *	−0.238 **	−0.342	1

* $p < 0.05$; ** $p < 0.01$ (all two-tailed).

4.2.4. Comparison with Other PREMIS Versions

The PREMIS for Pharmacists was compared to the factor structure of PREMIS previously identified in samples of physicians and health care students. The background scales of Perceived Preparation and Perceived Knowledge function similarly in the pharmacist sample as they did in all three of the previous studies. The same factor analytic strategy of the items related to opinions of IPV and IPV screening that was used in all three of the previous studies was utilized in this study. Several of the same factors were identified (Preparation, Legal Requirements, Alcohol and Drugs, Constraints). While the Opinions scale did find several of the same factors, there were a number of differences between the PREMIS for Pharmacists and the other studies. First, the PREMIS for Pharmacists identified a single factor for self-efficacy and workplace-efficacy, whereas the previous studies found these to be two separate factors. Second, the number of items in some of the scales was not identical. For example, the preparation scale had fewer items in the PREMIS for Pharmacists (3 items) compared to the physician PREMIS (5 items) and the student and Greek physician versions (4 items each). Finally, several of the factors identified in the original instrument (victim understanding and victim autonomy) and in the other adaptations of the instrument (IPV screening) were not found in the PREMIS for Pharmacists.

5. Discussion

The PREMIS for Pharmacists instrument was adapted and evaluated in a national random sample of practicing community pharmacists. This new measure, the PREMIS for Pharmacists, was found to be a valid tool that can be used with pharmacists to assess baseline knowledge, attitudes, behaviors, and intentions regarding IPV-related care. This measure would therefore provide a valid method to assess the potential impact of education and training programs related to IPV.

Importantly, a similar, but not identical, factor structure was found in the PREMIS for Pharmacists compared to previous studies with PREMIS in other, nonpharmacist populations. The background scales, including Perceived Preparation, Perceived Knowledge, and Actual Knowledge, translated well to the pharmacy setting. The factor structure of the opinions component of the instrument found four of the original factors (Preparation, Legal Requirements, Alcohol and Drugs, and Constraints). However, the pharmacy version found a single factor, which we labeled Workplace and Self-Efficacy, that was split into two separate factors (Workplace Issues and Self-Efficacy) in the previous studies. One reason for this finding may be related to the self-reported level of training and clinical experience with IPV and IPV screening. The pharmacists reported less training and experience compared to the other health care provider populations. The lack of knowledge and awareness of the details of the challenges related to IPV screening may have made it difficult for pharmacists to tease apart the efficacy issues related to themselves as clinicians as compared to their work environments. If educational and training initiatives for pharmacists increase, this may change and the factor structure should be re-evaluated. It is also interesting to note that the Victim Understanding and Victim Autonomy scales were not found in the PREMIS for Pharmacists. Both of these scales had low reliability in the previous studies and it was recommended that they be further explored. This is another example of how the lack of pharmacists' training and exposure to IPV screening recommendations and IPV screening programs may have impacted this finding. These results indicate that pharmacists do not have well-formed clinical opinions regarding IPV victims in general and educational and training initiatives may impact this.

There are several limitations to the current study. First, this survey covered a sensitive topic and this may have reduced response rate and may also have resulted in individuals responding with what they perceived to be more socially desirable responses. Second, the response rate to this survey was low, which may impact the generalizability of the results. Further, this was a cross-sectional survey study and as such, test–retest reliability could not be evaluated. Given that this was an online survey study, only participants with internet access could participate. Selective participation is an additional risk that could bias the results. The sample was drawn from a panel of pharmacists, further limiting the generalizability of the results.

Future studies are needed to further test the PREMIS for Pharmacists, especially test–retest reliability assessments, assessment in other pharmacy populations (e.g., pharmacy students, hospital pharmacists), as well as investigation of whether the instrument is able to detect improvement after IPV-related training. Additionally, given that pharmacists are the most accessible members of the health care team from both a cost and access perspective, the potential to expand screening to the pharmacy environment warrants further study. This new tool could help identify pharmacists' readiness to detect and support patients who may be experiencing IPV. In this manner, pharmacists, like other health care practitioners, could play a crucial frontline role in helping to identify individuals exposed to IPV and providing assistance and referrals.

6. Conclusions

Intimate partner violence is highly prevalent and has a negative impact on health and health behaviors, including medication adherence. Pharmacists receive minimal training regarding IPV and no instrument has been available to assess their readiness to care for these patients or the impact of potential IPV educational initiatives. This study demonstrated that the PREMIS for Pharmacists could fill this void. As with the original PREMIS and the Health Care Student PREMIS, the PREMIS for Pharmacists can be utilized in a variety of ways. The instrument can be used to conduct needs assessments to tailor education and training initiatives for pharmacists, as a pre- and posttest to evaluate the impact of training, and to identify differences between pharmacists who have participated in training and those who have not. The PREMIS for Pharmacists provides a key component in efforts to engage pharmacists in addressing the public health challenge of intimate partner violence.

Author Contributions: M.B., D.W.-S., E.H., and Y.Y. conceived and designed the study; M.B., E.H., and D.W.-S. developed the survey and collected the data; M.B and Y.Y. analyzed the data; M.B., D.W.-S., E.H., and Y.Y. wrote the paper.

Funding: This research received no external funding.

References

1. Breiding, M.J.; Smith, S.G.; Basile, K.C.; Walters, M.L.; Chen, J.; Merrick, M.T. Prevalence and Characteristics of Sexual Violence, Stalking, and Intimate Partner Violence Victimization-National Intimate Partner and Sexual Violence Survey, United States, 2011. *MMWR Morb. Mortal. Wkly. Rep.* **2014**, *63*, 1–18.
2. Bonomi, A.E.; Anderson, M.L.; Rivara, F.P.; Thompson, R.S. Health outcomes in women with physical and sexual intimate partner violence exposure. *J. Womens Health* **2007**, *16*, 987–997. [CrossRef] [PubMed]
3. Bonomi, A.E.; Anderson, M.L.; Rivara, F.P.; Thompson, R.S. Health Care Utilization and Costs Associated with Physical and Nonphysical-Only Intimate Partner Violence. *Health Serv. Res.* **2009**, *44*, 1052–1067. [CrossRef] [PubMed]
4. Coker, A.L.; Davis, K.E.; Arias, I.; Desai, S.; Sanderson, M.; Brandt, H.M.; Smith, P.H. Physical and mental health effects of intimate partner violence for men and women. *Am. J. Prev. Med.* **2002**, *23*, 260–268. [CrossRef]
5. Coker, A.L.; Hopenhayn, C.; DeSimone, C.P.; Bush, H.M.; Crofford, L. Violence against Women Raises Risk of Cervical Cancer. *J. Womens Health* **2009**, *18*, 1179–1185. [CrossRef] [PubMed]
6. Lopez, E.J.; Jones, D.L.; Villar-Loubet, O.M.; Arheart, K.L.; Weiss, S.M. Violence, coping, and consistent medication adherence in HIV-positive couples. *AIDS Educ. Prev. Off. Publ. Int. Soc. AIDS Educ.* **2010**, *22*, 61–68. [CrossRef] [PubMed]
7. Tjaden, T.; Thoennes, N. *Full Report of the Prevalence, Incidence, and Consequences of Violence against Women*; US Department of Justice: Washington, DC, USA, 2000.

8.   American College of Obstetricians and Gynecologists. ACOG issues technical bulletin on domestic violence. American College of Obstetricians and Gynecologists. *Am. Fam. Phys.* **1995**, *52*, 2387–2388.

9.   American Medical Association. American Medical Association Diagnostic and Treatment Guidelines on Domestic Violence. *Arch. Fam. Med.* **1992**, *1*, 39–47.

10. American Nurses Association. Position statement on physical violence against women. *Am. Nurse* **1992**, *24*, 8.

11. Bunn, M.Y.; Higa, N.A.; Parker, W.J.; Kaneshiro, B. Domestic violence screening in pregnancy. *Hawaii Med. J.* **2009**, *68*, 240–242. [PubMed]

12. Daugherty, J.D.; Houry, D.E. Intimate partner violence screening in the emergency department. *J. Postgrad. Med.* **2008**, *54*, 301–305. [CrossRef] [PubMed]

13. McGrath, M.E.; Hogan, J.W.; Peipert, J.F. A prevalence survey of abuse and screening for abuse in urgent care patients. *Obstet. Gynecol.* **1998**, *91*, 511–514. [PubMed]

14. O'Reilly, R.; Beale, B.; Gillies, D. Screening and Intervention for Domestic Violence during Pregnancy Care: A Systematic Review. *Trauma Violence Abuse* **2010**, *11*, 190–201. [CrossRef] [PubMed]

15. Plichta, S.B. Intimate partner violence and physical health consequences: Policy and practice implications. *J. Interpers. Violence* **2004**, *19*, 1296–1323. [CrossRef] [PubMed]

16. O'Doherty, L.; Hegarty, K.; Ramsay, J.; Davidson, L.L.; Feder, G.; Taft, A. Screening women for intimate partner violence in healthcare settings. *Cochrane Database Syst. Rev.* **2015**, CD007007. [CrossRef] [PubMed]

17. American Society of Health-System Pharmacists. ASHP Statement on the Role of Health-System Pharmacists in Public Health. *Am. J. Health. Syst. Pharm.* **2008**, *65*, 462–467. [CrossRef]

18. Grabenstein, J.D.; Guess, H.A.; Hartzema, A.G.; Koch, G.G.; Konrad, T.R. Effect of vaccination by community pharmacists among adult prescription recipients. *Med. Care* **2001**, *39*, 340–348. [CrossRef] [PubMed]

19. Dent, L.A.; Harris, K.J.; Noonan, C.W. Randomized Trial Assessing the Effectiveness of a Pharmacist-Delivered Program for Smoking Cessation. *Ann. Pharmacother.* **2009**, *43*, 194–201. [CrossRef] [PubMed]

20. Doucette, W.R.; Witry, M.J.; Farris, K.B.; Mcdonough, R.P. Community Pharmacist–Provided Extended Diabetes Care. *Ann. Pharmacother.* **2009**, *43*, 882–889. [CrossRef] [PubMed]

21. Mehuys, E.; Van Bortel, L.; De Bolle, L.; Van Tongelen, I.; Annemans, L.; Remon, J.-P.; Giri, M. Effectiveness of a community pharmacist intervention in diabetes care: A randomized controlled trial. *J. Clin. Pharm. Ther.* **2011**, *36*, 602–613. [CrossRef] [PubMed]

22. Hogue, M.D.; Grabenstein, J.D.; Foster, S.L.; Rothholz, M.C. Pharmacist Involvement with Immunizations: A Decade of Professional Advancement. *J. Am. Pharm. Assoc.* **2006**, *46*, 168–182. [CrossRef]

23. Pande, S.; Hiller, J.E.; Nkansah, N.; Bero, L. The effect of pharmacist-provided non-dispensing services on patient outcomes, health service utilisation and costs in low- and middle-income countries. *Cochrane Database Syst. Rev.* **2013**. [CrossRef] [PubMed]

24. Awaisu, A.; Alsalimy, N. Pharmacists' involvement in and attitudes toward pharmacy practice research: A systematic review of the literature. *RSAP* **2015**, *11*, 725–748. [CrossRef] [PubMed]

25. DiPietro Mager, N.A.; Ochs, L.; Ranelli, P.L.; Kahaleh, A.A.; Lahoz, M.R.; Patel, R.V.; Garza, O.W.; Isaacs, D.; Clark, S. Partners in Public Health: Public Health Collaborations With Schools of Pharmacy, 2015. *Public Health Rep.* **2017**, *132*, 298–303. [CrossRef] [PubMed]

26. Hilverding, A.T.; DiPietro Mager, N.A. Pharmacists' attitudes regarding provision of sexual and reproductive health services. *J. Am. Pharm. Assoc.* **2017**, *57*, 493–497. [CrossRef] [PubMed]

27. Cerulli, C.; Cerulli, J.; Santos, E.J.; Lu, N.; He, H.; Kaukeinen, K.; White, A.M.; Tu, X. Does the Health Status of Intimate Partner Violence Victims Warrant Pharmacies as Portals for Public Health Promotion? *J. Am. Pharm. Assoc.* **2010**, *50*, 200–206. [CrossRef] [PubMed]

28. Martín-Baena, D.; Talavera, M.; Montero-Piñar, I. Interpersonal Violence and Health in Female University Students in Spain. *J. Nurs. Scholarsh.* **2016**, *48*, 561–568. [CrossRef] [PubMed]

29. Stene, L.E.; Jacobsen, G.W.; Dyb, G.; Tverdal, A.; Schei, B. Intimate partner violence and cardiovascular risk in women: A population-based cohort study. *J. Womens Health* **2013**, *22*, 250–258. [CrossRef] [PubMed]

30. Mazer, M.; Bisgaier, J.; Dailey, E.; Srivastava, K.; McDermoth, M.; Datner, E.; Rhodes, K.V. Risk for cost-related medication nonadherence among emergency department patients. *Acad. Emerg. Med.* **2011**, *18*, 267–272. [CrossRef] [PubMed]

31. Maxwell, L.; Devries, K.; Zionts, D.; Alhusen, J.L.; Campbell, J. Estimating the Effect of Intimate Partner Violence on Women's Use of Contraception: A Systematic Review and Meta-Analysis. *PLoS ONE* **2015**, *10*. [CrossRef] [PubMed]

32. Mcfarlane, J.; Symes, L.; Frazier, L.; Mcglory, G.; Henderson-Everhardus, M.C.; Watson, K.; Liu, Y. Connecting the Dots of Heart Disease, Poor Mental Health, and Abuse to Understand Gender Disparities and Promote Women's Health: A Prospective Cohort Analysis. *Health Care Women Int.* **2010**, *31*, 313–326. [CrossRef] [PubMed]

33. Hatcher, A.M.; Smout, E.M.; Turan, J.M.; Christofides, N.; Stöckl, H. Intimate partner violence and engagement in HIV care and treatment among women: A systematic review and meta-analysis. *AIDS* **2015**, *29*, 2183–2194. [CrossRef] [PubMed]

34. Short, L.M.; Alpert, E.; Harris, J.M.; Surprenant, Z.J. A Tool for Measuring Physician Readiness to Manage Intimate Partner Violence. *Am. J. Prev. Med.* **2006**, *30*, 173–180. [CrossRef] [PubMed]

35. Connor, P.D.; Nouer, S.S.; Mackey, S.T.N.; Tipton, N.G.; Lloyd, A.K. Psychometric Properties of an Intimate Partner Violence Tool for Health Care Students. *J. Interpers. Violence* **2011**, *26*, 1012–1035. [CrossRef] [PubMed]

36. Papadakaki, M.; Prokopiadou, D.; Petridou, E.; Kogevinas, M.; Lionis, C. Defining physicians' readiness to screen and manage intimate partner violence in Greek primary care settings. *Eval. Health Prof.* **2012**, *35*, 199–220. [CrossRef] [PubMed]

37. Willis, G. *Cognitive Interviewing*; Sage Publishing: Thousand Oaks, CA, USA, 2005.

38. Dillman, D.A.; Smyth, J.D.; Christian, L.M. *Internet, Phone, Mail, and Mixed-Mode Surveys: The Tailored Design Method eBook: Don A. Dillman, Jolene D. Smyth, Leah Melani Christian*, 4th ed.; Wiley: Hoboken, NJ, USA, 2014.

39. Tinsley, H.E.; Tinsley, D.J. Uses of factor analysis in counseling psychology research. *J. Couns. Psychol.* **1987**, *34*, 414–424. [CrossRef]

40. Thompson, B. *Exploratory and Confirmatoy Factor Analysis*; American Psychological Association: Washington, DC, USA, 2004.

41. Shaffer, J.A.; DeGeest, D.; Li, A. Tackling the problem of construct proliferation: A guide to assessing the discriminant validity of conceptually related constructs. *Organ. Res. Methods* **2016**, *19*, 80–110. [CrossRef]

42. Flake, J.K.; Pek, J.; Hehman, E. Construct validation in social and personality research: Current practice and recommendations. *Soc. Psychol. Personal. Sci.* **2017**, *8*, 370–378. [CrossRef]

3

Students' Satisfaction with a Web-Based Pharmacy Program in a Re-Regulated Pharmacy Market

Maria Gustafsson [1,*], Sofia Mattsson [1] and Gisselle Gallego [2]

[1] Department of Pharmacology and Clinical Neuroscience, Umeå University, SE-90187 Umeå, Sweden; sofia.mattsson@umu.se

[2] School of Medicine, The University of Notre Dame, New South Wales 2010, Australia; gisselle.gallego@nd.edu.au

* Correspondence: maria.gustafsson@umu.se

Abstract: In response to the shortage of pharmacists in Northern Sweden, a web-based Bachelor of Science in Pharmacy program was established at Umeå University in 2003. In 2009, the Swedish pharmacy market was re-regulated from a state monopoly to an open market, but it is unknown what impact this has had on education satisfaction. The objectives of this study were to examine the level of satisfaction among graduates from a web-based pharmacy program and to describe what subjects and skills students would have liked more or less of in their education. A secondary objective was to compare the level of satisfaction before and after the Swedish pharmacy market was re-regulated. A cross-sectional survey was conducted in 2015 with all alumni who had graduated from the pharmacy program between 2006 and 2014 ($n = 511$), and responses to questions about graduates' satisfaction with the program were analyzed ($n = 200$). Most graduates (88%) agreed or strongly agreed that the knowledge and skills acquired during their education were useful in their current job. The graduates stated that they would have wanted more applied pharmacy practice and self-care counselling, and fewer social pharmacy and histology courses. Further, 82% stated that they would start the same degree program if they were to choose again today, and 92% agreed or strongly agreed that they would recommend the program to a prospective student. Graduates were more likely to recommend the program after the re-regulation ($p = 0.007$). In conclusion, pharmacy graduates were very satisfied with their education, and no negative effects of the re-regulation could be observed on program satisfaction.

Keywords: pharmacy education; web-based; student satisfaction; re-regulation

1. Introduction

Education satisfaction has been suggested to be an important influence on students' successful learning [1]. After completing their degree, graduates need to find their roles when practicing pharmacy. Discrepancies between expectations of job assignments and actual job assignments have been found in previous studies among pharmacists, and this might affect both education and job satisfaction [2,3].

In 2003, a web-based three-year Bachelor of Science in Pharmacy program was introduced at Umeå University. The program was initiated in response to the expressed request of Apoteket AB (the state-owned pharmacy monopoly at the time) because of their difficulties in recruiting pharmacists in the inland parts of Northern Sweden. The pharmacy program at Umeå University is web-based, and the education is mostly conducted through a virtual learning environment with regular online meetings between students and teachers and some mandatory meetings on campus in Umeå. During the on-campus meetings, the students engage in activities such as laboratory work, oral presentations, and role-play. The virtual learning environment contains recorded lectures, assignments, animations, and references to the literature. During the online meetings, the students and teachers discuss different topics concerning the specific course. The structure and content of the program has generally been the same over the years, besides regular revisions to keep the course material up to date. The courses constituting the program can be divided into three main areas—pharmaceutical chemistry, biomedical sciences, and pharmacy. After completing the bachelor's degree program, the students are eligible to apply to the Master of Pharmaceutical Science program in order to obtain a master's degree. This master's program was introduced at Umeå University in 2010.

In Sweden, the main place of work for graduates from the Bachelor of Science in Pharmacy program is at community pharmacies [4]. In 2009, the Swedish pharmacy market changed from a state-owned pharmacy monopoly (Apoteket AB) to an open pharmacy market in what is called the "re-regulation" of the Swedish market [5–7]. Because of the re-regulation, by the end of 2010 about 200 additional community pharmacies had opened across Sweden [4]. As a result, there was an increased demand for pharmacists [8–10], especially in areas of the country where there was a shortage of skilled personnel, such as Northern Sweden [11]. However, in 2011 the market appeared to become saturated, and some pharmacies announced redundancies and pharmacies were closed in response to poor financial results. Since the re-regulation, community pharmacies have worked on a retail supply model that focuses on the high throughput of prescriptions and the sale of non-prescription products [6,12]. As a consequence, new tasks have emerged for pharmacists, although the overall responsibilities are the same before and after the re-regulation. These new tasks might affect the skills and knowledge needed for pharmacists, and consequently the education needed to prepare them for these tasks.

Little is known about education satisfaction among pharmacy programs in Sweden. Hence, the main aim of this study was to examine the level of education satisfaction among pharmacy graduates at Umeå University and to describe what subjects and skills students would have liked more or less of in their education. A secondary objective was to compare the level of satisfaction before and after the re-regulation of the Swedish pharmacy market.

2. Materials and Methods

2.1. Survey Instrument

The study questionnaire was developed using information from the literature [13] as well as general student surveys from other departments within the university. The questionnaire consisted of 35 questions divided into the following five sections: (1) employment characteristics; (2) job satisfaction; (3) satisfaction with the education; (4) demographics; and (5) open-ended questions where the graduates were asked to provide further comments. The data used for this study contains information from Sections 3 and 4.

In Section 3, graduates were asked to express agreement or disagreement with two statements using a five-point Likert scale (1 = "strongly disagree" to 5 = "strongly agree"): (1) "The knowledge and skills you acquired during your training are useful in your current job" and (2) "I would recommend the program to a prospective student". Graduates were asked to respond to the question "If you had to choose today, would you start the same degree program?" using a five-point Likert scale (1 = No, I would not have started any education at all to 5 = Yes). Graduates were also asked if they believed their duties at work reflected their education (Yes/No). Those who chose "No" were asked to provide an explanation (open question). Graduates were also asked if they work in a sector that is completely outside their field. Those who chose "Yes" were asked why they chose to change careers after obtaining their pharmacy degree. In order to further explore how the knowledge and skills acquired during the education are useful in their current job, students were also asked two open-ended questions: "What in your education would you have liked more of?" and "What in your education would you have liked less of?" The responses to these questions were then categorized based on frequency. Only categories with more than 10 responses were included. The graduates could include subjects within the program as well as other subjects and skills (e.g., communication, laboratory work). Section 4 asked demographics questions concerning gender, age, income, marital status, and area of living.

2.2. Data Collection

A paper copy of the questionnaire was posted in May 2015 to people who graduated from the Bachelor of Science in Pharmacy program (a three-year web-based program) and/or the Master of Pharmaceutical Science program (a two-year web-based program) between 2006 and 2014 and who had a Swedish address in the university's administrative system ($n = 437$). The paper copy also had a link to an online version. To protect graduates' privacy, address labels were printed by the administrative department, and a research assistant was in charge of posting the envelopes. Those with no Swedish registered address ($n = 74$) were sent an email invitation asking if they wanted to participate or opt out from further communication regarding the survey. The contents of the paper version and the online version were identical. The link to the online version was active for two months (May and June 2015).

2.3. Data Analysis

Those who graduated before (2006–2009) and after (2010–2014) the re-regulation and those who were satisfied and not satisfied with their education were compared using the Pearson chi-square test and Student's t-test for dichotomous and continuous variables, respectively. Education satisfaction was measured with the response to the statement "I would recommend the program to a prospective student". The variables were dichotomized into "disagree" (Likert responses 1–3) and "agree" (Likert responses 4 and 5). Job satisfaction was measured with the question "All things considered, how often are you satisfied with your job?" and the answers were dichotomized into "not satisfied" (those who responded "never or rarely" and "sometimes satisfied") and "satisfied" (those who responded "satisfied most of the time" and "all of the time").

The answers to the questions regarding educational satisfaction among those who graduated before the re-regulation (2006–2009) and after the re-regulation (2010–2014) were compared, and a multivariate logistic regression model was constructed. The model had educational satisfaction as the dependent variable and included age and year of graduation (2006–2009 or 2010–2014) as independent variables. In the multivariate model, the variables were dichotomized into "disagree" (Likert responses 1–3) and "agree" (Likert responses 4 and 5) and into "no" (Likert responses 1–4) and "yes" (Likert response 5). In the analysis comparing year of graduation, 192 persons were included in the final analysis because data for eight respondents were missing.

Responses were collected and analyzed using SPSS version 23. A p-value of <0.05 was considered statistically significant. Open-ended responses were analyzed using a modified thematic analysis, which involved an open coding technique.

2.4. Ethics

No ethical committee approval was sought prior to beginning this research because it is not obligatory under Swedish law for this type of study. All data were anonymized before analysis. The participants in this study were informed about de-identification of the material and about the aim of the study, and they consented to the data being used for research purposes.

3. Results

Of 511 graduates, 222 graduates completed the survey for a response rate of 43%. In this study, only graduates from the Bachelor of Pharmaceutical Science program were analyzed, leaving a final sample of 200 graduates. Respondents graduating from the Master of Pharmaceutical Science program ($n = 21$) were excluded because this paper focuses on the education satisfaction among graduates from the bachelor program. This also includes graduates with both a bachelor and master's degree ($n = 9$). One respondent did not state the degree they received and was also excluded from further analysis. The characteristics of the respondents are shown in Table 1. The majority of respondents were female (96%), the mean age was 40.1 years, and most were employed at a community pharmacy (85%). The mean years in their current position was 3.7 years, and the majority (92%) were satisfied with their jobs. Respondents who graduated in 2006–2009 were older (43.0 years) compared to those who graduated in 2010–2014 (37.1 years), and there was a significant difference between years in current position of 5.2 years vs. 2.3 years. Among those who worked in a community pharmacy, most graduates were employed at Apoteket AB, and this was true for both groups. There was no statistically significant difference in job satisfaction between the two groups.

Table 1. Characteristics of the participants.

	Total Sample	Graduated 2006–2009	Graduated 2010–2014	p-Value
Total number of people n	200	96 *	96 *	
Women n (%)	191 (95.5)	96 (100)	88 (91.7)	0.004
Age mean ± SD	40.1 ± 8.8	43.0 ± 8.5	37.1 ± 8.6	<0.001
Current employment				
Community pharmacy n (%)	169 (84.5)	76 (79.2)	86 (89.6)	
Hospital pharmacy n (%)	5 (2.5)	3 (3.1)	2 (2.1)	
Pharmaceutical company n (%)	5 (2.5)	3 (3.1)	2 (2.1)	
County council n (%)	4 (2.0)	1 (1.0)	3 (3.1)	
Municipality n (%)	4 (2.0)	4 (4.2)	0 (0.0)	
Dose-dispensing pharmacy n (%)	3 (1.5)	2 (2.1)	0 (0.0)	
Others** n (%)	10 (5.0)	7 (7.3)	3 (3.1)	
Pharmacy				
Apoteket AB n (%)	45 (22.5)	23 (24.0)	20 (20.8)	
Kronans Apotek n (%)	40 (20.0)	21 (21.9)	18 (18.8)	
Apoteket Hjärtat n (%)	39 (19.5)	20 (20.8)	18 (18.8)	
Years in current position	3.7 ± 2.7	5.2 ± 2.7	2.3 ± 1.9	<0.001
All things considered, how satisfied are you with your job?				0.306
Satisfied n (%)	173 (91.5)	85 (89.5)	88 (93.6)	
Not satisfied n (%)	16 (8.5)	10 (10.5)	6 (6.4)	

* Data regarding graduation year for eight respondents was missing; Others** include drug product manufacturing, international clinical testing, medical technology, goods control at head office, teaching pharmaceutical technicians in training, university, and various work places.

The majority of graduates (88%) agreed or strongly agreed that the knowledge and skills acquired during the education were useful in their current job. The majority of the graduates (92%) agreed or strongly agreed that they would recommend the program to a prospective student (Table 2). Further, 82% stated that if they were to choose today, they would start the same pharmacy program. Of the graduates, 2.6% stated that they would have rather studied pharmacy at another university. A few graduates (8.3%) stated that they would have rather started another education program at the same university, and 2.1% would have chosen another educational area at a different university. Finally, 5.2% of the graduates would not have commenced any university studies at all if they were to choose today.

Table 2. Graduates' satisfaction with their education.

	Percentage of Graduates (%)				
	Strongly Disagree	Disagree	Neither Agree or Disagree	Agree	Strongly Agree
The knowledge and skills acquired during the education are useful in my current job (n = 217)	1.5%	5.2%	5.1%	**61.4%**	26.9%
I would recommend the program to a prospective student (n = 209)	2.0%	3.6%	2.6%	28.6	**63.3%**

There were no differences among graduates who were satisfied with their education and graduates who were not satisfied regarding age and gender (Table 3). Significantly more graduates among those who were satisfied with their education were also satisfied with their job ($p < 0.001$).

Table 3. Comparison between graduates satisfied and not satisfied with their education.

Total Number of People	Graduates Satisfied with Their Education $n = 180$	Graduates Not Satisfied with Their Education $n = 16$	p-Value
Age	40.0 ± 9.0	37.9 ± 7.6	0.294
Women n (%)	172 (95.6)	15 (93.8)	0.742
All things considered, how satisfied are you with your job?			<0.001
Satisfied	170 (95.5)	8 (53.3)	
Not satisfied	8 (4.5)	7 (46.7)	

Graduates reported that during their education they would have liked more of subjects such as applied pharmacy practice and self-care counselling and more training in skills such as communication. Other subjects mentioned included business administration, economics, sales, and leadership. Further, they wanted less of subjects such as social pharmacy and histology (Table 4).

Table 4. What subjects and skills graduates would like to have more or less of in their education.

Graduates n (%)	$n = 200$
What graduates would have liked more of in their education	
Applied pharmacy practice n (%)	35 (17.5)
Communication n (%)	25 (12.5)
Drug interactions n (%)	11 (5.5)
Other subjects within pharmacy * n (%)	34 (17.0)
Pathology n (%)	17 (8.5)
Pharmacology n (%)	23 (11.5)
Pharmacotherapy n (%)	12 (6.0)
Self-care counselling n (%)	30 (15.0)
Subjects not within pharmacy ** n (%)	12 (6.0)
What the graduates would have liked less of in their education	
Chemistry n (%)	14 (7.0)
Histology n (%)	24 (12.0)
Social pharmacy n (%)	16 (8.0)
Statistics n (%)	12 (6.0)

* Includes: clinical pharmacy, drug knowledge, adverse reactions, legislation, good manufacturing practice, generic substitution, pharmacokinetics, pharmacodynamics, anatomy, cytostatics, extemporaneous compounding, therapy recommendations, drugs and the elderly, skin care, drug evaluation, dose assessment, parallel imported drugs, contraindications, drug dispensing, toxicology, microbiology, and pharmaceutics. ** Includes: sales, promotion, business administration, economics, psychology, behavioral science, crisis management, and work environment.

The majority of the participants (75%) thought that their duties at work reflected their education. Graduates who answered "no" to this question were asked to provide further comments. From the analysis of these open-ended responses, two broad themes were identified: (1) I learned about this but have not had any use of this knowledge, and (2) This was not included in the program, but I need it at work.

Theme 1: I learned about this but have not had any use of this knowledge.

Some of the graduates explained that they have more knowledge than they need in their current job, which is exemplified by this comment:

"The program gives much deeper and more detailed knowledge than what is needed in order to handle prescriptions at a pharmacy".

Another graduate mentioned:

"Everything you learn about, for example, pharmacodynamics, pharmacokinetics and general chemistry, you unfortunately never use at a community pharmacy … This knowledge, that you knew really well, is forgotten … Very sad".

These comments highlight how some of the knowledge that the graduates gained might not be used and/or applied in their current jobs. In addition, some respondents mentioned that they would like to use their knowledge more, and they also felt that the knowledge they have is not requested, as exemplified by this quote:

"The boring thing is that when you work at a community pharmacy there are few people who ask for our competence. Neither employers nor customers are especially interested in what we know".

A common reason for the mismatch between their education and their current job was that some graduates perceived that the current focus of community pharmacies is on selling products. One of the graduates noted:

"Now it is only about selling products (outpatient care products) and earning money. You rarely get to use the knowledge you have. For example, giving advice and informing/discussing medicines with the customers. There is no time for that".

Theme 2: This was not included in the program, but I need it at work.

Some of the graduates mentioned that some subjects within the pharmacy degree were missing. For example, they would have liked more practical knowledge in areas such as patient counselling and therapeutics, but less focus on chemistry and basic science, as exemplified by these quotes:

"I think the program focused too much and in too much detail on chemistry at the expense of, for example, outpatient care and animal medicines, which we had on only one occasion".

"More practice, more about medicines and how they work in the body. More depth and a longer course".

Some respondents also mentioned competences outside the field of pharmacy, and particularly emphasized the lack of education regarding sales during the program; however, they did not say if they wanted more emphasis on knowledge of "how to sell".

"There is a lot of focus on sales at pharmacies, but we never heard anything about that in the program".

Another graduate mentioned:

"During my studies I did not learn to sell cosmetics and body lotion, which is something I am expected to do at work".

Graduates were also asked if they work in a sector that is completely outside of pharmacy, and nine (4.5%) answered yes to this question. These graduates were asked why they chose to change careers after obtaining their pharmacy degree. Most of the explanations provided were about job satisfaction. One of the graduates commented: "It's just stress. There are no opportunities for continuing professional development, and it is difficult to get a good working schedule." Another mentioned: "Working at a pharmacy did not live up to my expectations. I thought it was like working in any other store".

Two of the graduates mentioned that they could not get a permanent job in their hometown.

"I worked at a pharmacy for six months, had children, and then got a better job in my hometown in my previous profession".

In order to explore if graduates' satisfaction with their education had changed after the re-regulation, a regression analysis was performed. The analysis showed that a higher proportion of the respondents who graduated in 2010–2014 would recommend the program to a prospective student compared to respondents who graduated in 2006–2009 ($p = 0.007$) (Table 5). No other statistically significant differences regarding education satisfaction after the re-regulation were found in this analysis.

Table 5. Multivariate logistic regression including different questions regarding education satisfaction.

Total Number of People	Graduated before the Re-Regulation 2006–2009	Graduated after the Re-Regulation 2010–2014	Odds Ratio *	95% Confidence Interval	p-Value
The knowledge and skills acquired during the education are useful in my current job n (%)	81/95 (85.3)	86/94 (91.5)	2.437	0.901–6.588	0.079
I would recommend the program to a prospective student n (%)	82/94 (87.2)	91/94(96.8)	6.945	1.171–28.149	0.007
The duties at work reflect the education n (%)	70/95 (73.7)	76/96 (79.2)	1.851	0.888–3.860	0.100
If I had to choose today, I would start the same degree program n (%)	70/90 (77.8)	80/94 (85.1)	2.065	0.912–4.674	0.082

* Controlled for age.

4. Discussion

The main findings from this study are that pharmacy graduates were very satisfied with their education. Also, graduates stated that during their education they would have wanted more subjects such as applied pharmacy practice and self-care counselling, and fewer social pharmacy and histology courses. Further, people graduating after the re-regulation were more likely to recommend the program to a prospective student. That the vast majority of respondents were female and the mean age was 40 years is similar to what has been reported for the Swedish pharmacy workforce [7,13].

This study provided an opportunity for graduates to look back at their education and to consider if it provided the necessary skills and knowledge to perform their job. Most of the respondents stated that if they were to choose today, they would start the same degree program. Comparisons with other studies are somewhat difficult because different designs and questions are used; however, compared to one study from Australia, the results in the present study indicate a higher education satisfaction [14]. Further, a recent investigation from another university in Sweden found that almost half of the respondents three years after graduation from a Master of Science in Pharmacy program were not satisfied with their choice of education and would not choose the same education again [15]. In Sweden, there are two different professional degrees within pharmacy—prescriptionists (with a bachelor's degree) and pharmacists (with a master's degree). Both professional degrees have the same rights to dispense drugs in a community pharmacy. However, while prescriptionists mainly work in community pharmacies, pharmacists also work in other areas such as the pharmaceutical industry, universities, hospitals, and the government. The difference in education satisfaction between bachelor and master graduates could be due to a discrepancy in the students' expectations regarding their professional career. Because of the rather favorable labor market in community pharmacy at present, graduates with a master's degree often work there but might have a desire to work elsewhere within the pharmaceutical area, e.g., the pharmaceutical industry or a hospital pharmacy.

Because community pharmacy is the major workplace for the graduates, it was important to understand whether the graduates' education had responded to changes in the labor market. Graduates were positive about the knowledge and skills acquired and were willing to recommend the program to a prospective student. It is interesting to note how this is even higher after the re-regulation. Despite the changes in the pharmacy market, graduates would be willing to study pharmacy again. This might indicate that although the pharmacy market and the role of the pharmacist have changed, the education still succeeds in preparing the students for relevant job assignments. Another possible explanation is the increased number of community pharmacies with different owners [5], which has expanded the labor market and perhaps provided a greater variation regarding job assignments. The majority of the graduates thought that their duties at work reflected their education. However, one-third of the graduates considered that their knowledge was not being used and that they did things they had little or no training for. Business administration, economics, sales, and leadership were subjects mentioned by the graduates as missing in their education, subjects that might be of more importance for today's pharmacists compared to before the re-regulation. This is a reflection of how practice has become more commercial and how the vital source of revenue in community pharmacies has moved towards selling non-drug articles (for example, cosmetics and vitamins) [12]. Some graduates also commented on how their knowledge is not recognized, which could be due to a discrepancy between what community pharmacists do and what they want to do. This is found in both Nordic studies [2,3] as well as in Swedish settings [7].

Graduates in the present study wanted more pharmacy practice, self-care counselling, and communication training. This is probably a reflection of their duties at a community pharmacy. Usual work tasks at a community pharmacy are to serve at the counter or in the OTC self-selection department, advising customers [16]. A pharmacist should help patients choose the most effective, safe, and convenient pharmacotherapeutic option, and to be able to do this communication is important. Research has shown that improved communication can improve both satisfaction and adherence to prescribed therapy among patients [17,18].

Although the majority of the graduates work at community pharmacies, graduates from the Bachelor of Science in Pharmacy program can also work in other places such as the pharmaceutical industry and government agencies. Offering broad knowledge as well as expertise that addresses the labor market changes is a balancing act. There is a coexistence of different perspectives that needs to be considered when developing and changing higher education, and perhaps one way is to allow more dialogs in an external context.

The results of this study show that the re-regulation did not have a great impact on graduates' education satisfaction. Perhaps the education is broad enough to address the new labor market. It seems that Umeå University pharmacy graduates are satisfied with their education, but not with some of the tasks at their workplace.

One of the limitations of this study was that all graduates completing the survey are now working in a liberalized pharmacy market, and graduates' opinions about their education might be reflected by their current workplace, i.e., in the re-regulated pharmacy market. Further, some of the graduates might have experience with the former market, but the extent of this is not known. Also, years of work experience have not been corrected for, which might be a confounder. It would have been interesting to ask the graduates more detailed questions about how they have experienced the re-regulation in order to be able to compare the situation before and after, but this was beyond the scope of the study. There is also a risk of selection bias, and it cannot be excluded that students who are more positive about their education were more likely to complete the survey, which might influence the results.

5. Conclusions

This study provided an opportunity to investigate education satisfaction among graduates between 2006 and 2014. Pharmacy graduates were very satisfied with their education, and no negative effects of the re-regulation could be observed on program satisfaction. The subjects and skills the students would have liked more or less of in their education probably reflected their current duties at the community pharmacy.

Acknowledgments: Gisselle Gallego was supported by Carl Wilhelm Scheele, Visiting Professor from the Swedish Research Council. The funding body did not influence the data collection, analysis, the writing of the manuscript, or the decision to submit for publication.

Author Contributions: Gisselle Gallego and Sofia Mattsson contributed to study design; Maria Gustafsson and Sofia Mattsson analyzed the data; and Maria Gustafsson wrote the paper. All authors critically revised, contributed with comments, and approved the final version of the manuscript.

References

1. Susan, A.; Jennifer, R. Measuring customer satisfaction in higher education. *Qual. Assur. Educ.* **1998**, *6*, 197–204.

2. Svensberg, K.; Kälvemark Sporrong, S.; Håkonsen, H.; Toverud, E.L. Because of the circumstances, we cannot develop our role: Norwegian community pharmacists; perceived responsibility in role development. *Int. J. Pharm. Pract.* **2015**, *23*, 256–265. [CrossRef] [PubMed]

3. Olsson, E.; Kälvemark Sporrong, S. Pharmacists' experiences and attitudes regarding generic drugs and generic substitution: Two sides of the coin. *Int. J. Pharm. Pract.* **2012**, *20*, 377–383. [CrossRef] [PubMed]

4. The Swedish Pharmacy Association's Yearly Report 2010. Available online: http://www.sverigesapoteksforening.se/wp-content/uploads/AFP-Branschrapport.110504.pdf (accessed on 6 June 2017).

5. Wisell, K.; Winblad, U.; Sporrong, S.K. Stakeholders' expectations and perceived effects of the pharmacy ownership liberalization reform in Sweden: A qualitative interview study. *BMC Health Serv. Res.* **2016**, *16*. [CrossRef] [PubMed]

6. Balgård, M. The new pharmacy market in Sweden. *Eur. J. Hosp. Pharm.* **2012**, *19*, 23. [CrossRef]

7. Kvalitet Och Säkerhet på Arbetsmarknaden. Available online: http://www.regeringen.se/493a2f/contentassets/898886b519fa4630b9b576de75d5cbf9/kvalitet-och-sakerhet-pa-apoteksmarknaden-sou-2017_15.pdf (accessed on 6 June 2017). (In Swedish)

8. Olow, A.; Bergeå Nygren, N. Ostadigt nybygge—Många förklaringar till dålig start för kedjor. *Svensk Farmaci* **2011**, *6*, 7. (In Swedish)

9. Bergeå Nygren, N. Nedläggningar spås bli en del av vardagen—Turbulent apoteksmarknad att vänta. *Svensk Farmaci* **2011**, *6*, 4–5. (In Swedish)

10. Hed, F. Tuffare tider för apotekskedjorna. *Läkemedelsvärlden* **2011**, *8*, 11. (In Swedish)

11. Bergeå Nygren, N. Löneklipp med nytt apoteksjobb. *Svensk Farmaci* **2011**, *1*, 12–13. (In Swedish)

12. Bergeå Nygren, N. Backlash? *Svensk Farmaci* **2011**, *5*, 11–14. (In Swedish)

13. Statskontoret. En Omreglerad Apoteksmarknad. The Swedish Unions Report. Available online: http://www.statskontoret.se/upload/Publikationer/2013/201307.pdf (accessed on 6 June 2017). (In Swedish)

14. Shen, G.; Fois, R.; Nissen, L.; Saini, B. Course experiences, satisfaction and career intent of final year pre-registration Australian pharmacy students. *Pharm. Pract.* **2014**, *12*, 392. [CrossRef]

15. Bergeå Nygren, N. Många missnöjda med utbildningsval efter tre år. Available online: http://svenskfarmaci.se/arbetsliv/manga-missnojda-med-utbildningsval-efter-tre-ar/ (accessed on 6 June 2017). (In Swedish)

16. Westerlund, T.; Björk, H.T. Pharmaceutical care in community pharmacies: Practice and research in Sweden. *Ann. Pharmacother.* **2006**, *40*, 1162–1169. [CrossRef] [PubMed]

17. Kinnersley, P.; Stott, N.; Peters, T.J.; Harvey, I. The patient-centredness of consultations and outcome in primary care. *Br. J. Gen. Pract.* **1999**, *49*, 711–716. [PubMed]

18. Bultman, D.C.; Svarstad, B.L. Effects of pharmacist monitoring on patient satisfaction with antidepressant medication therapy. *J. Am. Pharm. Assoc.* **2002**, *42*, 36–43. [CrossRef]

4

Redesigning Journal Clubs to Staying Current with the Literature

Roland N. Dickerson *, G. Christopher Wood, Joseph M. Swanson and Rex O. Brown

Department of Clinical Pharmacy and Translational Science, University of Tennessee College of Pharmacy, 881 Madison Ave., Memphis, TN 38163, USA; cwood@uthsc.edu (G.C.W.); jswanson@uthsc.edu (J.M.S.); rbrown@uthsc.edu (R.O.B.)

* Correspondence: rdickerson@uthsc.edu

Abstract: Staying current with the literature is of paramount importance to the pharmacist engaged in an evidence-based clinical practice. Given the expanding roles and responsibilities of today's pharmacists combined with exponential growth in new medical and health sciences literature, staying current has become an extremely daunting task. Traditional journal clubs have focused upon their role as a training vehicle for teaching critical reading skills to residents. However, schools of pharmacy are now required to provide instruction in biostatistics, research design, and interpretation. We present a paradigm shift in the traditional journal club model whereby a collection of periodicals is screened and a short synopsis of the pertinent articles is provided. The associated tasks for screening and presenting of the primary literature are shared among a group of clinicians and trainees with similar practice interests resulting in a more reasonable workload for the individual. This journal club method was effective in identifying a significant majority of articles judged to be pertinent by independent groups of clinicians in the same practice arenas. Details regarding the shared core practice and knowledge base elements, journal club format, identification of journals, and evaluation of the success of the journal club technique are provided.

Keywords: education; pharmacy practice; learning; training; journal club; critical care; parenteral nutrition; enteral nutrition

1. Introduction

Journal clubs are commonplace in academic medical centers and hospitals in various fields of clinical practice including pharmacy. The first record of a medical journal club was attributed to Sir William Osler at McGill University in 1875 [1]. His intent for initiation of journal club was described as "for the purchase and distribution of periodicals to which he could not afford to individually purchase" [2]. The purpose of a journal club has traditionally been described as a vehicle to teach trainees critical reading skills [2–8], including analysis of study design, statistical inference, and evaluation of the author's interpretation of their findings. It also provides a forum for trainees to present the literature that they have read and interpreted. According to the Accreditation Council for Pharmacy Education's 2016 Accreditation Standards and Key Elements for the Professional Program in Pharmacy leading to the Doctor of Pharmacy degree, coursework that includes biostatistics, ethics, research design, and health information retrieval and evaluation are required elements of the Doctor of Pharmacy curriculum [9]. Thus, the historical intent of journal clubs (e.g., to develop critical reading skills in trainees) could be less emphasized and even argued that this purpose may be antiquated for the current pharmacy residency educational environment.

Staying current with the literature is an essential requirement for the pharmacist engaged in an evidence-based clinical practice. It has been suggested that the gap between implementation of new knowledge into clinical practice is a primary reason for the suboptimal provision of quality health care for some institutions [10]. However, due to expanding responsibilities among today's clinical pharmacy faculty and practitioners, combined with an exponential growth rate in the number of medical and health science publications [11], it becomes a daunting, if not overwhelming, task for one individual to consistently screen the abundant amount of journals to seek out those clinical studies, position papers, or clinical guidelines that may be incorporated into their evidence-based clinical practice [12]. Because of these expanding responsibilities, we have altered our journal club format from a detailed discussion of one or two articles to a methodology that allows bi-monthly screening of numerous journals pertinent to our clinical practice. We have embraced this altered format for at least the past several years within our journal club group based on the ideology of making a concerted effort to keep up to date with the literature. In addition, this format provides the opportunity for the mentoring of pharmacy residents via dialogic discussion of emerging innovative therapies. This paper reviews our current redesigned journal club format as well as the logistics to be considered in its implementation, and provides insight regarding its success in terms of staying current with the literature.

2. Shared Core Practice and Knowledge Base Elements of the Journal Club Participants

Five clinical faculty members with direct patient care responsibilities and three second post-graduate year (PGY2) pharmacy residents comprise the core of the journal club group. All faculty are within the same department at the University of Tennessee College of Pharmacy and are based at the same university-affiliated hospital (Regional One Health, formerly known as "The MED", in Memphis). Advanced clinical pharmacist activities are required via a contractual agreement between the College of Pharmacy and the hospital. Two faculty members have clinical responsibilities and coordinator duties for the Nutrition Support Service (NSS), another two faculty members provide critical care pharmacy services, and one faculty member shares responsibilities for both services. The NSS faculty members provide clinical services to adult patients throughout the entire hospital that require parenteral nutrition and to select complicated patients who require enteral nutrition. The critical care faculty members provide pharmacotherapy services to a Level 1 Trauma Intensive Care Unit (TICU) and its associated step-down unit. Most of the patients managed by the NSS are also trauma and surgical intensive care unit patients that frequently coincide with the population followed by the TICU faculty. The PGY2 pharmacy residents are required to complete four months of NSS experience and four months of TICU clinical pharmacy services with the remaining months dedicated to elective experiences, research, and miscellaneous activities. Thus, all clinical faculty and PGY2 trainees share a common thread of required knowledge and reading sources necessary for optimal performance of their respective duties. It would be intuitive that both NSS and TICU clinical pharmacy services could streamline their ability to stay current with the literature by sharing reading sources and communicating findings from pertinent articles with each other.

3. Specific Objectives for the Journal Club

The primary intent of our journal club is to stay current with new literature that may confirm, alter, or augment conventional practice in pharmacy nutrition support or pharmacy trauma intensive care. A second objective is to accomplish the task of screening and compiling pertinent studies on a consistent basis without burdening a sole person with the excessive workload. Third, this journal club methodology provides a forum for training pharmacy resident mentees via dialogic teaching of emerging innovative therapies, where perspective on the paper's application to clinical practice and what is currently known in the field can be provided. This model exemplifies one method on how to facilitate continued growth in knowledge of current literature for trainees to potentially emulate upon completion of their training.

4. Journal Club Participants and Format

The journal club process and organization are overseen by five clinical pharmacy faculty mentors. In addition to the faculty mentors, other active participants are also expected to screen journals, prepare materials for the journal club, and present papers at each session. These other participants include our three PGY2 critical care pharmacy residents and PGY1 pharmacy residents (or PGY2 pharmacy residents from another medical center hospital) enrolled in an elective NSS or TICU rotation. Students on Advanced Pharmacy Practice Experience (APPE) rotations for the month with the clinical faculty are also required to attend as non-presenting participants. Most journal club sessions are comprised of 12–15 attendees.

Journal club meetings are scheduled twice monthly on the second and fourth Tuesday of every month at 3 P.M. and is to last no longer than 1 h. This time was found to be conducive for attendance as the NSS and TICU pharmacy services tend to complete most of their clinical activities for the day by that time as clinical service responsibilities usually begin at 6 or 7 a.m. for each service. In addition, a consistent time and day facilitates the development of a routine, whereby the session is unlikely to be inadvertently forgotten and missed. The location of journal club meetings is also kept consistent and held in a conference room at the College of Pharmacy building, which is located adjacent to the hospital. The tables and chairs are arranged in a rectangular format to facilitate interactive communication among the participants. The presenter may be located within any location in the rectangle.

It has been suggested that journal clubs can encourage residents to regularly and critically read the medical literature but will not succeed if the journal club suffers from poor attendance or periodic abandonment [6]. Attendance is mandatory for the PGY2 pharmacy residents, PGY1 pharmacy residents in an elective TICU or NSS rotation, and APPE students. Attendance is not mandatory for faculty but strongly encouraged. Because faculty recognize the importance of journal clubs in their professional development as well as for the resident's growth, they consistently attend.

Twenty-nine journals are screened monthly (Table 1). The journals are then divided into four groups with approximately the same workload in terms of collective monthly publication rate for their respective journals. The "nutrition focused" journals are compiled into a single group and presentation of that material is assigned to a pharmacy resident on NSS that month or an NSS-oriented faculty member. The other three periodical groups comprise critical care, pharmacy, infectious disease, and medical journals and is assigned to a critical care faculty member or resident on a critical care rotation. Two participants are required to present at each journal club meeting with each having up to 30 min for their presentation. The presentation schedule is arranged biannually by the PGY2 residents and the number of presentations are equally distributed among all core journal club participants. This arrangement amounts to four or five required presentations by each full-time participant yearly.

Table 1. Organization of journals by presentation group *.

Group	Journals
A	Antimicrobial Agents & Chemotherapy, Chest, Critical Care Clinics, Emergency Medicine Clinics of North America, Journal of Trauma, Infectious Disease Clinics of North America, Medical Clinics of North America, New England Journal of Medicine, Surgical Clinics of North America
B	American Journal of Clinical Nutrition, Annals of Surgery, Clinical Nutrition, Current Opinion in Clinical Nutrition & Metabolic Care, JPEN Journal of Parenteral and Enteral Nutrition, Nutrition, Nutrition in Clinical Practice, Surgery
C	Annals of Pharmacotherapy, Critical Care, Critical Care Medicine, Current Opinion in Critical Care, Journal of the American Medical Association, Journal of Antimicrobial Chemotherapy
D	Annals of Internal Medicine, Clinical Infectious Diseases, Intensive Care Medicine, JAMA Internal Medicine, Journal of Critical Care, Pharmacotherapy

* Groups A and B are presented on the second Tuesday of the month; Groups C and D are presented on the fourth Tuesday of the month.

The scheduled presenter must screen the assigned journals and develop a packet of materials consisting of a face sheet, the table of contents for all assigned periodicals for the month, the first page of selected articles containing the abstract of the paper, and sometimes an entire article if the presenter considers the paper of pivotal importance. A truncated example of the journal club packet is provided in Appendix A. The face sheet contains a table containing the journal, its publication month/date, and titles of key papers selected by the presenter from those journals. The presenter is also expected to have read those key papers listed in the face sheet and be able to answer any inquiries the journal club participants may have. The current table of contents from each journal issue being presented are also provided to allow closer screening by all participants in the event a "pertinent article" was missed by the presenter. This scenario is more common among the trainee presenters as they do not have the depth of knowledge of the mentors and may not recognize an article as novel or controversial based on current information in the field. Because of the volume of material to be reviewed in thirty minutes, only a brief synopsis of those articles identified on the face sheet as "applicable to our clinical practice" can be given. The first page of the "key articles" is added to the packet of tables of contents so that the participant can read the abstract to ascertain if the full paper needs to be retrieved for closer evaluation. Additional time may be given for presentation of a paper deemed extremely important by the presenter. Under such conditions, the entire paper is usually added to the packet of materials. Only the primary literature is discussed. The preceptors will, at times, elaborate on a discussed manuscript. They will put the research in perspective based on their knowledge of the topic. This technique enhances the learning of those that are not experts in this area. For example, one preceptor might elaborate on the significance of a bacteremia study, since they personally conduct research in this area. They usually point out significant findings or deficiencies in the manuscript, based on their expertise in the field.

Reviews, guidelines, and position papers are not reviewed but may be provided on the face sheet and mentioned during the presentation to alert journal club attendees of its presence. The following month's presenters use the current month's face sheet to ascertain what issues of the assigned journals have already been evaluated so that a lapse in coverage in evaluating journal content can be avoided.

5. Identification of Journals

Our journal club's current periodicals identified for screening and presentation are listed in Table 1. Because our practices are intertwined between NSS and TICU with the trauma intensive care unit as the primary practice focus, most selected journals are applicable to both practice settings. Since a significant contribution of the TICU pharmacy practice entails antibiotic therapy, key infectious diseases journals are additionally included. The list of periodicals intentionally includes some journals that focus on providing state of the art reviews in various critical care and nutrition support arenas. The intent of including these journals is to facilitate a broader knowledgebase in the NSS and critical care practice arenas among the journal club attendees despite the unlikelihood of presentation of specific articles. It is also anticipated that journal club attendees may independently screen and read journals not listed in Table 1. Examples of this scenario would include journals associated with their organizational memberships or periodicals that are too specialized to meet the needs of all journal club participants, or those that do not consistently provide papers applicable to our practice group but are of scholarly interest to the individual. Approximately yearly, near the end of the residency cycle, the faculty mentors convene after a journal club session to discuss which journals lacked success in meeting our educational needs and whether any journals need to be added or deleted to our current screening list of periodicals.

6. Evaluation of Success of the Journal Club Technique

To evaluate the success of our journal club in identifying articles pertinent to our practice, we examined a series of publications which was intended to identify the most significant articles for pharmacy nutrition support and critical care pharmacy practice published from 2013 to 2017 [12–18] and compared them to our current list of periodicals screened by our journal club. The intent of these publication series was to assist the pharmacist engaged in nutrition support or critical care pharmacotherapy in staying current with the pertinent literature. For identification of papers deemed important to pharmacy nutrition support practice, eight board-certified pharmacists from differing institutions with advanced practice roles and direct patient care responsibilities contributed to the collective identification of papers. The authors had different practices with some having a diverse patient population, whereas others had a focused patient population (e.g., critical care, pediatrics, oncology, and long-term/home nutrition therapy). After an initial identification of over 100 articles published per year that may be important to pharmacy nutrition support practice, the group of authors significantly reduced the number of papers deemed to be of high importance as evidenced by the majority vote (defined as at five out of eight authors agreed that the paper was of high significance) [12–14]. On behalf of the Critical Care Pharmacotherapy Literature Update Group, comprised of over forty critical care pharmacists across the United States, the authors reviewed hundreds of articles annually with summaries disseminated nationally via a monthly newsletter and social media outlets. Articles selected for inclusion into the yearly paper indicating major publications were rated according to the Grading of Recommendation, Assessment, Development and Evaluation (GRADE) methodology [19] in addition to consideration of their applicability to reinforce or change current clinical practice in various critically ill subpopulations. These articles were published in a series of annual publications covering the years 2012–2015 [15–18].

Eighty-seven papers significant to pharmacy nutrition support practice were identified by the author group over the four-year observation period. Seventy-five articles were from periodicals included in our journal club. An additional three articles were from a journal that was not included in the screening list of periodicals but all faculty and PGY2 residents receive as part of their membership of the journal's sponsoring organization (Table 2). Seventy-eight out of eighty-seven papers or approximately 90% of significant papers deemed pertinent to pharmacy nutrition support practice could be potentially captured with our journal club methodology. For significant critical care pharmacotherapy papers, forty-four articles from thirteen different journals were reviewed by the Critical Care Pharmacy Literature Update Group (Table 3). Our journal club captured seven out of thirteen periodicals listed by the Critical Care group. Out of the total of forty-four identified papers from these thirteen journals that were identified by Critical Care Pharmacy Literature Update Group, our screening methodology captured 35 or 80% of them. Of the nine missed papers, seven were from cardiology journals. It is important to note that our specialized practice includes very little cardiology. Most patients with primary cardiac disorders are treated at another local hospital. The remaining journals that were not screened would be considered as low-yield journals for us throughout the year. These results indicate that a broad and appropriate selection of periodicals is of paramount importance to staying informed. Our methodology was an effective and efficient means to stay abreast of the majority of new knowledge applicable to our clinical practice.

Table 2. Evaluation of success of the journal club for identifying the most pertinent papers for pharmacy nutrition support practice from 2013 to 2016 [12–14].

Journal	Number of Significant Articles	Journal Screened?
Journal of Parenteral and Enteral Nutrition	27	Yes
Nutrition in Clinical Practice	10	Yes
Critical Care	7	Yes
Critical Care Medicine	7	Yes
Clinical Nutrition	7	Yes
Journal of the American Medical Association	5	Yes
New England Journal of Medicine	5	Yes
American Journal of Health-System Pharmacy	3	No *
American Journal of Clinical Nutrition	2	Yes
American Journal of Gastroenterology	2	No
Intensive Care Medicine	2	Yes
Annals of Intensive Care	1	No
Annals of Oncology	1	No

Table 2. *Cont.*

Journal	Number of Significant Articles	Journal Screened?
Annals of Surgery	1	Yes
British Medical Journal	1	No
Clinical Infectious Diseases	1	Yes
Diabetes Care	1	No
Journal of Pediatrics	1	No
Journal of Pediatric Surgery	1	No
Lancet	1	No
Nutrition	1	Yes
Pharmacotherapy	1	Yes

* All faculty members receive this journal as part of membership of the organization despite its not being listed in the journal club's screening list of journals.

Table 3. Evaluation of success of the journal club for identifying the most pertinent papers for pharmacy critical care practice from 2012 to 2015 [15–18].

Journal	Number of Significant Articles	Journal Screened?
New England Journal of Medicine	18	Yes
Critical Care Medicine	6	Yes
Journal of the American Medical Association	5	Yes
Journal of the American College of Cardiology	4	No
Circulation	2	No
Critical Care	2	Yes
American Journal of Health-System Pharmacy	1	No *
American Journal of Respiratory and Critical Care Medicine	1	Yes
Anesthesia and Analgesia	1	No
Clinical Infectious Diseases	1	Yes
Journal of Parenteral and Enteral Nutrition	1	Yes
Lancet	1	No
Stroke	1	No

* Guideline co-published in Critical Care Medicine. All faculty members receive this journal as part of membership of the organization despite its not being listed in the journal club's screening list of journals.

7. Conclusions

Staying current with the literature is a daunting but essential task for the pharmacist who is engaged in an evidenced-based clinical practice. Presented in this review is a method for redesigning journal clubs from the traditional technique of an in-depth analysis of one or two articles to a screening tool that effectively keeps pharmacists informed of current literature. This technique reduces workload of the individual by sharing duties among multiple pharmacists and provides a forum for faculty and senior clinicians to mentor their trainees. This methodological redesign of the traditional journal club is offered to others for consideration.

Acknowledgments: The assistance of Bradley A. Boucher for participation in the development and sustained activity of the journal club is acknowledged.

Author Contributions: Roland N. Dickerson conceived the project and prepared the first draft and subsequent revisions to the manuscript. G. Christopher Wood, Joe M. Swanson, and Rex O. Brown reviewed and made substantial contributions to the finalized version of the manuscript.

Appendix A. Journal Club Packet Example

1. The face or cover page would contain the following information for one group of journals in this format:

Journal Club
Group B Journals
9 May 2017 (*the date of the journal club presentation*)
Roland Dickerson, Pharm.D. (*the presenter*)

Table A1. Example of face page format and content.

Journal	Month	Selected Papers of Interest
JPEN	May	• Management of parenteral nutrition (tutorial) • Volume based enteral nutrition may improve caloric delivery but not clinical outcomes in critically ill patients • Hyperglycemia without DM during home PN • Prevention of CRBSI with catheter locks—home PN
Am J Clin Nutr	May	• None
Clin Nutr	April	• Previously done—next issue will be published in June
Nutrition	May	• Impact of nutrition support on clinical outcomes and cost effectiveness: prospective cohort with propensity score matching • Age dependent risk factors for malnutrition in trauma patients • Presence of validated malnutrition screening tool associated with better nutrition care
Nutr Clin Pract	April	• Proceedings of the 2016 International Protein Summit (Supplement)
Curr Opin Clin Nutr Metab Care	May	• Focus on muscle protein dynamics and pediatric nutrition • Vitamin D and muscle trophicity (review)
Ann Surg	May	• Pitfalls and bias in observational studies with propensity score analysis
Surgery	May	• None

2. The next set of pages are photocopies of all assigned journals' table of contents within the grouping for the month. The intent for providing the table of contents for all journals is for a second screening by the journal club participants to ensure all pertinent articles were identified (including those inadvertently omitted by the presenter).

3. The final set of pages are photocopies of the first page of the identified papers for each journal as outlined by the bullet points from the selected papers column on the face page. This gives the non-presenting journal club participant the ability to read the abstract to ascertain if retrieval of

the full paper for more in-depth reading is necessary. Sometimes, the journal club presenter may provide the entire paper in the packet if it is deemed of high importance to our practice.

References

1.   Linzer, M. The journal club and medical education: Over one hundred years of unrecorded history. *Postgrad. Med. J.* **1987**, *63*, 475–478. [CrossRef] [PubMed]
2.   Valentini, R.P.; Daniels, S.R. The journal club. *Postgrad. Med. J.* **1997**, *73*, 81–85. [CrossRef] [PubMed]
3.   Spillane, A.J.; Crowe, P.J. The role of the journal club in surgical training. *Aust. N. Z. J. Surg.* **1998**, *68*, 288–291. [CrossRef] [PubMed]
4.   Szucs, K.A.; Benson, J.D.; Haneman, B. Using a Guided Journal Club as a Teaching Strategy to Enhance Learning Skills for Evidence-Based Practice. *Occup. Ther. Health Care* **2017**, *31*, 143–149. [CrossRef] [PubMed]
5.   Linzer, M.; Brown, J.T.; Frazier, L.M.; DeLong, E.R.; Siegel, W.C. Impact of a medical journal club on house-staff reading habits, knowledge, and critical appraisal skills. A randomized control trial. *J. Am. Med. Assoc.* **1988**, *260*, 2537–2541. [CrossRef]
6.   Sidorov, J. How are internal medicine residency journal clubs organized, and what makes them successful? *Arch. Intern. Med.* **1995**, *155*, 1193–1197. [CrossRef] [PubMed]
7.   Hartzell, J.D.; Veerappan, G.R.; Posley, K.; Shumway, N.M.; Durning, S.J. Resident run journal club: A model based on the adult learning theory. *Med. Teach.* **2009**, *31*, e156–e161. [CrossRef] [PubMed]
8.   Alguire, P.C. A review of journal clubs in postgraduate medical education. *J. Gen. Intern. Med.* **1998**, *13*, 347–353. [CrossRef] [PubMed]
9.   Accreditation Council for Pharmacy Education. *Accreditation Standards and Key Elements for the Professional Program in Pharmacy Leading to the Doctor of Pharmacy Degree*; ("Standards 2016"); Accreditation Council for Pharmacy Education: Chicago, IL, USA, 2015; pp. 1–31. Available online: https://www.acpe-accredit.org/pdf/Standards2016FINAL.pdf (accessed on 21 September 2017).
10. Al Achkar, M. Redesigning journal club in residency. *Adv. Med. Educ. Pract.* **2016**, *7*, 317–320. [CrossRef] [PubMed]
11. Bornmann, L.; Mutz, R. Growth rates of modern science: A bibliometric analysis based on the number of publications and cited references. *J. Assoc. Inf. Sci. Technol.* **2015**, *66*, 2215–2222. [CrossRef]
12. Dickerson, R.N.; Kumpf, V.J.; Bingham, A.L.; Cogle, S.V.; Blackmer, A.B.; Tucker, A.M.; Chan, L.N.; Canada, T.W. Significant published articles for pharmacy nutrition support practice in 2016. *Hosp. Pharm.* **2017**, *52*, 412–421. [CrossRef]
13. Dickerson, R.N.; Kumpf, V.J.; Blackmer, A.B.; Bingham, A.L.; Tucker, A.M.; Ybarra, J.V.; Kraft, M.D.; Canada, T.W. Significant Published Articles for Pharmacy Nutrition Support Practice in 2014 and 2015. *Hosp. Pharm.* **2016**, *51*, 539–552. [CrossRef] [PubMed]
14. Dickerson, R.N.; Kumpf, V.J.; Rollins, C.J.; Frankel, E.H.; Kraft, M.D.; Canada, T.W.; Crill, C.M. Significant publications for pharmacy nutrition support practice in 2013. *Hosp. Pharm.* **2014**, *49*, 717–730. [CrossRef] [PubMed]
15. Day, S.A.; Cucci, M.; Droege, M.E.; Holzhausen, J.M.; Kram, B.; Kram, S.; Pajoumand, M.; Parker, C.R.; Patel, M.K.; Peitz, G.J.; et al. Major publications in the critical care pharmacotherapy literature: January-December 2014. *Am. J. Health-Syst. Pharm.* **2015**, *72*, 1974–1985. [CrossRef] [PubMed]
16. Rech, M.A.; Day, S.A.; Kast, J.M.; Donahey, E.E.; Pajoumand, M.; Kram, S.J.; Erdman, M.J.; Peitz, G.J.; Allen, J.M.; Palmer, A.; et al. Major publications in the critical care pharmacotherapy literature: January-December 2013. *Am. J. Health-Syst. Pharm.* **2015**, *72*, 224–236. [CrossRef] [PubMed]
17. Turck, C.J.; Frazee, E.; Kram, B.; Daley, M.J.; Day, S.A.; Horner, D.; Lesch, C.; Mercer, J.M.; Plewa, A.M.; Herout, P. Major publications in the critical care pharmacotherapy literature: February 2012 through February 2013. *Am. J. Health-Syst. Pharm.* **2014**, *71*, 68–77. [CrossRef] [PubMed]
18. Wong, A.; Erdman, M.; Hammond, D.A.; Holt, T.; Holzhausen, J.M.; Horng, M.; Huang, L.L.; Jarvis, J.; Kram, B.; Kram, S.; et al. Major publications in the critical care pharmacotherapy literature in 2015. *Am. J. Health-Syst. Pharm.* **2017**, *74*, 295–311. [CrossRef] [PubMed]
19. Guyatt, G.H.; Oxman, A.D.; Vist, G.E.; Kunz, R.; Falck-Ytter, Y.; Alonso-Coello, P.; Schünemann, H.J. GRADE: An emerging consensus on rating quality of evidence and strength of recommendations. *Br. Med. J.* **2008**, *336*, 924–926. [CrossRef] [PubMed]

5

Assessing the Understanding of Pharmaceutical Pictograms among Cultural Minorities: The Example of Hindu Individuals Communicating in European Portuguese

Lakhan Kanji, Sensen Xu and Afonso Cavaco * (iD)

Department of Social Pharmacy, Faculty of Pharmacy, University of Lisbon. Av. Prof. Gama Pinto, 1649-003 Lisboa, Portugal; lakhan@hotmail.com (L.K.); sensen.58@hotmail.com (S.X.)
* Correspondence: acavaco@ff.ulisboa.pt

Abstract: One of the sources of poor health outcomes is the lack of compliance with the prescribed treatment plans, often due to communication barriers between healthcare professionals and patients. Pictograms are a form of communication that conveys meaning through its pictorial resemblance to a physical object or an action. Pharmaceutical pictograms are often associated with a better comprehension of treatment regimens, although their use is still subject to limitations. The main goal of this study was to examine the potential understanding of pharmaceutical pictograms by a cultural minority when providing patient information while comparing the effectiveness of two reference systems (United States Pharmacopeia USP and International Pharmacy Federation FIP) for this purpose. A self-administered questionnaire was developed comprising 30 pictograms, 15 selected from the United States Pharmacopeia Dispensing Information and the equivalent from the International Pharmaceutical Federation. The questionnaire comprised plain instructions, socio-demographic data, self-reported language fluency and pictogram labels in Portuguese presented to conveniently selected members of the Hindu community of Lisbon (Portugal) until reaching a quota of 50. Participants showed difficulties in understanding some pictograms, which was related to the self-reported reduced fluency in Portuguese. Overall, the interpretation of USP pictograms was better than FIP ones, as well as for pictograms composed of multiple images, presenting a negative reading, or when conveying information unrelated to medication instructions. Even using internationally validated pictograms, added care should be taken when community pharmacists use such communication resources with cultural minorities. It is important not to disregard other forms of patient communication and information, considering pictograms as a complement to other forms of patient counselling.

Keywords: pharmaceutical pictograms; written health communication; Hindu community; USP; FIP PictoRx; Portugal

1. Introduction

It is well accepted that it is the responsibility of community pharmacists to actively contribute to the safe and effective use of medications [1,2]. While their primary mission is to assure the quality of the products dispensed, the current focus on pharmaceutical care practice adds a professional responsibility towards patient medication outcomes [3]. Community pharmacists are actively contributing to improving medication usage, including medication compliance, treatment effectiveness and adverse events monitoring [1,3]. Medication compliance can be defined as the extent to which a patient acts in accordance with the prescribed dosing regimen [4]. Inadequate compliance has important negative patient outcomes [5,6] and usually emerges from therapy costs and complexity of the regimen, being communication barriers between health professionals and patients also known to contribute to non-compliance [6].

Communication barriers may arise from speech or hearing impairments but are commonly a consequence of language issues related to schooling or literacy limitations [7]. Lack of therapy compliance is frequent for the elderly and those who do not speak the same language as the healthcare providers [8–11]. Despite efforts to implement Esperanto or basic English, communication issues persist based on language differences between communities including alphabet, lexical, syntactic and semantic variations, even between bordering counties [12]. To overcome communication issues, information can be conveyed using pictures, symbols, audiotapes or interpreters [9]. One widely known resource, frequently considered a beneficial solution, is the use of pictograms.

1.1. What are Pictograms?

Pictograms are graphic representations of objects or actions conveying a meaning which should be independent of any particular culture or language [12]. They are frequently used to quickly transmit important information such as the male or female gender (e.g., toilets info), safety hazards (e.g., health precautions) or road information (e.g., prohibitions and warnings). Although each cultural environment may promote differences in signs relevance [12,13], a basis for the use of pictograms is their universal interpretation, i.e., they should offer the same meaning regardless of language, culture or education [9,14].

Pictograms have been used to give instructions or warnings regarding health products usage [10,14]. Characteristics such as visual intricacy, concreteness, simplicity, the shape and color of the illustrations can help clarify the information conveyed or, if not well designed, misguide its assimilation [15–17]. As familiarity also plays a role in understanding visual aids, pictogram testing is required to determine its appropriateness [16,18]. Given most pictograms have been designed within Western societies, caution is suggested when using them in cross-cultural contexts [9,19,20].

Pharmaceutical pictograms are useful tools to reinforce both comprehension and recall of medicines-related information, attract attention and reduce misunderstandings regarding a drug treatment [13,15]. Attributes such as the design of the frames, marks expressing negation (e.g., crosses or strikethroughs), specific human body parts, and marks for pain and movement can lead to a decline in comprehension [21]. Pharmaceutical pictograms have been developed and disseminated by a few different organizations such as the Risk-benefit Assessment of Drugs-Analysis and Response (RAD-AR) Council of Japan pictograms, the United States Pharmacopeia Dispensing Information pictograms (USP) and the International Pharmaceutical Federation (FIP) pictograms [22]. The USP pictograms have been widely used in Western societies, although published studies regarding their usability and legibility in different settings revealed potential limitations for culturally diverse populations (e.g., South African) [9–11,23,24]. The FIP pictograms developed in June 2009 were last updated 7 February 2017, according to the website (https://www.fip.org/pictograms, accessed November 2017). This update fixed issues with the language and added Turk and Malayan, which suggest a greater potential to suit multi-cultural societies.

In Portugal, the legibility of USP pictograms was studied by Soares (2012) [25] using the overall Lisbon population. Patients' ability to understand a set of 15 pictograms was measured according to the International Standards Organization (ISO) 3864, which considers as legible the icons presenting over 67% of correct results. Only 10 pictograms were able to achieve the legibility threshold, thus suggesting limitations in USP understanding by the Portuguese population. This was particularly relevant with low literacy and foreign communities, those justifying the development of pictograms [25]. Despite the economic recession, the influx of foreign populations has been constant in mainland Portugal. For instance, the Hindu community has been growing in Lisbon with 6160 emigrants who were born in India (before 2010), as well as from other countries such as Mozambique, Pakistan and Bangladesh [26]. Cultural minorities, who are not well versed in Portuguese, often face communication issues with treatment adherence. The use of pictograms by community pharmacy practitioners may contribute to improving adherence if the pictograms are comprehensible by all patients.

1.2. Study Objectives

The aim of this study was to investigate if pharmaceutical pictograms, specifically United States Pharmacopeia (USP) and the International Pharmaceutical Federation (FIP), were understandable by a Hindu-based population living abroad thus defining a feasible form of pharmaceutical communication with culturally diverse populations in Portugal. Besides the cultural sensitivity of both USP and FIP, pictograms design and other characteristics which may contribute to an enhanced meaning discernment were also investigated.

2. Materials and Methods

The present study followed a cross-sectional design, using a survey approach.

2.1. Study Participants

This study was conducted with a convenience sample of 50 Hindu individuals living in Lisbon and Tagus Valley regions of Portugal. These individuals were selected from two different Hindu temples, the Radha Krishna Temple and the Shiv Temple in Lisbon, between March and August 2017, by direct invitation from the field researcher. The inclusion criteria considered people aged over 18 years, from both genders, with different levels of education and income. Individuals who lived in India, Pakistan and/or Bangladesh (major Hindu nationalities living in Portugal) for less than five consecutive years, declaring to be unable to read Portuguese, or presenting any limitations that might prevent them from interpreting the pictograms, were excluded from the study. The selected participants responded to the questionnaire, after voluntarily signing the informed consent. From all approached and able to participate, a drop out of 18 participants was registered before achieving the 50 participants quota. The study followed all ethical research principles, particularly concerning participants' full anonymity and data confidentiality, having received ethical approval by the Faculty of Pharmacy Ethical Committee, as well as with respect for the principles stated in the current Portuguese law of personal data protection.

2.2. Questionnaire

The research questionnaire consisted of three sections. The first one comprised participants' socio-demographic data i.e., age, gender, place of birth and citizenship, level of schooling and its location, time living in Portugal, household income, employment status, and healthcare-related variables. While most of these variables were evaluated through closed multiple-choice questions, a Likert-scale was used for participants' self-assessment of their perceived Portuguese proficiency, running from 0 (null aptitude) to 10 (native speaker). This variable was dichotomized in poor and good self-perceived Portuguese fluency, respectively ≤ 5 and >5 points, defining subsample B and subsample A, respectively.

The next section comprised 30 pictograms, 15 selected from the USP set and 15 from the FIP offline non-USA MEPS set. Both sets were obtained from the official websites, accessed in January 2017 (respectively, https://www.usp.org/download-pictograms and https://www.fip.org/www/?page=meps_pict_download_eu). The 15 USP pictograms were those used in previously published papers [24,25,27], 7 reported to be difficult to interpret and 8 more often correctly interpreted. The 15 FIP pictograms were those that conveyed an equal or similar meaning to the selected USP ones. It was checked if the pictograms comprised the graphics features of more than one illustration, non-affirmative marks (e.g., prohibition), and information such as warnings and precautions, besides directions. The pictograms were randomly sequenced in the questionnaire.

Each pictogram was followed by 3 descriptions, one correct and two incorrect options, written in plain European Portuguese. The pictograms correct option was obtained from the direct translation of each USP pictogram label. To develop the two incorrect options, a pilot study was conducted interviewing face-to-face 5 individual members of the Hindu community who speak and write both Portuguese and Hindi fluently. Each pictogram was shown and their interpretations noted. If their interpretation matched the correct label, two other possible options were requested, making sure those were incorrect in wording and/or meaning. If not matching the original description only one alternative interpretation was requested. This procedure produced two incorrect, but credible options, within cultural sensitivity. An informal consensus on the most suitable wrong options to use in the study was reached by the research team, which included two members of cultural minorities living in Lisbon, one from the Hindu community. The pilot study also confirmed the ease of use and completeness of the questionnaire for the members of the community.

Participants filling-in the questionnaire were asked to mark the option they considered to be correctly describing each pictogram. Each correct answer was scored with 3 points, while an incorrect answer would 1 point. A standardized final score between 1 and 3 points was obtained for all questionnaires. In the last section participants were asked about previous experiences with pictograms and to give feedback on the pictograms relevance as a patient information tool. Although this was a self-administered questionnaire, a field researcher was always present during questionnaire completion to answer any participants' voluntary doubts.

2.3. Data Analysis

The analysis started by detailing pictograms classification according to the three previous graphical features, i.e., being composed of either single or multiple image, the presence or absence of any negation mark (e.g., cross or strike) and disclosing directions (e.g., how to take or apply the medication) or relaying other medication information (e.g., contraindications or side-effects). The analysis included the whole set of 30 pictograms of the USP and FIP subsets (15 + 15) i.e., no paired comparisons were intended, although equivalent pictograms from both sets were chosen.

Questionnaire data were analyzed using the IBM SPSS software, version 24. The statistics performed included descriptive results, Students' t-test, Persons' Chi-Square, non-parametric ANOVA tests and Pearson linear correlations. A confidence level equivalent to $p < 0.05$ was used in all tests.

3. Results

3.1. Socio-Demographic Data

The sample comprised mostly males (62%), with an age range between 23 and 63 years of age. Thirty-six of them declared having an Indian passport (72%), while the rest declared being citizens from Pakistan, Bangladesh or Mozambique, the last being included after confirming their main language and culture was Hindu and having lived for at least five consecutive years in that country. Overall, 44% of the respondents have lived in Portugal for up to five years, 26% between 5 and 20 years and 30% lived there for more than 20 years. Almost half (46%) of the participants had more than 12 years of education, with 66% completing their education in India, 12% studied in Portugal and the remainder studied in Pakistan, Bangladesh or Mozambique. Table 1 presents participants' education, self-perceived Portuguese (PT) proficiency and time spent in Portugal across gender and citizenship.

Twenty-two (44%) participants rated their Portuguese fluency as 5 or below, while 28 (56%) rated their fluency as 6 or above. Hence, participants were divided into two subsamples: A speakers ($n = 28$) and B speakers ($n = 22$). The amount of time the respondents have lived in Portugal and their education level were positively associated with their self-perceived Portuguese fluency (respectively, Chi^2 = 6.445, $p = 0.04$ and Chi^2 = 5.547, $p = 0.019$). There was no significant association with the location where the participants acquired their Portuguese language skills, nor associations with other background variables, such as the reported household income (68% under 1000€ per month), employment status (all declared to have a job), and the healthcare provider, e.g., choosing a community pharmacist when afflicted by a minor ailment (72%) and having access to a general practice (GP) physician (64%).

If presenting an ill-health condition, 52% of the participants said they would also seek traditional Hindu medical care. Only one participant admitted having a chronic condition and 39 (78%) reported taking medicines less than once a month.

Table 1. Participants' demographics ($n = 50$) including variables associated with Portuguese fluency.

		Education (Years)		Self-Perc. PT Proficiency		Time Living in PT (Years)		
		≤ 9	>9	≤ 5	>5	≤ 5	≤ 20	>20
Gender	Male	15	16	15	16	15	8	8
	Female	12	7	7	12	7	5	7
	Total	27	23	22	28	22	13	15
Nationality	Portuguese	11	11	6	16	2	5	15
	Hindu	11	10	11	10	14	7	0
	Pakistani	5	0	4	1	4	1	0
	Bangladesh	0	2	1	1	2	0	0
	Total	27	23	22	28	22	13	15

3.2. Pictograms Data

The percentage of correct answers obtained for each individual pictogram are displayed in Table 2. Participants' average score was 1.83 ($\sigma = 0.34$), ranging from 1.27 (the lowest score) to 2.67 (the highest). The most frequently correctly interpreted pictograms were #27, correctly interpreted by 70% of the participants, and #15 by 66% both from the UPS set. The worst interpreted pictograms were #9 (USP), with 45 (90%) participants missing the correct label and #18 (FIP) with 41 (82%) participants missing the correct label option.

Table 2. Pictograms used, meaning and number of correct answers per pictogram ($n = 50$).

Pictogram Id	Images	Pictogram Meaning	Correct Answers Counts (%)
#1 (FIP)		Take this medicine in the morning, afternoon and at night	19 (38%)
#2 (USP)		Do not take this medicine if pregnant	24 (48%)
#3 (FIP)		If this medicine makes you dizzy, do not drive	25 (50%)

Table 2. *Cont.*

Pictogram Id	Images	Pictogram Meaning	Correct Answers Counts (%)
#4 (FIP)		Take this medicine with an empty stomach	19 (38%)
#5 (USP)		Store this medicine in the fridge	24 (48%)
#6 (USP)		Keep this medicine out of the reach of children	32 (64%)
#7 (FIP)		Do not drink alcoholic beverages during treatment with this medicine	15 (30%)
#8 (USP)		Do not break the tablets nor open the capsules	20 (40%)
#9 (USP)		Take this medicine 3 times per day	5 (10%)
#10 (FIP)		Do not take this medicine if breastfeeding	17 (34%)
#11 (USP)		Take this medicine with meals	20 (40%)

Table 2. *Cont.*

Pictogram Id	Images	Pictogram Meaning	Correct Answers Counts (%)
#12 (FIP)		Insert the medicine in the vagina	23 (46%)
#13 (USP)		Do not take this medicine with meals	26 (52%)
#14 (FIP)		This medicine can cause sleepiness	18 (36%)
#15 (USP)		Do not take this medicine if breastfeeding	33 (66%)
#16 (USP)		Do not drink alcoholic beverages during treatment with this medicine	23 (46%)
#17 (USP)		Wash your hands before and after applying this medicine on the ear	24 (48%)
#18 (FIP)		Keep this medicine out of the reach of children	9 (18%)
#19 (FIP)		Store this medicine in the fridge	18 (36%)

Table 2. *Cont.*

Pictogram Id	Images	Pictogram Meaning	Correct Answers Counts (%)
#20 (FIP)		Shake this medicine before using	26 (52%)
#21 (FIP)		Do not break the tablets nor open the capsules	26 (52%)
#22 (FIP)		Do not take this medicine if pregnant	14 (28%)
#23 (FIP)		Take this medicine with meals	12 (24%)
#24 (USP)		Drink this medicine with an extra glass of water	12 (24%)
#25 (USP)		Shake this medicine before using	22 (44%)
#26 (FIP)		Apply one drop of this medicine on the left and on the right ears	18 (36%)

Table 2. *Cont.*

Pictogram Id	Images	Pictogram Meaning	Correct Answers Counts (%)
#27 (USP)		Wash your hands before and after applying this medicine on the vagina	35 (70%)
#28 (USP)		This medicine can cause sleepiness	26 (52%)
#29 (USP)		If this medicine makes you dizzy, do not drive	17 (34%)
#30 (FIP)		Take this medicine with water	17 (34%)

USP—United States Pharmacopeia; FIP—International Pharmacy Federation.

No significant linear correlation was found between participants' age and the total score. A significant negative correlation existed between the total score and the time spent outside Portugal ($r = -0.584$, $p < 0.001$) corroborated by the positive correlation for the total score and the time lived in Portugal ($r = 0.385$, $p = 0.006$). No significant differences were found between; male and female participants, the level or place of schooling, or income and employment status. A statistically significant difference was found between those having good Portuguese fluency (A participants) and poor fluency (B participants) ($t = -3.008$, $p = 0.004$). Only one participant acknowledged having had previous contact with pictograms. Thirty-eight (76%) participants considered them to be helpful for correctly understanding treatment plans.

The average USP and FIP pictograms scores were, respectively, 1.92 ($\sigma = 0.37$) and 1.74 ($\sigma = 0.37$). The USP set had a statistically significantly higher score ($t = -3.40$, $p = 0.001$) compared to the FIP. Testing the self-reported language ability (subsamples A and B) against the USP and FIP average scores confirmed differences within both pictorial sets (respectively, $t = -2.98$, $p = 0.004$ and $t = -2.53$, $p = 0.01$). The poorer Portuguese speaking participants (subsample B) showed average scores for USP of 1.75 ($\sigma = 0.36$) and for FIP of 1.59 ($\sigma = 0.33$), a difference that was significantly lower ($t = -2.27$, $p = 0.03$). Several other variables (e.g., pictograms relevance, household income, minor ailments behavior, and having a GP) were tested against participants' average scores within all sample and subsamples and no significant associations were found.

3.3. Pictogram Design Data

Mean scores and standard deviations were calculated according to pictograms dichotomous graphical classifications. These were compared using Students' *t*-test for the entire sample as well as subsamples A and B. The results are presented in Table 3.

Table 3. Means and standard deviation according to pictograms design.

		Entire Sample		Subsample A		Subsample B	
		Average	σ	Average	σ	Average	σ
Images	1	1.68	0.43	1.79	0.46	1.55	0.36
	>1	1.92	0.35	2.05	0.29	1.75	0.34
Negation marks	Present	1.87	0.45	2.06	0.39	1.62	0.39
	Absent	1.80	0.32	1.86	0.32	1.72	0.31
Text	Directions	1.80	0.34	1.88	0.35	1.71	0.31
	Other info	1.86	0.43	2.04	0.37	1.62	0.39

There were 12 (40%) pictograms consisting of a single image and 18 (60%) with multiple images, the latter achieving a significantly higher total score (All: $t = -3.91$, $p = 0.001$; A: $t = -3.09$, $p = 0.005$; B: $t = -2.62$, $p = 0.016$). Thirteen (43%) pictograms had negation marks, with only a significantly higher mean interpretation score found between A participants and the entire sample (A: $t = -3.35$, $p = 0.002$) for multiple images. Sixty percent of pictograms had medication directions, while 40% had other information. As with non-affirmative signs, only the subsample A had significantly better interpretation of other information (A: $t = -2.42$, $p = 0.022$).

4. Discussion

Pharmaceutical pictograms are widely accepted as an important resource that provide patients with information regarding their drug therapies and believed to meaningfully contribute to safer and more effective medication use. The present study addressed the comprehension of well-known pharmaceutical pictograms by a population that does not necessarily share the cultural and linguistic background of the native population, thus requiring additional resources for effective communication.

In the present study, participants' self-reported Portuguese fluency was found to be associated with their schooling, as well as with the time spent in Portugal, but not related to the country of formal education. On the other hand, their pictogram comprehension was significantly related to the time participants have lived in and out of Portugal. In this sense, participants' Portuguese literacy might have been developed from an informal daily usage of the language, which suggests potential language limitations regarding less frequent and more specific contexts, such as being ill and using medication. The present study population could be an adequate means to study the usefulness of pharmaceutical pictograms.

4.1. Pictograms Comprehension

This study found only one pictogram (#27) out of 30 that could be immediately used in pharmacy practice, according to the ISO-3864 legibility criteria, i.e., using the 67% correct interpretation cut-off. This was lower than expected, given previous results from participants living in Portugal [25]. One cause might be the interpretation issues with reading Portuguese when choosing from the pictogram 3 label options. In fact, there was a clear association between the self-reported Portuguese fluency and average scores: the poor language proficiency group always scored worse. This confirms the common belief that effective communication issues resulting from language barriers, which frequently emerge within culturally diverse populations, may not be overcome without the effort to explain pictograms. These signs on their own might not be enough to guarantee appropriate patient information and the expected medication usage. Practitioners should keep in mind that pictograms comprehension was also independent of variables such as the frequency of using community pharmacies (for solving minor health ailments) or being in contact with a GP. Having more or less interaction with healthcare providers does not guarantee better or worse understanding of pharmaceutical pictograms, assuming the absence of translators in community pharmacies. The Hindu cultural minority, as many other minorities living in Portugal, will not necessarily be better informed just by using pictograms and hoping they will do their job. Moreover, no associations were found between different comprehension scores and appreciation of pictograms relevance, which were considered helpful to understand medication regimens. Thus, pharmaceutical pictograms are an important tool in patient counselling, although their full success requires further attention regarding the actual level of comprehension achieved by a certain population.

4.2. SP and FIP Comparison

FIP MEPS pictograms are a set of illustrations issued in 2009, more than one decade after the USP set released in 1997. FIP, a world-wide organization, released a pictogram software update on 7 February 2017 that fixed some language issues and included Turkish and Malayan as languages. Even if developers warn of cultural sensitivity issues, it was expected the pictograms would relay information more precisely. However, this was not confirmed: the average total comprehension score obtained with USP pictograms was significantly higher than the correspondent FIP result. This is also true when the individuals rated their Portuguese fluency as poor. This indicates that USP pictograms could be better suited to the Hindu population living in Lisbon than the FIP set, knowing pharmacists can access both freely.

4.3. Pictograms Design

The present study findings were not always in line with previous studies, acknowledging different research settings. The use of single images did not seem to be preferable to multiple images [17,20]. One possible explanation may be the use of several sequential frames helping the participant to better infer the meaning of subsequent images. Negatively marked pictograms were more easily interpreted, which also differs from previously published literature [18,21]. However, interpreting negative marks well (as well as medication-related information content) was achieved by those who considered themselves fluent in Portuguese. This could be a cultural feature from this sample, where these pictograms may resemble other common signs of caution to which Hindus are more sensitive. Finally, pictograms illustrating medication directions may convey more information than pictograms with warnings or precautions thus increasing complexity leading to diminished understanding among the sampled population. All these results are in line with previous findings mentioning that culture-specific and education level-specific pictograms may be essential for the effective communication of health information [28].

4.4. Study Limitations

Some resistance to full participation was found during the fieldwork. Bulky questionnaires with a high number of pages because of the room need for the pictures seemed to discouraged participants from completing them. As mentioned earlier, 18 selected participants dropped out before achieving the 50 participants quota, even with support from the field researcher where requested. During the pre-test, participants took an average of 11 min to complete the questionnaire but during data gathering people often took longer, mainly due to poorer understanding of the questions or to external interferences (e.g., others waiting). This apparent reluctance in completing the survey may also result from the infrequent contact due to disbelief in pictograms by community pharmacies. Using an interview approach instead of a self-administered questionnaire may have improved participation, although impact on findings is not possible to assess.

More importantly, participants showed some difficulties in reading and understanding the written information, including the wording of the options for each pictogram. While assuring a more genuine background (i.e., Portuguese is the dominant language in healthcare provision), it was not possible to control for the effects of functional cognitive abilities and literacy. No structured and independent assessment of Portuguese speaking proficiency was conducted which possibly contributed to less accurate reading of the options per pictogram and answering. This was minimized by translating questions to Hindu only when necessary, avoiding introducing undue variation in survey administration and additional response bias.

Extending the present results to all Hindu communities in Lisbon or Portugal, or other culturally diverse sub-populations, should be done with care since no representativeness or external validation was achieved in this study, resulting from anticipated time constraints. Finally, no qualitative approach was taken to investigate the reasons underlying such diverse interpretation on paired pictograms (e.g., #1 and #9 or #7 and #16), which adds further caution if the present findings are to be directly used in practice, even within the Hindu community.

5. Conclusions

Pictograms are potentially a good way to pass on treatment directions and precautions, in particular to culturally challenging populations, such as the Hindu Community in Portugal. Nevertheless, this study indicated that pictograms may fail their mission. Thus, it is recommended that prior to generalized usage, pictograms are tested with local populations. If local refinements are not possible, usage warnings should be issued by the responsible health authorities, alerting professionals to use them with attention.

Further field studies with pharmaceutical pictograms in Portuguese community pharmacies are needed to improve the validation and usefulness of this tool. Pictograms do not replace pharmacist–patient communication, but they cannot be ignored as an information resource in Portuguese pharmacy practice.

Acknowledgments: No sources of funding were used.

Author Contributions: A.C. conceived and designed the survey; L.K. and S.X. performed the data collection; L.K., S.X. and A.C. analyzed the data; and L.K. and A.C. wrote the paper.

References

1. O'Loughlin, J.; Masson, P.; Déry, V.; Fagnan, D. The role of community pharmacists in health education and disease prevention: A survey of their interests and needs in relation to cardiovascular disease. *Prev. Med.* **1999**, *28*, 324–331. [CrossRef] [PubMed]
2. Van Grootheest, A.C.; de Jong-van den Berg, L.T. The role of hospital and community pharmacists in pharmacovigilance. *Res. Soc. Adm. Pharm.* **2005**, *1*, 126–133. [CrossRef] [PubMed]
3. Bryant, L.J.; Coster, G.; Gamble, G.D.; McCormick, R.N. General practitioners' and pharmacists' perceptions of the role of community pharmacists in delivering clinical services. *Res. Soc. Adm. Pharm.* **2009**, *5*, 347–362. [CrossRef] [PubMed]
4. Cramer, J.A.; Roy, A.; Burrell, A.; Fairchild, C.J.; Fuldeore, M.J.; Ollendorf, D.A.; Wong, P.K. Medication compliance and persistence: Terminology and definitions. *Value Health* **2008**, *11*, 44–47. [CrossRef] [PubMed]
5. Balkrishnan, R.; Rajagopalan, R.; Camacho, F.T.; Huston, S.A.; Murray, F.T.; Anderson, R.T. Predictors of medication adherence and associated health care costs in an older population with type 2 diabetes mellitus: A longitudinal cohort study. *Clin. Ther.* **2003**, *25*, 2958–2971. [CrossRef]
6. Ho, P.M.; Rumsfeld, J.S.; Masoudi, F.A.; McClure, D.L.; Plomondon, M.E.; Steiner, J.F.; Magid, D.J. Effect of medication nonadherence on hospitalization and mortality among patients with diabetes mellitus. *Arch. Intern. Med.* **2006**, *166*, 1836–1841. [CrossRef] [PubMed]
7. Barros, I.M.; Alcântara, T.S.; Mesquita, A.R.; Santos, A.C.; Paixão, F.P.; Lyra, D.P. The use of pictograms in the health care: A literature review. *Res. Soc. Adm. Pharm.* **2014**, *10*, 704–719. [CrossRef] [PubMed]
8. Ng, A.W.; Chan, A.H.; Ho, V.W. Comprehension by older people of medication information with or without supplementary pharmaceutical pictograms. *Appl. Ergon.* **2017**, *58*, 167–175. [CrossRef] [PubMed]
9. Kassam, R.; Vaillancourt, L.R.; Collins, J.B. Pictographic instructions for medications: Do different cultures interpret them accurately? *Int. J. Pharm. Pract.* **2004**, *12*, 199–209. [CrossRef]
10. Yasmin, R.; Shakeel, S.; Iffat, W.; Hasnat, S.; Quds, T. Comparative Analysis of Understanding of Pictograms in Pharmacy and non-Pharmacy Students. *Intl. J. Sci. Basic Appl. Res.* **2014**, *13*, 197–204.

11. Barros, I.M.; Alcântara, T.S.; Mesquita, A.R.; Bispo, M.L.; Rocha, C.E.; Moreira, V.P.; Junior, D.P.L. Understanding of pictograms from the United States Pharmacopeia Dispensing Information (USP-DI) among elderly Brazilians. *Patient Prefer Adher.* **2014**, *8*, 1493–1501.

12. Kolers, P. Some formal characteristics of pictograms. *Am. Sci.* **1969**, *57*, 348–363.

13. Dowse, R.; Ehlers, M. Medicine labels incorporating pictograms: Do they influence understanding and adherence? *Patient Educ. Couns.* **2005**, *58*, 63–70. [CrossRef] [PubMed]

14. Fonseca, R. Reading Pictograms and Signs—The Need for Visual Literacy. Master's Thesis, University of Stavanger, Stavanger, Norway, 2011. Available online: https://brage.bibsys.no/xmlui/handle/11250/185313 (accessed on 1 September 2017).

15. Davies, S.; Haines, H.; Norris, B.; Wilson, J.R. Safety pictograms: Are they getting the message across? *Appl. Ergon.* **1998**, *29*, 15–23. [CrossRef]

16. McDougall, S.J.; Curry, M.B.; de Bruijn, O. Measuring symbol and icon characteristics: Norms for concreteness, complexity, meaningfulness, familiarity, and semantic distance for 239 symbols. *Behav. Res. Methods Instrum. Comput.* **1999**, *31*, 487–519. [CrossRef] [PubMed]

17. Rogers, Y. Icon Design for the User Interface. In *International Reviews of Ergonomics*; Oborne, D.J., Ed.; Taylor & Francis: London, UK, 1989; pp. 129–155.

18. Wolf, J.S.; Wogalter, M.S. Test and development of pharmaceutical pictorials. *Proc. Interface* **1993**, *93*, 187–192.

19. Foster, J.J.; Afzalnia, M.R. International assessment of judged symbol comprehensibility. *Int. J. Psychol.* **2005**, *40*, 169–175. [CrossRef]

20. Lee, S.; Dazkir, S.S.; Paik, H.S.; Coskun, A. Comprehensibility of universal healthcare symbols for wayfinding in healthcare facilities. *Appl. Ergon.* **2014**, *45*, 878–885. [CrossRef] [PubMed]

21. Montagne, M. Pharmaceutical pictograms: A model for development and testing for comprehension and utility. *Res. Soc. Adm. Pharm.* **2013**, *9*, 609–620. [CrossRef] [PubMed]

22. Health Sciences Library. Health Literacy and Patient Education Guide: Pictograms. 2017. Available online: http://hslibraryguides.ucdenver.edu/c.php?g=259516&p=1732398 (accessed on 22 August 2017).

23. Dowse, R.; Ehlers, M.S. The evaluation of pharmaceutical pictograms in a low-literate South African population. *Patient Educ. Couns.* **2001**, *45*, 87–99. [CrossRef]

24. Dowse, R.; Ehlers, M. Pictograms for conveying medicine instructions: Comprehension in various South African language groups. *S. Afr. J. Sci.* **2004**, *100*, 678–693.

25. Soares, M.A. Legibility of USP pictograms by clients of community pharmacies in Portugal. *Int. J. Clin. Pharm.* **2013**, *35*, 22–29. [CrossRef] [PubMed]

26. Instituto Nacional de Estatística. Censos—Resultados Definitivos. Região Lisboa—2011. Available online: http://censos.ine.pt/xportal/xmain?xpid=CENSOS&xpgid=ine_censos_publicacao_det&contexto=pu&PUBLICACOESpub_boui=156651739&PUBLICACOESmodo=2&selTab=tab1&pcensos=61969554 (accessed on 17 December 2016).

27. Yu, B.; Willis, M.; Sun, P.; Wang, J. Crowdsourcing participatory evaluation of medical pictograms using Amazon Mechanical Turk. *J. Med. Internet Res.* **2013**, *15*, e108. [CrossRef] [PubMed]

28. Richler, M.; Vaillancourt, R.; Celetti, S.; Besançon, L.; Arun, K.; Sebastien, F. The use of pictograms to convey health information regarding side effects and/or indications of medications. *J. Commun. Healthc.* **2012**, *5*, 200–226. [CrossRef]

6

Does Competency-Based Education Have a Role in Academic Pharmacy?

Melissa S. Medina

College of Pharmacy, The University of Oklahoma, 1110 N Stonewall Ave, Oklahoma City, OK 73117, USA; Melissa-medina@ouhsc.edu

Academic Editor: Jeffrey Atkinson

Abstract: Competency-based Education (CBE) is an educational model that allows students to learn and demonstrate their abilities at their own pace. CBE is growing in popularity in undergraduate educational programs and its role in pharmacy education in the United States (US) is under review. In comparison, medical education is utilizing competency-based approaches (such as competencies and Entrustable Professional Activities) to ensure that students possess the required knowledge, skills, and attitudes prior to graduation or program completion. The concept of competency-based approaches is growing in use in pharmacy education in the US, but the future related to aspects of this concept (e.g., mandatory Entrustable Professional Activities) is not certain. A review of pharmacy education's evolution in the US and a comparison of competency-related terms offers insight into the future use of competency-based approaches and CBE in pharmacy education in the US through the lens of benefits and challenges.

Keywords: competence; pharmacy; healthcare; program outcomes; education; standards

---

1. Introduction

In the United States (US), medical education has increased its interest in Competency-based Education (CBE) over the past several years, which has piqued interest in pharmacy. Formally, a CBE program is an educational model that removes traditional semester timeframes, allowing students to learn at their own pace and demonstrate what they know through assessments developed by the program [1]. Relatedly, competency-based approaches (including assessment of competencies) have been used in educational programs such as pharmacy, as seen in the 2016 Accreditation Council for Pharmacy Education (ACPE) Standards program outcomes which use the term competencies in relationship to outcomes [2,3]. It is important to note that a competency-based approach and competencies in pharmacy education are different than formal CBE, which removes semester timeframes. In order to understand the future of CBE in pharmacy education in the US, it is important to reflect on the past and present of pharmacy education; define the terminology related to CBE and competencies, and evaluate how other health professions (such as medical education) address CBE and competencies, which can offer insight into future directions for pharmacy education.

2. History of Pharmacy Education Standards

In the US in the 19th century, there was no legal requirement to learn the pharmacy profession through formal education and the apprenticeship model was the dominant training method [4]. State universities were the first to design formal pharmacist education models, starting in 1868 at the University of Michigan, where students enrolled in full-day courses over four terms (3-months long each) and no prior pharmacy work experience was required for admittance and in 1892, the University of Wisconsin established a four-year program [4]. During the 20th and 21st centuries, the Flexner report precipitated changes to the content and length of the pharmacy curriculum, mode of delivery, required prerequisites, and the degree earned [4,5]. There was also little uniformity in pharmacy licensure and no program accrediting bodies until 1932 when ACPE was founded [4].

The US Department of Education (USDE) now recognizes ACPE as the organization that evaluates the quality of professional degree programs leading to the Doctor of Pharmacy degree, the standard entry level degree. To receive accreditation, Doctor of Pharmacy programs must meet expectations outlined in the 2016 ACPE Accreditation standards [2]. During the 20th and 21st centuries ACPE has overseen many changes in pharmacy education such as the length of the program from 4 to 6 years and the entry level degree from Bachelor of Science to Doctor of Pharmacy. Recently, major changes have occurred regarding how programs are delivered and there are now accelerated 3-year programs, online programs, and multi-site campuses that are connected through synchronous video-streaming. These changes to program delivery have resulted in changes to the accreditation standards, with the most recent update occurring in 2016 [2]. The reverse is also true, where changes in the accreditation standards have required changes to pharmacy curricula. The 2016 ACPE standards include emphasis on an affective domain (standard 4) based on the 2013 CAPE outcomes revision [2]. The growing importance of interprofessional education is seen in standard 11 [2] and the administration of the Pharmacy Curriculum Outcomes Assessment (PCOA) in the pre-advanced pharmacy practice experience (Pre-APPE) is delineated in standard 12 [2]. Standard 10 outlines Curriculum Design, Deliver, and Oversight requirements and states that the minimum curriculum duration is a minimum of four years of full–time study or the equivalent [2,6]. Standard 10.3 (knowledge application) and Standard 10.4 (skill development) indicate that students must demonstrate their competencies in both knowledge and skills and as a result, assessment of these competencies has grown in importance [2]. These significant events are outlined in Figure 1.

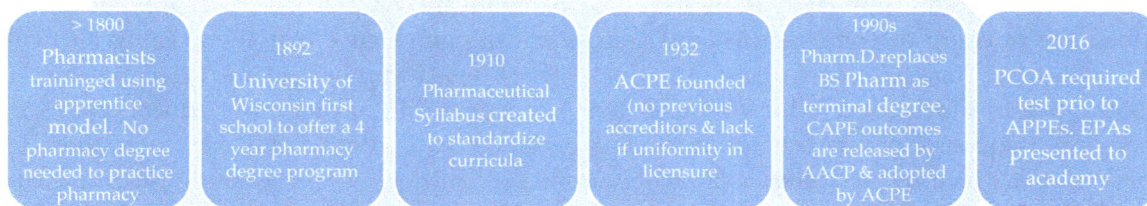

Figure 1. Timeline of Significant Pharmacy Curriculum Events in the US. ACPE = Accreditation Council for Pharmacy Education. AACP = American Association of Colleges of Pharmacy. CAPE = Center for the Advancement of Pharmacy Education outcomes; which are revised every 7 years (current version is 2013). PCOA = Pharmacy Curriculum Outcomes Assessment. APPE = Advanced Pharmacy Practice Experiences. EPA = Entrustable Professional Activities.

3. Definitions of Competency-Based Education (CBE) and Competency-Based Approaches

The growing importance of assessment has increased the terminology and concepts related to assessment. One of these newer concepts that has arisen in higher education is the term competency-based education. Higher education has historically used time (e.g., semesters and credit hours-formally known as the Carnegie Unit) as the yardstick for determining readiness, which arose in the early 1900s and formed the basis for program design, accreditation, and funding [1,7]. CBE in contrast emphasizes directly measuring how much students have learned (learning-based system) instead of how long they have spent learning (time–based system), which allows students to move at their own pace [1]. CBE programs are aimed at nontraditional students who need more flexible options to earn their first or second degree or update their skills [1]. These programs are more than just on-line programs because the focus instead turns to allowing students to demonstrate their achievement of required competencies which may have been gained during previous work experience, therefore allowing the more flexible awarding of credit in comparison to credit hours [7]. In CBE, students demonstrate mastery of explicit and measurable knowledge, skill, and attitude outcomes (competencies) and receive individualized support that is tailored to their specific developmental needs [7]. Students progress in the program by demonstrating they have mastered the knowledge and skills (competencies) for a course regardless of time, meaning they could take more or less time [8], therefore studying and learning at their own pace. CBE allows students to accelerate through what they already know and spend more time on what they do not know, which means students can accelerate (or delay) their progress toward a degree [8]. A comparison of traditional versus CBE can be seen in Table 1.

Table 1. Comparison of traditional vs. competency based education.

Curricular Concept	Traditional Instruction	CBE
Structure	Time-based, semesters and credit hours	Learner-centered; Competency-based
Teaching mode	Group learning, emphasis on knowledge	Individualized, tailored, emphasis on abilities or competencies
Pace	Faculty-paced; all students move together through content at same time; structured	Self-paced; movement through content determined by individual student's competency attainment; flexible
Assessment method	Summative, high stakes	Mastery-learning, performance-based
Program completion time	Finish when all required courses are passed	Finish when mastery of competencies demonstrated

In comparison to CBE, which focuses on changing the structure and time requirements of educational programs, ultimately changing curricula, there are competency-based approaches that embed the teaching of competencies and assessment of competence into the existing curricula and traditional time-based structure [3]. Competency-based approaches are currently used in undergraduate and medical education and their use is growing in pharmacy education [3,9,10]. Therefore, the future of competency-based approaches is now. Within this approach, there are competencies, which are predefined abilities or outcomes of a curriculum [10]. There is also competence that can be thought of as progression toward professional expertise or demonstration of a predefined skill or knowledge level that is multi-dimensional, dynamic, contextual, and developmental [10]. Competencies describe qualities of professionals and measuring professional competence can be difficult [11]. One way that medicine has evaluated competencies of their students or trainees within the medical curricula is to use Entrustable Professional Activities (EPAs) [12] and pharmacy education has focused recent attention on EPAs as well [3]. The terms EPA and competencies should not be used interchangeably because EPAs are descriptors of work and translate competencies in professional practice whereas competencies describe physicians [11,12]. Outlining core EPAs is a way to ensure that students are practice ready upon graduation [3] which is an aim of the 2016 ACPE Accreditation Standards [2]. EPAs reflect the level of supervision required for students (e.g., direct vs. distant supervision) and are aimed at establishing the level of proficiency that is required for professional practice upon completion of training or graduation [11]. When an EPA is first learned and practiced, the level of supervision needed may be high, which would be considered developmentally appropriate and expected for early leaners [3,11].

Competency-based approaches as described above are currently in use and development. In the future, although the EPAs are not officially required in the ACPE standards 2016, it is possible they will follow the path of the CAPE Outcomes and become adopted in the standards [2,6]. It is also possible that in the future, EPAs may set the stage for required mandatory skills-based examinations (such as Objective Structured Clinical Exams), similar to the PCOA exam The ACPE standards 2016 have become more prescriptive in this version related to assessment as a way for programs to increase their transparency while working on continuous quality improvement [2]. Key elements in Section 3 require formative and summative assessments as well as mandatory, standardized, and comparative assessments [2]. This section also discusses student achievement and readiness to "enter APPE, provide direct patient care in a variety of settings, and contribute to an Interprofessional collaborative patient care team" [2] (p. 25). The assessment standards offer colleges and schools of pharmacy more guidance on how they should demonstrate that their students have learned and achieved the educational outcomes and as a result, an OSCE-like exam based on competencies and EPAs is possible.

While competency-based approaches are emerging in current pharmacy curricula with attention on EPAs, the appeal is that the competency based assessment can provide a mechanism to prevent students from graduating from a pharmacy program unless they have demonstrated the predefined and expected level of competence for program outcomes [3]. This appeal is a subtle yet important distinction because in its current and near future use EPAs require students to demonstrate and achieve OR remediate deficient knowledge and skills prior to graduation within the existing curricular structure. Students can take more time if needed but it must be completed within the allotted timeframe and academic standing policies. EPAs do not currently allow an open-ended and limitless timeframe. Although competency-based approaches are used in medicine and pharmacy, it is unclear what the future holds for formal CBE. There are benefits and challenges to the design.

4. Benefits and Challenges of CBE in Pharmacy Education

Frank and colleagues [10] described benefits to medical education and these benefits can be extrapolated to pharmacy education. (1) Defines consistent competencies and milestones. CBE would help pharmacy educators define competencies expected of graduates and developmental milestones prior to graduation, better ensuring that all students possess the same level of baseline skills upon graduation; (2) Determines acceptable levels of performance for competencies and milestones. CBE would promote a national discussion of what constitutes an acceptable level of evidence of abilities; such as when are students expected to demonstrate novice, competent, proficient, or expert performance for specific competencies. This would better align faculty expectations so that one faculty member does not expect a higher or lower level than another faculty member; (3) Outlines acceptable assessment methods and tools for assessing the competencies. CBE would shape what assessments best measure the outcomes of specific competencies. It would also better ensure that assessment of graduates' abilities would not vary as a result of programmatic, regional, or local differences; (4) Offers flexibility in learning. CBE would offer students a more flexible timeframe to demonstrate competencies and therefore allow them to progress at their own rate, which is more learner centered and personalized [10].

There are challenges associated with CBE in pharmacy education which can be inferred from medicine [10]. (1) Presents IPPE and APPE logistical concerns. The biggest challenge to using CBE is that moving students through time-based curricula is efficient and manageable. For example, it is unclear how programs will accommodate students on introductory and advanced pharmacy practice experiences (IPPE and APPE) when the prescribed number of weeks is removed but preceptor laws remain and some sites can only accommodate a limited number of students; (2) Complicates faculty time allocation. When students complete course content at different times, it is unclear how faculty would handle assessment of knowledge, skills, and attitudes in an efficient manner. There is an efficiency to administering exams to an entire class during a set time block. It is possible that faculty would spend a majority of their time assessing knowledge, skills, and attitudes on an individual basis for the didactic portion of the program, leaving little time to teach and assess on IPPE and APPEs as well as fulfill other parts of the tripartite mission; (3) Makes managing poor student performance and progression difficult. Pharmacy curricula are designed to have courses and content build upon each other. While students can self-pace, much of the course work is lock-step in nature. It is not clear how programs will manage students completing prescriptive course work at different rates. In addition, many programs have some rate of attrition due to poor performance. Academic standing committees would need to establish time limits and maximum number of attempts for students to complete competencies, which could be logistically difficult to manage. CBE is also less structured by design, which may lead to more student dismissals as a result of weak students who may not manage their time well. The structure offered in time-based curricula can benefit academically at-risk students, whereas the lack of structure in CBE may hurt that category of students; (4) Creates a narrow focus of curricula. A focus on completing competencies can shift attention from the big picture of how content within a curriculum builds up and advances to a more fragmented picture of small units of performance and "jumping through hoops" which can frustrate faculty and students [10]. Focus can also shift from learning goals to performance goals, which are indicative of a fixed mindset where students are more likely to cheat, give up when faced with failure, and focus on receiving validation from others instead of striving for competence and mastery [13,14]; (5) Shifts attention from knowledge to skills. Previous complaints have arisen that pharmacy is too content heavy and that students may enter professional practice lacking skills. Shifting to CBE may create an imbalance in the opposite direction where skills are more valued than knowledge, emphasizing the role of the pharmacist as a technician versus a health-care provider and problem-solver.

5. Discussion

Overall, CBE is an instructional model that is built on eliminating time-based curricula. Based on this definition, the use of CBE in US pharmacy education is unclear. A review of the literature suggests the CBE definition is applied broadly and the future of the concept competency-based approaches (e.g., EPAs) where attention is placed on students demonstrating competencies during the traditional time-limited and structured program is currently being implemented and grown in pharmacy education. There are still areas of future uncertainty related to competency-based approaches such as mandatory EPAs and required national OSCE assessments in ACPE program accreditation. The future of formal CBE in pharmacy education has benefits and challenges. CBE appears to be difficult to implement, especially in a political climate where colleges and universities are asked to do more with less money and resources. While the pharmacy academy may benefit from ensuring that students can meet specific competencies at predefined levels along the expert-novice continuum, removing time-based curricula may not be feasible in the immediate future.

References

1. Kamenetz, A. NPR-Education, Higher Education: Competency-Based Education: No More Semesters? Available online: http://www.npr.org/sections/ed/2014/10/07/353930358/competency-based-education-no-more-semesters (accessed on 13 December 2016).
2. Accreditation Council for Pharmacy Education. Accreditation Standards and Key Elements for the Professional Program in Pharmacy Leading to the Doctor of Pharmacy Degree, 2015. Available online: https://www.acpe-accredit.org/standards/ (accessed on 13 December 2016).
3. Pittenger, A.L.; Chapman, S.A.; Frail, C.K.; Chapman, S.A.; Moon, J.Y.; Undeberg, M.R.; Orzoff, J.H. Entrustable professional activities for pharmacy practice. *Am. J. Pharm. Educ.* **2016**, *80*, 57. [CrossRef] [PubMed]
4. Mrtek, R.G. Contemporary pharmaceutical education in these United States-An interpretive historical essay of the twentieth century. *Am. J. Pharm. Educ.* **1976**, *40*, 339–365. [PubMed]
5. Flexner, A. *Medical Education in the United States and Canada: A Report to the Carnegie Foundation for the Advancement of Teaching*; Carnegie Foundation for the Advancement of Teaching: New York, NY, USA, 1910.

6.   Medina, M.S.; Plaza, C.M.; Stowe, C.D.; Robinson, E.T.; DeLander, G.; Beck, D.E.; Melchert, R.B.; Supernaw, R.B.; Roche, V.F.; Gleason, B.L.; et al. Center for the Advancement of Pharmacy Education (CAPE) 2013 educational outcomes. *Am. J. Pharm. Educ.* **2013**, *77*, 162. [CrossRef] [PubMed]

7.   Competency Works: Learning from the Cutting Edge. Available online: http://www.competencyworks. org/about/competency-education/ (accessed on 13 December 2016).

8.   Mendenhall, R. What Is Competency-Based Education? 2012, Huffington Post. Available online: http://www.huffingtonpost.com/dr-robert-mendenhall/competency-based-learning-_b_1855374.html (accessed on 13 December 2016).

9.   Fain, P. Competency-Based Education Arrives at Three Major Public Institutions. Inside Higher Ed. Available online: https://www.insidehighered.com/news/2014/10/28/competency-based-education-arrives-three-major-public-institutions (accessed on 13 December 2016).

10.   Frank, J.R.; Snell, L.S.; Cate, O.T.; Holmboe, E.S.; Carraccio, C.; Swing, S.R.; Harris, P.; Glasgow, N.J.; Campbell, C.; et al. Competency-based medical education: Theory to practice. *Med. Teach.* **2010**, *32*, 638–645. [CrossRef] [PubMed]

11.   Ten Cate O. Nuts and bolts of entrustable professional activities. *J. Grad. Med. Educ.* **2013**, *5*, 157–158. [CrossRef] [PubMed]

12.   Ten Cate O. Entrustability of professional activities and competency-based training. *Med. Educ.* **2005**, *39*, 1176–1177. [CrossRef] [PubMed]

13.   Dweck, C.S. Can personality be changed? The role of beliefs in personality and change. *Curr. Direct. Psychol. Sci.* **2008**, *17*, 391–394. [CrossRef]

14.   Murphy, M.C.; Dweck, C.S. A culture of genius: How an organization's lay theories shape people's cognition, affect, and behavior. *Personal. Soc. Psychol. Bull.* **2010**, *36*, 283–296. [CrossRef] [PubMed]

7

Regional Variation in Pharmacist Perception of the Financial Impact of Medicare Part D

Shamima Khan [1,*] ⓘ, Joshua J. Spooner [2] and Harlan E. Spotts [3]

[1] CRE Services, Inc., 1560 Broadway, Suite 812, New York, NY 10036, USA
[2] College of Pharmacy and Health Sciences, Western New England University, 1215 Wilbraham Road, Springfield, MA 01119, USA; jspooner@wne.edu
[3] College of Business, Western New England University, 1215 Wilbraham Road, Springfield, MA 01119, USA; hspotts@wne.edu
*   Correspondence: s_nsk@yahoo.com

Abstract: The objective of this study was to perform a nationwide investigation of the financial performance of community pharmacies in the United States since the inception of Medicare Part D. A nationwide, cross-sectional survey of pharmacists was conducted in 2013. The 43-item online survey collected information about demographics, financial implications of Part D on community pharmacy and patients, provision of Medication Therapy Management (MTM) services and opinions about Medicare Part D 2010 updates. The adjusted response rate was 22.3% (419/1885). A majority of respondents (75.6%) reported a stable or increased prescription volume since 2006 but only 40.4% indicated that the financial performance of their pharmacy as either excellent or good during the same period. Owners and part-owners of rural independent pharmacies were more likely to report a below average or poor financial performance (75.0%). The provision of MTM services was not related to the financial performance of the pharmacy. Nearly half (44.7%) of pharmacy owners or part-owners indicated that they were considering selling their pharmacy, with most (94.1%) reporting that their decision to sell was due to the Part D financial pressures. However, the decision to sell was not related to the change in financial performance since 2006 or the volume of prescriptions dispensed.

Keywords: Medicare Part D; pharmacy; rural pharmacy; pharmacy closure

1. Introduction

The United States Medicare system (a federally administered national health insurance plan for seniors and the disabled) was vastly changed following the passage of the Medicare Prescription Drug, Improvement and Modernization Act in 2003, resulting in the establishment of new Medicare Advantage plans, expansion of allowable contributions and employer participation in health savings accounts and the establishment of a Medicare prescription drug benefit—Medicare Part D—in January 2006 [1,2]. While many individuals enrolling in Medicare Part D ("Part D") had prescription drug coverage through a commercial or state Medicaid plan prior to Part D's implementation, the estimated 3.4 million enrollees who lacked previous prescription coverage experienced a significant 60% reduction in their out of pocket (OOP) payments for prescription drugs and a resultant 24% increase in medication utilization in the first year of the program [3]. Longitudinal surveys have found a high degree of satisfaction among Part D from its inception to the present time [4,5].

While Part D has provided a net benefit to enrollees and is perceived positively by many physicians [2,6], the community pharmacist—especially independent pharmacy owners—have not fared as well under Part D. From the point of initial rollout, Part D plans utilized a variety of third party prescription plan controls inherent in commercial or state Medicaid plans, namely formulary restrictions and prior authorization requirements, reduced prescription dispensing payment rates and delays in receiving payment [2,7–13]. Pharmacists were also tasked with addressing patient enrollment issues [8]; none of these issues had existed previously for the high-margin "cash customer" (individuals without a prescription drug benefit). The changes imparted by Part D occurred at a time when the pharmacy business environment itself was undergoing a market shift. An increasingly mature market, retail pharmacy has been evolving into a duopoly controlled by major chains in an effort to maintain financial viability through operational efficiencies [14]. The commodity-like nature of filling prescriptions and governmental and commercial insurance industry cost controls were responsible for increased financial pressure on pharmacies. While traditional chain pharmacies and pharmacies within supermarkets and mass merchandising stores were able to withstand these pressures, many independent pharmacies did not survive this period; over 1400 independent pharmacies (6% of independent pharmacies nationwide) closed between 2006 and 2010 [14–17].

In an era of low rates of payment for dispensing prescriptions (with mean dispensing fees paid by health insurers currently 28% lower than they were in 1995) [18,19], pharmacists have been advised to seek alternative revenue streams and reduce their dependence on prescription gross margins as the driver of profitability [20]. One provision of the Medicare Modernization Act was the requirement that Part D prescription drug plans and Medicare Advantage prescription drug plans provide medication therapy management (MTM) programs as part of the benefit. MTM programs were created "to assure . . . that covered part D drugs are appropriately used to optimize therapeutic outcomes through improved medication use and to reduce the risk of adverse events, including adverse drug interactions." [21] (p. 2086). While the Act defines basic elements of the program and who should be targeted for services, it also gave plans a large degree of flexibility for the design and implementation of the MTM program. While the Medicare Modernization Act specifically mentioned pharmacists as a provider of MTM services, the Act does not require the provider of such services be community pharmacist; few health plans are utilizing community pharmacists to provide MTM services, opting to provide these services via telephone or mail despite evidence suggesting superior prescription drug cost savings with face to face services [22,23]. Further, the rate at which community pharmacies are reimbursed for MTM services by plans does not cover the costs of delivering the service, [24] challenging the assumption that MTM services can stabilize a pharmacy's balance sheet.

These changing pharmacy market dynamics have significantly impacted rural pharmacies. Rural pharmacies are more likely to be independently owned [25]. Due to physician scarcity, rural pharmacists often serve as first contact providers and may be the only source of healthcare in isolated rural communities [26–28]. The rate of rural pharmacy closures increased following the establishment of Part D; [17] these closures may leave residents without convenient access to pharmacy services and can significantly impact the population's ability to obtain a number of essential health services [29]. Pharmacists practicing in rural independent pharmacies work longer hours and receive less compensation than those practicing in urban or suburban areas, making the ownership of a rural independent pharmacy less appealing to recent pharmacy graduates [26,29].

The impact of Part D on community pharmacy has been studied previously [9–13,17,30]. While these studies demonstrated financial instability within community pharmacy since the inception of Part D, these investigations were limited to a single state or region, or were retrospective in nature. This study sought to expand previously conducted research by including chain and independent pharmacies located in rural, urban and suburban settings across the country. The purpose of this study is to perform a nationwide investigation of the financial performance of community pharmacies in the United States since the inception of Part D.

2. Materials and Methods

A nationwide cross-sectional survey of practicing pharmacists was conducted between April and July 2013 using an internet-based survey platform (SurveyMonkey, San Mateo, CA, USA). To ensure proper representation of practicing pharmacists, a third-party vendor was selected to provide the principal investigator (PI) with a unique count of available email addresses of pharmacists practicing in independent (1 to 3 locations) and chain (4 or more locations) pharmacies. The total number of email addresses for pharmacists practicing in independent and community pharmacies were 35,911 and 51,677, respectively. To ensure proper representation from each state and Washington DC, a sample size determination, using a confidence interval of 95% and confidence level of 3, established an ideal sample size to be 17,920 and 21,221 for pharmacists practicing in independent and chain pharmacies, respectively [31]. However, budgetary constraints allowed us to send the email broadcasts (cover email and a link to the survey instrument) to a total of 7828 pharmacists (3584 practicing in independent and 4244 practicing in chain pharmacies). These email addresses were randomly selected by the third-party vendor. Following sample selection, the third-party vendor sent the introductory invitation and survey link by email broadcast to the entire sample of 7828 with four iterations. The researchers (including the PI) did not have access to the email addresses and, as such, were unable to contact the non-responding pharmacists. However, after the first introductory email broadcast, 3 consecutive email broadcasts occurred at approximately one month intervals (April 2013 (1st broadcast), May 2013, June 2013 and July 2013), which provided pharmacists ample time to respond. Survey participation was both voluntary and anonymous.

The survey instrument was developed following a thorough literature review, the results of a focus group study and two previously published multi-state, multi-region surveys of pharmacist opinions about Part D [9–11]. The survey included multiple choice questions, ranked ordered questions, 5-point Likert type scales and categorical scales. As the vast majority of the questions included in this survey were selected from a previously validated instrument [10,11], no pilot testing was conducted. The final instrument consisted of a total of 43 questions in multiple categories:

1. Financial Performance of Pharmacy since 2006
2. Considerations regarding the sale of the pharmacy
3. Providing Medication Therapy Management
4. Concerns about Part D 2010 Updates

The study was approved by Western New England University (WNEU) Institutional Review Board and was funded by WNEU College of Pharmacy.

Descriptive statistics (frequency counts and percentages) were used to report demographic data, outcomes data and other variables of interest. Univariate comparisons (i.e., Chi-square [χ^2] analyses) were used to explore relationships between respondent demographics and variables of interest. Systematic comparisons in terms of pharmacists' primary role and geographic locations of practice were explored. The outcomes of interest reported in this publication are: the financial performance of the pharmacy since the initiation of Part D; the volume of prescriptions dispensed since the initiation of Part D and for the two years prior to the completion of the survey; the dispensing of 90-days' supply of medications under Part D; Part D prescription switching at the time of dispensing; respondent opinions about reimbursement received; the provision of MTM; the viability of the respondent's pharmacy; and respondent opinions about the Part D 2010 updates. All demographic data in relation to practice location were analyzed; practice locations (rural/suburban/urban) were self-reported by the participants. We specifically examined relationships between providing MTM services (which was reimbursed by at least 1 Part D plan) and other variables of interest. Subsequently, we isolated all pharmacy owners- and part-owners and conducted sub-group analyses.

The primary outcome was an excellent or good financial performance of the pharmacy since the inception of Part D. This outcome was dichotomized: pharmacists who responded that the financial performance of their pharmacy has been excellent or good were compared to pharmacists who reported that the financial performance of their pharmacy was average, below average, or poor. A logistic regression model examined the relationship between the financial performance of the respondent's pharmacy and select demographic characteristics: practice site ['chain & other' versus 'independent'], primary role as a pharmacist, percentage of prescriptions received electronically, number of years in community pharmacy practice, percentage of patients enrolled in Part D and the number of prescriptions dispensed per weekday at the primary practice site.

Statistix® Version 8.2 was used to conduct all statistical analyses [32].

3. Results

3.1. Survey Responses

Surveys were distributed via email to 7828 pharmacists, with 1885 determined by the third-party vendor to have reached the intended recipient. Of these, 419 responded, yielding an adjusted response rate of 22.3%. Four respondents were excluded from analyses because they were not a pharmacist (3 respondents were pharmacy technicians, 1 was a non-pharmacist pharmacy owner); an additional 9 respondents were excluded because their primary practice site did not accept Part D plans. The final sample size was 406. More than half of the respondents (56.6%) were practicing in independent pharmacies, of which 18.1% were owners and 4.0% were part-owners (data not shown). Respondents from urban locations were more likely to be practicing at an independent pharmacy setting compared to suburban and rural respondents ($P = 0.0003$). Among the respondents, 60.5% were male, 55.7% were between the ages of 51 to 70 years of age and 74.4% had practiced in community pharmacy as Registered Pharmacists (RPh) for more than 15 years (Table 1). Nearly 30% of respondents had more than 50% of their patients enrolled in Part D; respondents in rural practice settings were more likely to reach this threshold compared to suburban and urban counterparts ($P = 0.0268$).

Table 1. Respondent demographics and practice characteristics.

	Total (n = 419)	Rural (n = 84)	Suburban (n = 163)	Urban (n = 131)
Male	60.5%	53.6%	60.7%	64.6%
Age (>40 years)	80.4%	76.2%	81.5%	81.7%
Primary Region of Practice (via US Census Bureau designation)				
Northeast	16.6%	27.3%	16.9%	7.8%
Midwest	31.9%	35.1%	29.2%	35.9%
South	39.5%	28.6%	40.9%	44.5%
West	11.9%	9.1%	13.0%	11.7% *
Primary Type of Practice Site				
Independent (1 store to 3 stores)	56.6%	51.8%	49.4%	71.8%
Chain (≥4 stores) and Other §	43.4%	48.2%	50.6%	28.2% **
Work Status (Full-Time)	82.0%	82.1%	80.1%	83.9%
Work Status (Part-Time 30 h or less)	18.0%	17.9%	19.9%	16.1%
Terminal Degree				
Doctor of Pharmacy	26.9%	29.3%	25.5%	26.7%
Bachelor of Science	69.9%	64.6%	71.4%	71.8%
Other	3.2%	6.1%	3.1%	1.5%
Primary Role as a Pharmacist				
Staff Pharmacist	40.1%	40.5%	52.8%	22.1%
Pharmacist-in-Charge/Pharmacy Manager/Part of Upper Level Pharmacy Management (District Manager)/Other	37.9%	40.5%	34.4%	41.2%
Community Pharmacy Part-Owner/Owner	22.0%	19.0%	12.9%	36.6% ***
Years of community pharmacy practice as a Registered Pharmacist				
15 years or less	25.6%	36.9%	24.4%	19.2%
More than 15 years	74.4%	63.1%	75.6%	80.8% ****
Number of prescription dispensed in a typical day				
0 to 300/weekday	67.1%	71.4%	59.9%	73.8%
>300/weekday	32.9%	28.6%	40.1%	26.2%
>50% of patients enrolled in Medicare Part D	29.4%	38.6%	25.8%	28.2% *****

Table 1. *Cont.*

	Total (*n* = 419)	Rural (*n* = 84)	Suburban (*n* = 163)	Urban (*n* = 131)
Percentage of prescriptions received electronically				
Zero	1.1%	0	0.6%	2.3%
1% to 25%	32.3%	27.4%	29.4%	38.9%
26% to 50%	44.4%	51.2%	45.4%	38.9%
>50%	22.2%	21.4%	24.5%	19.8%

Percentages do not always sum to 100% because of missing data; Number of responses to the item of interest (*n*) varies because of missing data; § other included hospital outpatient pharmacies, rehabilitation facilities and long-term care pharmacies; * χ^2 = 16.63, *P* = 0.011; ** χ^2 = 16.38, *P* = 0.0003; *** χ^2 = 37.17, *P* < 0.00001; **** χ^2 = 8.57; *P* = 0.0138; ***** χ^2 = 7.24; *P* = 0.0268.

3.2. Financial Performance Since 2006

Less than half of the respondents (40.4%) indicated that the financial performance of their pharmacy since 2006 has been either excellent or good and 22.7% reported that it was either below average or poor. There were no geographic differences in the percentage of respondents reporting the financial performance of their pharmacy as excellent or good (rural: 39.3% suburban: 44.7%; urban: 36.9%; *P* = 0.3842), though a higher percentage of those practicing in rural locations reported a below average or poor financial performance (28.6% vs. 20.5% and 22.3%, respectively; *P* = 0.3534 (Figure 1)). Nevertheless, a majority (54.9%) reported an increase in the volume of prescription dispensed since 2006 (Figure 2). Over the two year period prior to the survey completion (years 2011 to 2013), a slightly lower percentage (41.5%) indicated an increase in prescription volume dispensed. The change in prescription volume since 2006 did not vary based upon geographic location.

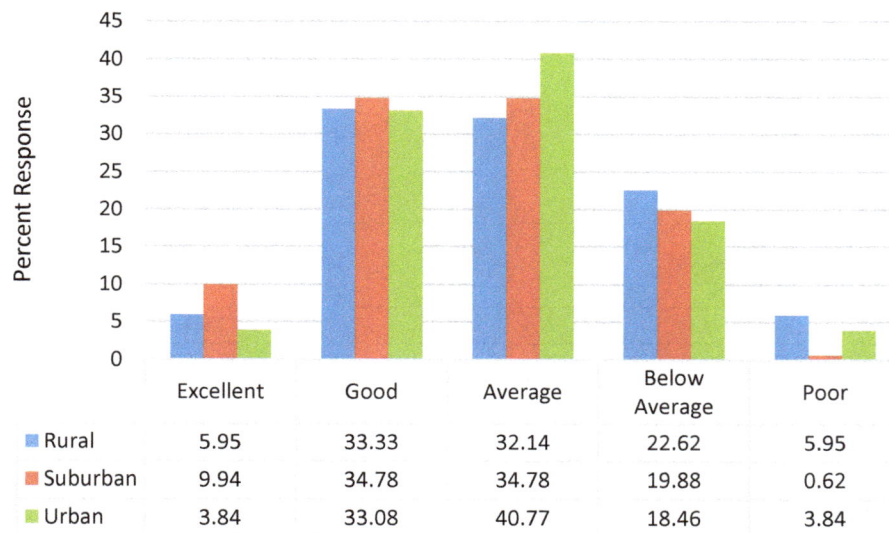

	Excellent	Good	Average	Below Average	Poor
Rural	5.95	33.33	32.14	22.62	5.95
Suburban	9.94	34.78	34.78	19.88	0.62
Urban	3.84	33.08	40.77	18.46	3.84

Figure 1. Pharmacy Financial Performance since 2006.

Pharmacists practicing at different capacities viewed the financial performance of their pharmacies since 2006 differently. Owners and part-owners of community pharmacies were less likely to view their pharmacies financial performance as excellent or good (20.9%, Figure 3) compared to mid to upper level pharmacy managers and staff pharmacists (39.7% and 51.9%, respectively; *P* = 0.0001). Several factors influenced the likelihood that the respondents either reported that the financial performance of their pharmacy as either excellent or good. Compared to pharmacists who practiced in an independent location, pharmacists who practiced in a 'chain or other location' were almost twice as likely to report the financial performance of their pharmacy as excellent or good. Pharmacists who practiced in pharmacies that received prescriptions electronically were less likely to report that the financial performance of their pharmacy as excellent or good as opposed to pharmacists who practiced in pharmacies that received none of their prescriptions electronically (Table 2). Pharmacists who practiced in pharmacies that dispensed more than 300 prescriptions per weekday were more than 3 times more likely to report that the pharmacy's financial performance since 2006 as excellent or good as opposed to pharmacists who practiced in pharmacies that dispensed less than 100 prescriptions per weekday (Table 2).

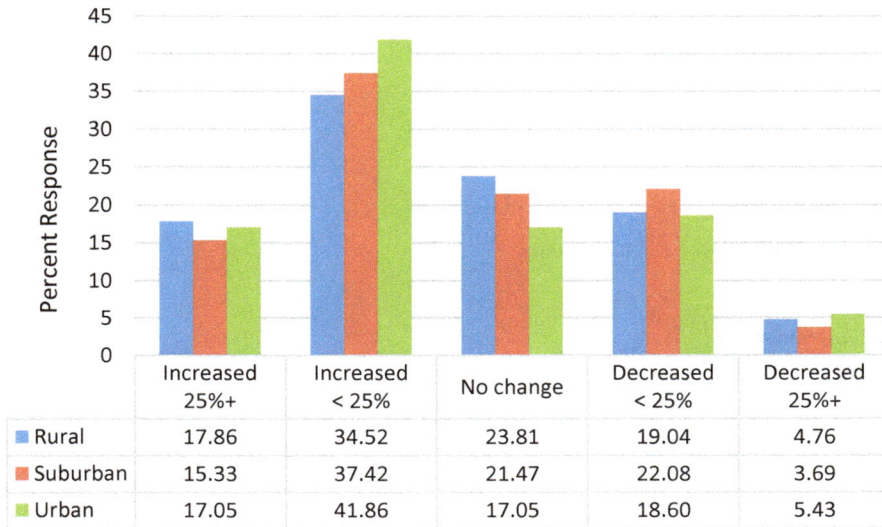

	Increased 25%+	Increased < 25%	No change	Decreased < 25%	Decreased 25%+
Rural	17.86	34.52	23.81	19.04	4.76
Suburban	15.33	37.42	21.47	22.08	3.69
Urban	17.05	41.86	17.05	18.60	5.43

Figure 2. Change in Prescription Volume since 2006.

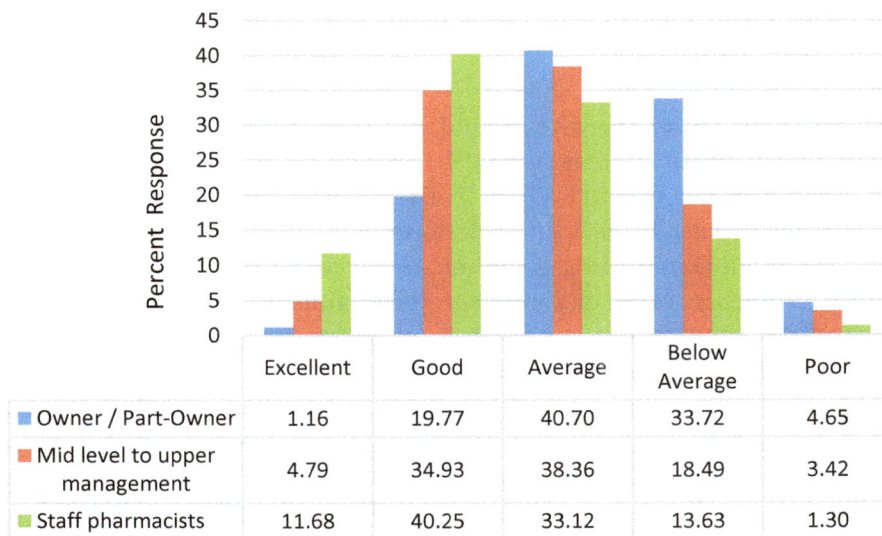

	Excellent	Good	Average	Below Average	Poor
Owner / Part-Owner	1.16	19.77	40.70	33.72	4.65
Mid level to upper management	4.79	34.93	38.36	18.49	3.42
Staff pharmacists	11.68	40.25	33.12	13.63	1.30

Figure 3. Pharmacy financial performance since 2006, stratified by employment role.

Table 2. Factors influencing financial performance of the pharmacy.

Factor	Odds Ratio	95% CI	P value
Primary Practice Site *	**1.84**	**1.10 to 3.08**	**0.0211**
Primary Practice location **			
Rural	0.75	0.40 to 1.42	0.3834
Suburban	0.86	0.50 to 1.49	0.5900
Number of years in community practice	0.64	0.38 to 1.07	0.0892
Percentage of Part D patients	0.88	0.53 to 1.46	0.6116
Percentage of Prescriptions Received Electronically ***			
1% to 25%	**0.06**	**0.00 to 0.80**	**0.0329**
26% to 50%	0.10	0.01 to 1.33	0.0812
>50%	**0.06**	**0.00 to 0.81**	**0.0343**
Primary Role ****			
Pharmacist-in-charge, Pharmacy Manager, Part of Upper Level Management and Other	0.65	0.39 to 1.09	0.1013
Community Pharmacy Owner and Part-Owner	**0.38**	**0.18 to 0.79**	**0.0090**
Prescription Volume †			
100 to 300 per weekday	2.08	0.78 to 5.54	0.1421
301 to 500 per weekday	**2.95**	**1.02 to 8.58**	**0.0465**
>500 per weekday	**3.30**	**1.08 to 10.02**	**0.0356**

† Reference category less than 100 prescriptions dispensed per weekday; * Dichotomized as independent pharmacy = 0; ** Reference category urban location; *** Reference category: 0% or None; **** Reference category: staff pharmacist. Bold rows indicate statistical significance. Subgroup Analyses: Pharmacy Owners & Part-Owners.

The vast majority of respondents (91.7%) reported that they dispensed 90-day supply of medication at least some of the time, which may have accounted for some of the slowing in the volume of prescriptions dispensed. Work-flow factors imparted by Part D may also have affected pharmacy performance; 27.8% of the pharmacists reported that at least 40% of the Part D prescriptions they received were switched at the point of dispensing and 4.7% reporting that at least 70% were switched at the point of dispensing, creating work-flow disruption and costing time and money.

Although less than half of the owners and part-owners (44.7%) indicated that they were considering selling their pharmacy, nearly all (94.1%) reported that their decision to sell was due to the financial pressure exerted by Part D (Table 3). Despite this attestation, the decision to sell did not appear to be significantly related to the financial performance of the pharmacy since Part D inception in 2006, the volume of prescriptions dispensed, the volume or prescription dispensed in the last two years prior to the survey completion, or the dispensing of 90-day supplies of prescriptions. No demographic variables exerted a statistically significant relationship on respondents who were considering the selling their pharmacy with one exception: work status. Almost half (48.1%) of the owner or part-owners who were working full-time were considering selling their pharmacy, as opposed to none of the owners or part-owners working part-time ($\chi^2 = 6.01$, $P = 0.0142$). Rural pharmacy owners and part-owners were least likely to report considering the sale of the pharmacy (31.3% vs. 40.0% of suburban and 51.1% urban owners and part owners), despite being more likely to report a below average or poor financial performance for the pharmacy since 2006 (75.0% vs. 23.8% of suburban and 31.3% of urban owners and part owners ($\chi^2 = 15.91$, $P = 0.0437$).

Table 3. Subgroup analyses: pharmacy owners & part-owners.

	All	Rural	Suburban	Urban
Primary region of practice *				
Northeast	13 (14.9%)	5 (38.5%)	5 (23.8%)	1 (2.1%)
Mid-West	26 (29.9%)	3 (23.1%)	8 (38.1%)	14 (29.2%)
South	42 (48.3%)	4 (30.8%)	7 (33.3%)	29 (60.4%)
West	6 (6.9%)	1 (7.7%)	1 (4.8%)	4 (8.3%)
Percent of prescriptions received electronically **				
None	2 (2.2%)	0	0	2 (4.2%)
1% to 50%	71 (79.8%)	14 (87.5%)	12 (57.1%)	42 (87.5%)
>50%	16 (18.0%)	2 (12.5%)	9 (42.9%)	4 (8.3%)
Pharmacy's financial performance since 2006 ***				
Excellent	1 (1.2%)	0	0	1 (2.1%)
Good	17 (19.8%)	2 (12.5%)	3 (14.3%)	12 (25.0%)
Average	35 (40.7%)	2 (12.5%)	13 (61.9%)	20 (41.7%)
Below average	29 (33.7%)	10 (62.5%)	5 (23.8%)	13 (27.1%)
Poor	4 (4.7%)	2 (12.5%)	0	2 (4.2%)
Prescription volume dispensed (past 2 years prior to survey completion) ****				
Decreased	30 (33.3%)	8 (50.0%)	4 (20.0%)	15 (33.3%)
Increased	39 (43.3%)	7 (43.8%)	7 (35.0%)	20 (44.4%)
Remained the same	21 (23.3%)	1 (6.3%)	9 (45.0%)	10 (22.2%)
Provide MTM which is reimbursed by at least one Part D plan *****	55 (64.0%)	6 (37.5%)	13 (65.0%)	34 (75.6%)
Number of prescription dispensed in a typical day of practice ******				
0 to 300/weekday	63 (75.0%)	8 (50.0%)	16 (76.2%)	39 (83.0%)
>300/weekday	21 (25.0%)	8 (50.0%)	5 (24.8%)	8 (17.0%)
Considerations regarding the sale of the pharmacy				
Respondent considering sale of the pharmacy	38 (44.7%)	5 (31.3%)	8 (40.0%)	24 (51.1%)
The decision to sell is influenced by the financial pressure exerted by Part D	32 (94.1%)	5 (100%)	6 (75.0%)	20 (83.3%)
Considering sale and have identified a potential buyer	14 (36.8%)	1 (20.0%)	4 (50.0%)	8 (33.3%)
Another community pharmacy located within 1 to 10 mile radius of the pharmacy considered for sale	33 (86.8%)	5 (100%)	7 (87.5%)	20 (83.3%)

* $\chi^2 = 16.51$, $P = 0.0113$; ** $\chi^2 = 13.53$, $P = 0.009$; *** $\chi^2 = 15.91$, $P = 0.0437$; **** $\chi^2 = 8.36$, $P = 0.0791$; ***** $\chi^2 = 7.56$, $P = 0.0228$; ****** $\chi^2 = 6.94$, $P = 0.0310$.

3.3. MTM Services

Although two-thirds of the pharmacists reported providing MTM services at their primary practice sites, fewer (57.3%) reported that they were providing MTM services reimbursed by at least one Part D plan. While rural pharmacies were less likely to provide MTM (62.3%) compared to suburban and urban pharmacies (67.8% and 73.2%, respectively), rural pharmacies were more likely to provide MTM services reimbursed by at least one Part D plan (59.5%) than suburban pharmacies (54.0%) and similar to urban pharmacies (60.3%). None of these differences reached statistical significance. No relationships between providing MTM services and the financial performance of the pharmacy were observed (data not shown). Almost four-fifths of the pharmacists who were less than 40 years of age were providing MTM services, which was being reimbursed by at least one Part D plan as opposed to half of the pharmacists who were over the age of 40 years (Table 4). A statistically significant relationship between increased volume of prescriptions being dispensed (64.9%) and providing MTM services which were reimbursed by at least one Part D plan was observed (Table 4).

Table 4. Provision of Medication Therapy Management (MTM) and reimbursement by Medicare Part D.

	Do You Provide MTM Reimbursed by at Least one Part D Plan at Your Primary Practice Site?	
	Yes	No
All	220 (57.3%)	164 (42.7%)
Geographic location		
Rural	50 (59.5%)	34 (40.5%)
Suburban	88 (54.0%)	75 (46%)
Urban	79 (60.3%)	52 (39.7%)
Age ($\leq$40 years)	57 (26.3%)	17 (10.6%)
Age (>40 years) *	160 (73.7%)	143 (89.4%)
Years of community pharmacy practice **		
15 years or less	67 (31.0%)	29 (18.2%)
More than 15 years	149 (69.0%)	130 (81.8%)
For the past 2 years, volume of prescription dispensed has ***		
Increased	98 (48.3%)	53 (33.5%)
Remained the same	62 (30.5%)	55 (34.8%)
Decreased	43 (21.2%)	50 (31.6%)

* χ^2 = 14.28, P = 0.0002; ** χ^2 = 7.85, P = 0.0051; *** χ^2 = 8.88, P = 0.0118.

3.4. Part D 2010 Updates

We asked 3 specific questions targeting Part D 2010 updates, two of which were specifically related to the financial performance of the pharmacy and the third was indirectly related. Even though 85.1% of the pharmacists reported that they thought different pharmacies received different reimbursement for the fulfillment of their Part D prescription medications, only 16.1% felt that the new Center for Medicare and Medicaid Services (CMS) reporting requirement (required to report the actual price paid to the pharmacy) would have a positive financial impact on community pharmacies. The majority (68.7%) reported that it would be much easier to provide MTM services due to opt-out enrollment system. No statistically significant relationships were observed between these update related questions and all other variables (data not shown).

4. Discussion

Based on a thorough literature review, we believe that this is the first nationwide study conducted in the United States to understand the impact of Part D on community pharmacy. Previous analyses were regional in scope and primarily focused on rural independent pharmacies [12,13,17,30]. Contrary to previous analyses, we found the financial performance of community pharmacies nationwide since 2006 has been mixed, with pharmacists practicing at chain locations nearly twice as likely to report a better financial performance for their pharmacy compared to those at independent locations. It is possible that survivors bias, due to the number of independent pharmacy closures from 2006 onwards [33,34], may be underestimating the magnitude of the difference in the changes in financial performance between chain pharmacies and independent pharmacies since the introduction of Part D.

This study found that the financial performance of a community pharmacy is directly tied to the volume of prescriptions dispensed, as pharmacists who practiced in stores that dispensed 300 or more prescriptions per weekday were approximately 3 times more likely to report that the pharmacy's financial performance as excellent or good as opposed to pharmacists who practiced in pharmacies that dispensed less than 100 prescriptions per weekday. The literature supports this direct relationship between volume and financial performance, albeit the magnitude of the effect being minor. An increase in annual prescription volume of 1000 prescriptions (approximately 20 prescriptions per week) has been associated with 0.4 percentage point increase in the likelihood of reporting a good or very good financial performance [35]. While Part D has contributed to an increase in prescription drug utilization nationwide [17], the increase has not been uniformly distributed; nearly one quarter of respondents reported a drop in prescription volume since 2006. Similar to a previous regional analysis [10,11], respondents reported that Part D created work-flow disruptions, costing both money and time.

Similar to previous research, we found that pharmacists practicing in rural locations were more likely to report a 'below average' or 'poor' financial performance since 2006 [12,17,30]. We also found a higher percentage of patients receiving Part D benefits in rural pharmacies and changes in reimbursement rates for these patients may have left these pharmacies more vulnerable to changes in reimbursement rates.

The community pharmacy industry in the United States has undergone tremendous change over last 10 years. Independent community pharmacies tend to be commonly located in rural areas, while chain community pharmacies are more concentrated in urban areas [36]. Further, as noted by Hoffman et al. (2016) rural pharmacies have declined in number between 2011 and 2016 [36]. This trend is expected to continue, as consumers can fill prescriptions at large chain pharmacies, independent pharmacies, mass merchandisers, supermarkets, warehouse stores and mail-order pharmacies. Retail pharmacy industry consolidation has resulted in a small number of large retailers controlling over 60 percent of total industry revenues [36] and the partial purchase of Rite Aid by Walgreens further consolidates industry dominance as it moves towards a duopoly controlled by Walgreens and CVS. Characteristic of mature industries, the pace of consolidation appears to be accelerating, with continued acquisition of smaller pharmacies by larger chains in an effort to expand geographic reach [36]. This consolidation is also fueled by pressure to improve financial performance in an environment characterized by "anemic" reimbursement rates [37]. The current industry trends lead to the conclusion that independent pharmacies will become fewer in number as large chain pharmacies assume greater industry dominance. Even that conclusion may appear null and void, given the most recent purchase of PillPack by Amazon [38], which has created a new market scenario for mail-order pharmacies. This purchase has sent shock waves through the industry; as reported by *Wall Street Journal*, Walgreens, CVS Health and Rite Aid (as well as the wholesalers) lost $22 billion in market value following this acquisition [39]. The implications for chain pharmacies have been immediately obvious, though implications for rural pharmacies are not as visible immediately. Financial performance pressures have stimulated the consolidation to streamline operations for cost savings and increase market shares that help to negotiate better drug price reimbursement rates with PBMs [25], a business strategy that is not available to the independent community pharmacy.

In 2015 there were approximately 22,160 independent community pharmacies, with 1800 as the sole provider in their rural community [40]. This is characteristic of past research reporting that counties within the United States with more lower-income and elderly residents had a higher proportion of independent community pharmacies [41]. Community pharmacies have been under increasing financial pressure due to the complexity of working with Part D plans, low reimbursement rates and lag in payments, so much so that their future viability as sole retail providers was in question [42]. This is important, as independent community pharmacies have been relied upon by consumers in underserved rural areas and the inner city [43].

Given this unsatisfactory situation, almost half of independent pharmacy owners and part-owners reported a desire to sell, the vast majority of whom cited financial pressure exerted by Part D as the reason for considering the sale. However, our analyses failed to connect an owner's or part-owner's decision to sell to the financial performance of the pharmacy, or the volume of prescriptions dispensed. When stratified by geographic location, rural pharmacy owners were most likely to report dispensing more than 300 prescriptions per weekday but were more likely than their urban or suburban counterparts to report the financial performance of the pharmacy since 2006 as below average or poor. As such, it is unclear as to the extent that financial pressures exerted by Part D continues to influence the interest in the sale or closure of independent pharmacies nationwide. Others have speculated that non-financial factors were leading to the sale or closure of rural independent pharmacies [44]. Our research supports others' beliefs that the decision to continue to operate an independent pharmacy is based upon the owner's perception of their financial position rather than the actual financial performance of the pharmacy [35]. These findings indicate a further need to conduct additional research to understand the challenges of owning and operating an independent community pharmacy independent of financial performance.

More than half of the pharmacists reported providing MTM services at their pharmacy, and these pharmacies were more likely to report an increase in prescription volume compared to those that did not. Nonetheless, the provision of MTM services did not result in a better financial performance. Given the voluntary and optional nature of MTM, there must be a self-perceived need of beneficiaries to obtain and benefit from these services [45]. However, rural older adults face unique challenges in accessing MTM services [33] and find it more challenging to comprehend the complexities of Part D [46]. Additionally, the earlier successes of MTM do not appear to be resonating in current clinical practice. A recent systematic review and meta-analysis reported insufficient evidence to demonstrate MTM interventions on many outcomes, including drug therapy problems, adverse drug events, disease-specific morbidity, disease specific or all-cause mortality and impairments [47]. When compared to usual care, MTM interventions were somewhat successful in improving a few measures of medication-related problems and health care use and costs (lowered odds of hospitalization and hospital costs); however, MTM interventions failed to improve patient satisfaction and health related quality of life [48]. This finding is in contrast to earlier literature, where the MTM-style interventions of the Asheville and Hickory Projects were associated with improvements in outcomes for various chronic diseases while reducing total health care costs [48–50]. Two tenets of the Asheville and Hickory Projects—use of specially trained pharmacists and a reduction in prescription co-payment—are absent from most current MTM programs. In this study, the majority of respondents were older pharmacists with Bachelors in Science in Pharmacy as their terminal degree. Targeted training of this group of older pharmacists may lead to the realization of better MTM outcomes for both patients and pharmacy owners.

Similar to previous research demonstrating more service orientation amongst rural pharmacists [51], our study found similar percentages of both rural and urban pharmacists providing MTM services which were reimbursed by at least one Part D plan. However, we found that rural pharmacy owners and part owners were less likely than their urban and suburban counterparts to provide MTM services that were reimbursed by Part D plans. Given the disparities in disease burden among rural older residents, a high prevalence of chronic illnesses and shortage of primary health providers [51], we believe that pharmacists practicing in rural locations have an important role to play in terms of improving the overall situation for older rural adults and pharmacy owners and part owners in rural areas have an opportunity to be more engaged in the care of their Part D patients.

While this survey determined whether or not respondents were providing MTM services at their pharmacy, the volume of MTM services provided was not captured. Community pharmacies face several barriers to offering MTM services, including staffing issues, physical barriers within the pharmacy itself and a lack of dedicated space for patient care areas; these barriers may be more pronounced within independent community pharmacies [12]. It remains unclear as to whether these barriers have been addressed in the decade since the opportunity for pharmacies to offer MTM services through Part D were first offered; additional research on this topic would be warranted.

There are several limitations to this research which merit mention. This study has a low unadjusted response rate, with a final response rate of 419. However, the response rate for this study was comparable to a recently published online survey which appeared in the *Journal of Managed Care Pharmacy* [52] and we believe can be considered representative of the population studied. Other limitations included the authors' inability to contact the non-responders directly (as e-mail addresses were controlled by the third-party vendor) and the use of a mailing list that included both business and personal email accounts. Amongst the respondents, we received an over-representation of practicing pharmacists from urban independent locations; as such, these respondents were more likely to be owners or part-owners of the pharmacy and more likely to have been in practice for more than 15 years. Nonetheless, since the survey participants were selected randomly from a national database of pharmacists, we believe the sample adequately represents pharmacists practicing in various states and settings across the country. Compared to the American Association of Colleges of Pharmacy (AACP) recent national survey of the pharmacist workforce [53], our respondent sample matched up well for many demographic variables, including age (73% of the AACP respondents >40 years of age vs. 80% of our sample) and full-time work status (82% for both surveys excluding retired and unemployed). Due to the intentional over-sampling of recent graduates (within 1–3 years of graduation) within the AACP survey [53], our respondent sample differed in a few demographic variables, including an overrepresentation of males (60% vs. 47%), those practicing with a terminal BSPharm degree (70% vs. 52%) and individuals practicing in independent pharmacies (57% vs. 22%). Nonetheless, the marginal response rate and the low response rate from the west coast limit the generalizability of the results. As with any survey, the results of this study are subject to non-response bias (with the worst performing pharmacies since the introduction of Part D ceasing operations) and social-desirability response bias.

5. Conclusions

Though a majority of community pharmacist respondents reported an increase in volume of prescription dispensed since 2006, less than the majority reported that their pharmacy experienced a favorable financial performance during the same timeframe. The provision of MTM services was not related to better pharmacy financial performance. Nearly half of pharmacy owners or part-owners indicated that they were considering selling their pharmacy, with most reporting that their decision to sell was due to the Part D financial pressures. However, the decision to sell was not related to the change in financial performance since 2006 or the volume of prescriptions dispensed.

Author Contributions: S.K. led on project conceptualization and administration, methodology creation, data collection, data input and statistical analyses and is the primary author of the paper. J.J.S. led on writing the various drafts of the paper and contributed to the statistical analyses. H.E.S. contributed to writing of the paper and statistical analyses. All authors read and approved the final version of this manuscript.

Funding: This research received no external funding.

Acknowledgments: The authors of this study would like to thank Thomas J. Moore, Media and Simulation Operations Manager at the College of Pharmacy and Health Sciences at Western New England University, for his technical assistance.

References

1. Schneeweiss, S.; Patrick, A.R.; Pedan, A.; Varasteh, L.; Levin, R.; Liu, N.; Shrank, W.H. The effect of Medicare Part D coverage on drug use and associated cost sharing among seniors without prior drug benefits. *Health Aff.* **2009**, *28*, W305–W316. [CrossRef] [PubMed]
2. Pitts, B.; Dominelli, A.; Khan, S. Physician patient communication concerning Part D in two Midwestern states. *P&T* **2007**, *32*, 544–551.
3. IMS Health. *Medicare Part D: The First Year*; Plymouth Meeting; IMS: Danbury, CT, USA, 2007.
4. Montgomery, L.; Lee, C. Success of drug plan challenges Democrats. *Washington Post*, 26 November 2006.
5. Medicare Today. Senior Satisfaction Survey: 2007–2016. Available online: http://medicaretoday.org/resources/senior-satisfaction-survey/ (accessed on 6 October 2016).
6. Epstein, A.J.; Rathmore, S.S.; Alexander, G.C.; Ketcham, J.D. Primary care physicians views of Medicare Part D. *Am. J. Manag. Care* **2008**, *14*, SP5–SP13. [PubMed]
7. Khan, S.; Sylvester, R.; Scott, D.; Pitts, B. Physicians' opinions about responsibility for patient out-of-pocket costs and formulary prescribing in two Midwestern states. *J. Manag. Care Pharm.* **2008**, *14*, 780–789. [CrossRef] [PubMed]
8. Spooner, J.J. A bleak future for independent community pharmacy under Medicare Part D. *J. Manag. Care Pharm.* **2008**, *14*, 878–881. [CrossRef] [PubMed]

9.   Khan, S. Urban and Suburban Community Pharmacists' Experiences with Part D—A Focus Group Study. *J. Pharm. Technol.* **2012**, *28*, 249–257. [CrossRef]

10.   Khan, S. What can pharmacists' do about the Medicare Part D Donut hole and Reimbursement? A six-state survey. *Aging Clin. Exp. Res.* **2014**, *27*, 373–381. [CrossRef] [PubMed]

11.   Khan, S. Medicare Part D: Pharmacists and Formularies—Whose Job is it to Address Copays? *Consult. Pharm.* **2014**, *29*, 602–613. [CrossRef] [PubMed]

12.   Radford, A.; Slifkin, R.; Fraser, R.; Mason, M.; Mueller, K. The experience of rural independent pharmacies with Medicare part D: Reports from the field. *J. Rural Health* **2007**, *23*, 286–293. [CrossRef] [PubMed]

13.   Bono, J.D.; Crawford, S.Y. Impact of Medicare Part D on independent and chain community pharmacies in rural Illinois—A qualitative study. *Res. Soc. Adm. Pharm.* **2010**, *6*, 110–120. [CrossRef] [PubMed]

14.   Stern, C. CVS and Walgreens are Completely Dominating the US Drugstore Industry. Available online: http://finance.yahoo.com/news/cvs-walgreens-completely-dominating-us-211840229.html (accessed on 30 November 2016).

15.   *NCPA-Pfizer Digest 2007*; National Community Pharmacists Association: Alexandria, VA, USA, 2007.

16.   *NCPA Digest 2011*; National Community Pharmacists Association: Alexandria, VA, USA, 2011.

17.   Klepser, D.G.; Xu, L.; Ullrich, F.; Mueller, K.J. Trends in community pharmacy counts and closures before and after the implementation of Medicare part D. *J. Rural Health* **2011**, *27*, 168–175. [CrossRef] [PubMed]

18.   Retail Brand Reimbursement (Table 4). In *The Prescription Drug Benefit Cost and Plan Design Survey Report*; Takeda Pharmaceuticals North America: Osaka, Japan, 2003.

19.   Average dispensing fee by pharmacy channel (Table 25). In *The 2014–2015 Prescription Drug Benefit Cost and Plan Design Report*; Takeda Pharmaceuticals USA: Boston, MA, USA, 2014.

20.   Urick, B.Y.; Urmie, J.M.; Doucette, W.R.; McDonough, R.P. Assessing changes in third-party gross margin for a single community pharmacy. *J. Am. Pharm. Assoc.* **2014**, *54*, 27–34. [CrossRef] [PubMed]

21.   U.S. Government Printing Office. Public Law 108–173. The Medicare Prescription Drug, Improvement, and Modernization Act of 2003. Available online: https://www.gpo.gov/fdsys/pkg/PLAW-108publ173/html/PLAW-108publ173.htm (accessed on 4 October 2016).

22.   Winston, S.; Lin, Y.S. Impact on drug cost and use of Medicare part D of medication therapy management services delivered in 2007. *J. Am. Pharm. Assoc.* **2009**, *49*, 813–820. [CrossRef] [PubMed]

23.   MacIntosh, C.; Weiser, C.; Wassimi, A.; Reddick, J.; Scovis, N.; Guy, M.; Boesen, K. Attitudes toward and factors affecting implementation of medication therapy management services by community pharmacists. *J. Am. Pharm. Assoc.* **2009**, *49*, 26–30. [CrossRef] [PubMed]

24.   Cook, D.M.; Mburia-Mwalili, A. Medication therapy management favors large pharmacy chains and creates potential conflicts of interest. *J. Manag. Care Pharm.* **2009**, *15*, 495–500. [CrossRef] [PubMed]

25.   Fraher, E.P.; Slifkin, R.T.; Smith, L.; Randolph, R.; Rudolf, M.; Holmes, G.M. How might the Medicare Prescription Drug, Improvement, and Modernization Act of 2003 affect the financial viability of rural pharmacies? An analysis of pre implementation prescription volume and payment sources in rural and urban areas. *J. Rural Health* **2005**, *21*, 114–121. [CrossRef] [PubMed]

26.   Hilsenrath, P.; Woelfel, J.; Shek, A.; Ordanza, K. Redefining the role of the pharmacist: Medication therapy management. *J. Rural Health* **2012**, *28*, 425–430. [CrossRef] [PubMed]

27.   Khan, S.; Snyder, H.W.; Rathke, A.M.; Scott, D.M.; Peterson, C.D. Is there a successful business case for telepharmacy? *Telemed. J. Health* **2008**, *14*, 235–244. [CrossRef] [PubMed]

28.   Nattinger, M.; Ullrich, F.; Mueller, K.J. Characteristics of Rural Communities with a Sole, Independently Owned Pharmacy. *Rural Policy Brief.* **2015**, *6*, 1–4.

29.   Scott, D.M. Assessment of pharmacists' perception of patient care competence and need for training in rural and urban areas in North Dakota. *J. Rural Health* **2010**, *26*, 90–96. [CrossRef] [PubMed]

30.   Radford, A.; Lampman, M.; Richardson, I.; Rutledge, S. *Profile of Sole Community Pharmacists' Prescription Sales and Overall Financial Position*; NC Rural Health Research & Policy Analysis Center: Chapel Hill, NC, USA, 2009.

31.   Creative Research Systems. Sample Size Calculator. Available online: https://www.surveysystem.com/sscalc.htm (accessed on 31 May 2018).

32.   Analytical Software. Statistix 10: Data Analysis Software for Researchers. Available online: https://www.statistix.com/ (accessed on 31 May 2018).

33. Weigel, P.; Ullrich, F.; Mueller, K. Demographic and economic characteristics associated with sole county pharmacy closures, 2006–2010. *Rural Policy Brief.* **2013**, *15*, 1–4.
34. Ullrich, F.; Mueller, K.J. Update: Independently owned pharmacy closures in rural America, 2003–2013. *Rural Policy Brief.* **2014**, *7*, 1–4.
35. Radford, A.; Slifkin, R.; King, J.; Lampman, M.; Richardson, I.; Rutledge, S. The relationship between the financial status of sole community independent pharmacies and their broader involvement with other rural providers. *J. Rural Health* **2011**, *27*, 176–183. [CrossRef] [PubMed]
36. Hoffman, E. *Pharmacies & Drug Stores in the US, Industry Report;* IBIS World: Los Angeles, CA, USA, 2016.
37. PwC Health Research Institute. The Pharmacy of the Future: Hub of Personalized Health. Available online: http://pwchealth.com/cgi-local/hregister.cgi/reg/pwc-hri-pharmacy-of-the-future-united-states.pdf (accessed on 30 November 2016).
38. Terlep, S.; Stevens, L. Amazon Buys Online Pharmacy PillPack for $1 Billion. Available online: https://www.wsj.com/articles/amazon-to-buy-online-pharmacy-pillpack-1530191443 (accessed on 3 July 2018).
39. Kim, T. Walgreen, CVS and Rite-Aid Lose $11 Billion in Value after Amazon Buys Online Pharmacy PillPack. Available online: https://www.cnbc.com/2018/06/28/walgreens-cvs-shares-tank-after-amazon-buys-online-pharmacy-pillpack.html (accessed on 3 July 2018).
40. National Community Pharmacists Association. Independent Pharmacy Today. Available online: http://www.ncpanet.org/home/independent-pharmacy-today (accessed on 7 June 2017).
41. Brooks, J.M.; Doucette, W.R.; Wan, S.; Klepser, D.G. Retail pharmacy market structure and performance. *Inquiry* **2008**, *45*, 75–88. [CrossRef] [PubMed]
42. Radford, A.; Mason, M.; Richardson, I.; Rutledge, S.; Poley, S.; Mueller, K.; Slifkin, R. Continuing effects of Medicare Part D on rural independent pharmacies who are the sole retail provider in their community. *Res. Soc. Adm. Pharm.* **2009**, *5*, 17–30. [CrossRef] [PubMed]
43. National Community Pharmacists Association. NCPA Statement on CVS-Target Deal. Available online: http://www.ncpanet.org/newsroom/details/2015/06/15/ncpa-statement-on-cvs-target-deal (accessed on 7 June 2017).
44. Todd, K.; Westfall, K.; Doucette, B.; Ullrich, F.; Mueller, K. Causes and consequences of rural pharmacy closures: A multi-case study. *Rural Policy Brief.* **2013**, *11*, 1–4.
45. Law, A.V.; Okamoto, M.P.; Brock, K. Perceptions of Medicare Part D enrollees about pharmacists and their role as providers of medication therapy management. *J. Am. Pharm. Assoc.* **2008**, *48*, 648–653. [CrossRef] [PubMed]
46. Henning-Smith, C.; Casey, M.; Moscovice, I. Does the Medicare Part D Decision-Making Experience Differ by Rural/Urban Location? *J. Rural Health* **2017**, *33*, 12–20. [CrossRef] [PubMed]
47. Viswanathan, M.; Kahwati, L.C.; Golin, C.E.; Blalock, S.J.; Coker-Schwimmer, E.; Posey, R.; Lohr, K.N. Medication therapy management interventions in outpatient settings: A systematic review and meta-analysis. *JAMA Intern. Med.* **2015**, *175*, 76–87. [CrossRef] [PubMed]
48. Cranor, C.W.; Bunting, B.A.; Christensen, D.B. The Asheville Project: Long-term clinical and economic outcomes of a community pharmacy diabetes care program. *J. Am. Pharm. Assoc.* **2003**, *43*, 173–184. [CrossRef]
49. Bunting, B.A.; Smith, B.H.; Sutherland, S.E. The Asheville Project: Clinical and economic outcomes of a community-based long-term medication therapy management program for hypertension and dyslipidemia. *J. Am. Pharm. Assoc.* **2008**, *48*, 23–31. [CrossRef] [PubMed]
50. Bunting, B.A.; Lee, G.; Knowles, G.; Lee, C.; Allen, P. The Hickory Project: Controlling healthcare costs and improving outcomes for diabetes using the Asheville project model. *Am. Health Drug Benefits* **2011**, *4*, 343–350. [PubMed]
51. Gadkari, A.S.; Mott, D.A.; Kreling, D.H.; Bonnarens, J.K. Pharmacy characteristics associated with the provision of drug therapy services in nonmetropolitan community pharmacies. *J. Rural Health* **2009**, *25*, 290–295. [CrossRef] [PubMed]

52. Nemlekar, P.; Shepherd, M.; Lawson, K.; Rush, S. Web-based survey to assess the perceptions of managed care organization representatives on use of copay subsidy coupons for prescription drugs. *J. Manag. Care Pharm.* **2013**, *19*, 602–608. [CrossRef] [PubMed]
53. Midwest Pharmacy Workforce Consortium. Final Report of the 2014 National Sample Survey of the Pharmacist Workforce to Determine Contemporary Demographic Practice Characteristics and Quality of Work-Life. American Association of Colleges of Pharmacy. Available online: http://www.aacp.org/resources/research/pharmacyworkforcecenter/Documents/PWC-demographics.pdf (accessed on 1 November 2016).

8

Clozapine Patients at the Interface between Primary and Secondary Care

Marita Barrett [1,*], Anna Keating [1], Deirdre Lynch [1], Geraldine Scanlon [2], Mary Kigathi [2], Fidelma Corcoran [2] and Laura J. Sahm [3,4]

[1] Pharmacy Department, Cork University Hospital, Cork T12 DC4A, Ireland; anna.keating@hse.ie (A.K.); deirdrem.lynch@hse.ie (D.L.)
[2] Adult Mental Health Unit, Cork University Hospital, Cork T12 DC4A, Ireland; geraldine.scanlon@hse.ie (G.S.); mary.kigathi@hse.ie (M.K.); fidelma.corcoran@hse.ie (F.C.)
[3] School of Pharmacy, University College Cork, Cork T12 YN60, Ireland; l.sahm@ucc.ie
[4] Pharmacy Department, Mercy University Hospital, Cork T12 WE28, Ireland
*   Correspondence: maritabarrett@gmail.com

Abstract: Patients receiving clozapine must undergo routine blood monitoring to screen for neutropenia, and to monitor for potential agranulocytosis. In Cork University Hospital, Cork, Ireland, clozapine is dispensed in the hospital pharmacy and the pharmacists are not aware of co-prescribed medicines, potentially impacting upon patient safety. The aim of this study was to examine the continuity of care of patients prescribed clozapine. A retrospective audit was conducted on patients attending the clozapine clinic at Cork University Hospital and assessed patients' (i) independent living, (ii) co-prescribed medicines and (iii) knowledge of their community pharmacists regarding co-prescribed clozapine. A list of prescribed medicines for each patient was obtained, and potential drug-drug interactions between these medicines and clozapine were examined using Lexicomp® and Stockley's Interaction checker. Secondary outcomes included patients' physical health characteristics, and a review of co-morbidities. Data were collected between the 29 May 2017 and 20 June 2017. Local ethics committee approval was granted. Patients were eligible for inclusion if they were receiving clozapine treatment as part of a registered programme, were aged 18 years or more, and had the capacity to provide written informed consent. Microsoft Excel was used for data analysis. Of 112 patients, (33% female; mean age (SD) 43.9 (11.3) years; 87.5% living independently/in the family home) 86.6% patients reported that they were taking other prescribed medicines from community pharmacies. The mean (SD) number of co-prescribed medicines in addition to clozapine was 4.8 (4) per patient. Two thirds of community pharmacists were unaware of co-prescribed clozapine. Interactions with clozapine were present in all but 3 patients on co-prescribed medicines ($n = 97$). Lexicomp® reported 2.9 drug-drug interactions/patient and Stockley's Interaction Checker reported 2.5 drug-drug interactions/patient. Secondary outcomes for patients included BMI, total cholesterol, and HbA_{1c} levels, which were elevated in 75%, 54% and 17% respectively. Patients prescribed clozapine did not receive a seamless service, between primary and secondary care settings. Community pharmacists were not informed of clozapine, prescribed for their patients, in two thirds of cases. Patients in this study were exposed to clozapine-related drug-drug interactions and hence potential adverse effects. This study supports reports in the literature of substandard management of the physical health of this patient group. This study shows that there is an opportunity for pharmacists to develop active roles in the management of all clozapine-related effects, in addition to their traditional obligatory role in haematological monitoring. This study supports the need for a clinical pharmacist to review inpatients commencing on clozapine, monitor for drug-drug interactions and provide counselling.

Keywords: Clozapine; Pharmacy; drug-drug interactions; patient safety

1. Introduction

Clozapine is the medication of choice for Treatment Resistant Schizophrenia; as its efficacy is superior to other antipsychotic agents [1]. Despite the benefits of clozapine therapy, it is underutilised due to safety concerns and strict monitoring requirements. Patients prescribed clozapine must have their bloods monitored routinely to screen for neutropenia, and to monitor for potential agranulocytosis. Monitoring is carried out in secondary care in some countries including Ireland, often from designated clozapine clinics. Hospital pharmacists supply clozapine only after obtaining a valid prescription and blood result.

The life expectancy of people with schizophrenia is 20% lower than the general population. Men with this diagnosis die, on average, 20 years earlier than those without schizophrenia [2]. Most of the increased mortality is due to higher levels of cardiovascular disease (CVD) and physical health problems [2]. The incidence of obesity, type 2 diabetes mellitus (T2DM) and hyperlipidaemia is higher than in the general population. Hyperlipidaemia is up to five times higher in those prescribed antipsychotics than in those who are not, and over half of these have low High Density Lipoprotein Cholesterol (HDL-C) and raised triglycerides [3]. This increases the risk of developing metabolic syndrome. Unemployment, tobacco use and alcohol misuse contribute to this increased CVD risk, in addition to the metabolic effects of antipsychotic agents; in particular clozapine [2,3]. Patients prescribed clozapine, with co-morbidities, whether clozapine-induced or not, will also be prescribed and taking other medications. These are prescribed by General Practitioners (GPs) and dispensed by community pharmacists, thus adding to their burden by attending multiple healthcare professionals (HCPs) at different locations, including both hospital and community pharmacies [4]. There is evidence in the literature about the communication gap that exists between primary and secondary care services for patients prescribed clozapine [5]. Obtaining medicines from multiple sources leads to fragmented service delivery, compromises safe use of medicines and, exposes patients to an increased risk of drug-drug interactions (DDIs) and adverse effects [5,6]. There is little published on the consequences of disjointed pharmacy services for those patients who receive clozapine separate to their other medicines. Additionally, these patients may be at risk of the sequelae of poor communication between physicians in primary and secondary care services [7]. Consequently, errors may occur when patients transition between these services or there may be substandard management of clozapine-associated physical comorbidities as a result of ambiguity, between prescribers, as to where responsibility lies [2,8,9].

Many of clozapine's pharmacodynamic and pharmacokinetic interactions are reported in the literature [1,5]. Community pharmacists however, are unable to monitor for clozapine-related adverse effects or provide appropriate counselling to the patient, if they are unaware that it has been prescribed [5]. Polypharmacy (the prescribing of five or more medications) is increasing in patients with schizophrenia, another factor that contributes to DDIs and adverse drug events [10].

There are other models that manage clozapine therapy differently: In New Zealand and Australia, clozapine is now available from community pharmacies [4]. One benefit is that community pharmacists know all co-prescribed medicines, and can therefore monitor for interactions and counsel the patient appropriately [4]. Knowledge of co-prescribed clozapine means they are ideally positioned to monitor for associated side effects, provide advice on the management of these, and recommend alleviating treatments [4]. Whether clozapine is dispensed by hospital or community pharmacists, the literature agrees that patients prescribed clozapine should be provided with an integrated holistic pharmacy service [4,8,11,12].

In Cork University Hospital (CUH), Ireland, patients who require clozapine therapy are commenced as an inpatient in the Acute Mental Health Unit (AMHU) of the hospital. As the AMHU does not have a clinical pharmacist, patients' medicines are not reviewed by a clinical pharmacist prior to initiation. Once discharged, these patients receive clozapine from CUH pharmacy department, in the absence of any information regarding co-morbidities or concomitant medications. There is no formal system in place to inform community pharmacists of clozapine therapy. The aim of this study was to describe the impact of non-integration of pharmacy services, upon patient care.

This study examined:

- The prevalence of patients prescribed clozapine who were living in a community setting; their demographics, physical health characteristics, co-morbidities and co-medications.
- Community pharmacists' awareness of clozapine prescription for their patients as recorded in their Patient Medication Record (PMR). This is the unique record for each patient held by community pharmacies on their computer systems.
- Co-prescribed medicines in this cohort.
- DDIs between clozapine and co-prescribed medicines.

2. Methods

Permission for conducting this research study was granted by both, the Clinical Research and Ethics Committee (CREC) of the Cork Teaching Hospitals, and the Quality Department of CUH. All data were saved on a password-encrypted laptop. Research Setting and Participants: This study was carried out at the Clozapine Clinic, CUH. The Clozapine Clinical Nurse Specialists (CCNS) take routine bloods and records observations for patients prescribed clozapine. At initiation of the study, there were 141 adult patients registered. Patients were given information about the study. Written informed consent was obtained from patients willing to participate. Inclusion criteria: All patients aged 18 years or over, and registered with the Clozaril Patient Monitoring Service (CPMS) were included. Exclusion criteria: those who did not attend the clinic during the study period (29 May–20 June 2017), and those deemed by the CCNS to lack capacity to provide informed consent, were excluded from the study.

The following data were collected from participants:

- Patient characteristics: gender, weight, height and blood pressure
- Lifestyle factors: smoking status and living arrangements
- Co-prescribed medicines, and the name of the patient's community pharmacy

After the clinic, the following data were obtained for each study participant:

- Age
- Number of years taking clozapine as recorded on the CPMS website
- The total daily dose of clozapine as per the prescriptions for dispensing in the pharmacy department in CUH
- A list of medicines obtained from the nominated community pharmacy
- Community pharmacists were also asked:

  1. "Are you aware that Mr Y/ Ms X is receiving clozapine?"
  2. If yes, "Has this been documented in the patient's PMR?"
  3. "Is clozapine listed on prescriptions from the GP, for this patient?"

- For those that were inpatients during the study period (both newly initiated and long stay patients), the list of co-prescribed medicines was obtained from their inpatient medication prescription and administration record.
- An interaction check was undertaken between clozapine and all medicines, using Lexicomp® [13] and Stockley's Interaction Checker (SIC) [14]. Lexicomp® is a widely accessible drug interaction software program and studies show it provides the most competent, complete, and user-friendly applications [15]. SIC is a comprehensive and authoritative international reference book on DDIs. DDIs were graded as:

1.   Avoid Combination: Contra-Indicated (CI) /Life Threatening
2.   Consider Therapy Modification/Dose Adjustment
3.   Monitor Therapy

- Co-morbidities as documented in the patient's records sourced from the medical records department.
- Physical health characteristics including lipid profile and glycosylated haemoglobin (HbA_{1c}) were sourced from the laboratory within CUH (iLab), where they are measured on an annual basis.

All data obtained from the retrospective audit were entered into Microsoft Excel and descriptive statistics were performed.

3. Results

Of a total of 141 patients registered for clozapine therapy, five patients were deemed too unwell by the CCNS to participate, and 19 patients did not attend the clinic during the study period. Of 117 eligible patients, five patients did not agree to participate, leaving 112 patients, who agreed and provided written informed consent. The demographics of the participants are shown in Table 1. Table 2 details the frequency and type of co-morbidities of participants.

Table 1. Study Participant Demographics.

Study Participant Demographics	Variable	$n =$	%
Gender	Male	75	67
	Female	37	33
Age (years)	Mean (SD)	43.9 (11.3)	-
	Median	32	-
Patient type	Outpatient	104	92.9
	Inpatient	8	7.1
Daily dose of clozapine (mg)	Mean (SD)	350 ($\pm$136)	-
	Median	312.5	-
Duration prescribed clozapine (years)	<0.5	10	8.9
	$\geq$0.5–1	4	3.6
	>1–5	20	17.9
	>5–10	23	20.5
	>10	55	49.1
Clozapine Indication	TRS *	108	96.4
	Psychotic disorder in PD ~	2	1.8
	Not specified	2	1.8
Smoking status	Smoker	44	39
	Non-smoker	68	61
Ethnic Origin (as per CPMS)	Caucasian	111	99.1
	Asian	1	0.9
Living Arrangements	Independent /Family home	98	87.5
	Other (NH, H) #	14	12.5

* TRS = treatment resistant schizophrenia, ~PD = Parkinson's disease, # NH = Nursing Home, H = Hostel, supported accommodation, CPMS = clozaril patient monitoring service, SD = standard deviation, - = not applicable

Table 2. Frequency and type of co-morbidities of participants ($n = 112$).

Co-Morbidities of Participants	$n =$ *	%
Hypercholesterolemia/dyslipidaemia	35	31.3
T2DM [#]	21	18.8
Hypothyroidism	12	10.7
Hypertension	16	14.3
Gastrointestinal	43	38.4
(Constipation)	(13)	(30.2)
(GORD ~/dyspepsia)	(19)	(44.2)
(Both)	(11)	(25.6)
Respiratory (Asthma & COPD ≈)	15	13.4
Cardiovascular disease	9	8
Tachycardia	8	7.1
Known QT prolongation	2	1.8

* patients may have multiple co-morbidities. # T2DM = Type 2 Diabetes Mellitus, ~GORD = gastro oesophageal reflux disease, ≈ COPD = chronic obstructive pulmonary disease.

Community Pharmacy Awareness

The majority of patients prescribed clozapine reported that they were prescribed additional medicines in primary care ($n = 97$; 86.6%). Of these 97 patients, 89 had a regular community pharmacy that was contacted, the remaining eight patients did not record having a regular pharmacy. Pharmacists were aware of co-prescribed clozapine for thirty of these patients (33.7%), but for only 20, was this recorded in their PMR. The GP had clozapine on prescriptions for ten of these patients.

Drug-Drug Interactions

Patients ($n = 97$) were taking a total of 535 prescribed medicines in addition to clozapine. The mean number of co-prescribed medicines (not including clozapine) per patient was 4.8 (SD ± 4.) and ranged from zero to 21.

Medicines for each patient were checked for interactions with clozapine using two separate reference sources; Lexicomp® and SIC. Of those; 60% (322/535) of medicines had documented interactions with clozapine using Lexicomp® and, 51.5% (277/535) using SIC.

Figure 1 shows the categories of DDI with clozapine in this study group for both reference sources.

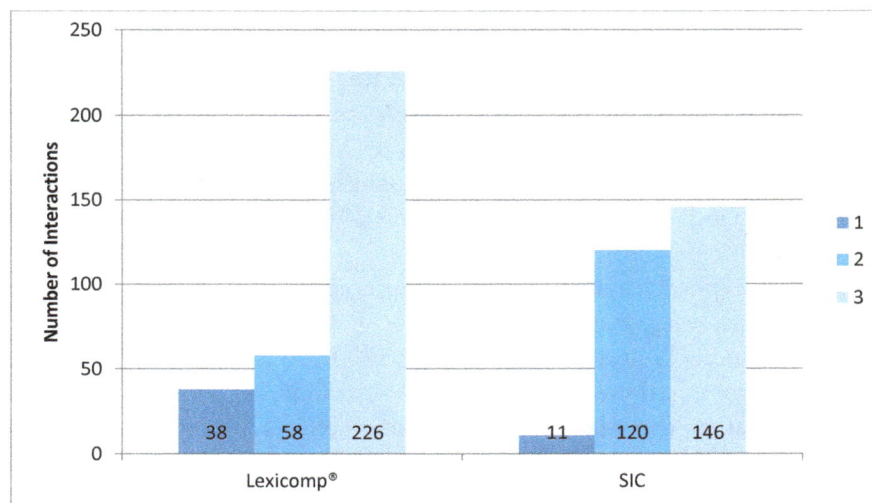

Figure 1. Drug-drug Interactions (DDIs) with Clozapine using Lexicomp and Stockley's Interaction Checker (SIC) (**1** = *Avoid Combination: Contra-indicated (CI) /life threatening*, **2** = *Consider Therapy Modification/Dose Adjustment*, **3** = *Monitor therapy*).

For those patients taking co-prescribed medicines ($n = 97$); Lexicomp® recorded 3.3 DDIs per patient and SIC recorded 2.9 DDIs per patient.

3.1. 'Avoid Combination: Contra-Indicated (CI) /Life Threatening' DDIs

The most frequently prescribed contra-indicated (CI) drugs were amisulpride (Lexicomp®) and domperidone (SIC) (Table 3). Both domperidone and flupentixol are classified as CI in both references. With regard to amisulpride, SIC does not classify it as CI with clozapine, but does advise that concurrent use might increase the risk of QT prolongation and torsade de pointes (TdP), and that there should be further monitoring in those at risk [14].

Table 3. Co-prescribed Contra-indicated (CI)/life-threatening medicines with clozapine.

Medicine	Contra-Indicated (CI)/Life-Threatening DDIs	
	Lexicomp ($n = 38$)	SIC ($n = 11$)
Amisulpride	16	-
Citalopram	7	-
Domperidone	4	4
Olanzapine	-	3
Fluoxetine	3	-
Quetiapine	2	-
Inhaled Antimuscarinics	3	-
Fluphenazine	-	2
Trimethoprim	-	1
Carbamazepine	1	-
Flupentixol	1	1
Phenytoin	1	-

3.2. 'Consider Therapy Modification/Dose Adjustment' DDIs

These interactions advise either therapy modification, a dose adjustment or close monitoring. Both Lexicomp® and SIC include benzodiazepines in this category (Table 4). SIC reports several cases describing severe hypotension, respiratory depression, and potentially fatal respiratory arrest in patients taking benzodiazepines and clozapine [14]. Dizziness and sedation are also increased. Lexicomp® also includes hypersalivation, unconsciousness and delirium as risks with concurrent use of clozapine and benzodiazepines [13]. 26.8% ($n = 30$) of patients in this study were taking a benzodiazepine with their clozapine.

SIC grades all anti-hyperglycaemic agents in this category as *"clozapine has been associated with glucose intolerance and therefore might affect diabetic control"* [14].

Many selective serotonin reuptake inhibitors (SSRIs) are included in this category, as they increase the risk of QT prolongation/TdP. In addition, sertraline, paroxetine and fluoxetine increase clozapine levels. Mirtazapine can cause additive sedative effects, blood dyscrasias and potentially fatal agranulocytosis with concurrent clozapine therapy [14].

Ciprofloxacin increases clozapine concentrations and cases of clozapine toxicity have been reported when taken concomitantly [14]. It also has QT prolonging effects, as have the macrolide antibiotics.

Table 4. Consider Therapy Modification/Dose Adjustment DDIs with Clozapine.

	Consider Therapy Modification/Dose Adjustment	
	Lexicomp ($n = 58$)	SIC ($n = 120$)
Anti-hyperglycaemic agents	-	34
Benzodiazepines	32	32
Zolpidem	1	-
SSRIs	3	19
Mirtazapine	-	4
Anti-Epileptic Drugs/Mood Stabilisers		
-Lithium	-	8
-Phenytoin	-	11
-Carbamazepine	-	1
Antipsychotics		
-Haloperidol	7	7
-Chlorpromazine	2	-
Antibiotics		
-Macrolides	4	-
-Ciprofloxacin	1	1
Anti-Parkinson's medicines		
-Carbidopa/levodopa	2	2
-Ropinirole	1	1
Analgesia		
-Codeine	3	-
-Tramadol	2	-
Omeprazole	-	8
Desmopressin	-	1
Memantine	-	1

3.3. 'Monitor therapy' DDIs

The recommendation for this category of DDIs is to monitor therapy and provide guidance. In this study, 70% of clozapine's DDIs fall in this category in Lexicomp® and 53% in SIC.

Medicines causing DDIs with clozapine listed in Lexicomp® include blood pressure lowering agents, antipsychotics, serotonin noradrenaline reuptake inhibitors (SNRIs) and some SSRIs and anticholinergic agents. These can have additive pharmacodynamics effects with clozapine. Other agents include anti-hyperglycaemic agents which may be antagonised by clozapine, and the proton pump inhibitor (PPI) omeprazole which may decrease serum concentration of clozapine. Similar agents are listed in SIC. Of note, SIC lists sodium valproate in this category. Valproate can have a minor effect on clozapine concentrations and advice is provided to monitor for the additive effects of weight gain and central nervous system depressant effects with concomitant clozapine. This is important as almost 22% of the study group were prescribed sodium valproate. Combined hormonal contraception is also in this category, as it can increase clozapine levels. Two patients were taking the oral contraceptive pill (OCP), and hence both will require monitoring if their OCP is discontinued.

Other findings in relation to co-prescribed medicines include 28% of patients were prescribed antiepileptic drugs (AED) or mood stabilizers (MS), 43% were prescribed another antipsychotic and 19% were taking both AED/MS and another antipsychotic in addition to clozapine. Another finding that has implications on clozapine is concomitant nicotine replacement therapy (NRT). Four patients were prescribed NRT, therefore highlighting changes in smoking status. Polycyclic aromatic hydrocarbons in cigarette smoke cause CYP1A2 enzyme induction which reduces clozapine levels. Cessation of smoking can increase plasma clozapine concentrations, thus leading to an increase in adverse effects [16].

Medical Complications/Adverse Effects

Body mass index (BMI) was within recommended target for just a quarter of patients ($n = 26$) (Table 5).

Table 5. BMI (kg/m^2).

BMI	($n = 112$)
$\leq$25	26
26–29	39
30–35	26
>35	19
Not done	2
Mean	29.8 ($\pm$6.16)

The documented prevalence of hypercholesterolemia/dyslipidaemia in the study group was estimated at over 30%. However, when the level of hypercholesterolemia and dyslipidaemia was assessed using the laboratory values recorded, this figure increased to 70%. Dyslipidaemia is defined as elevated total cholesterol (TC) >5 mmol/L OR elevated fasting triglycerides (TGs) >1.7 mmol/L OR elevated fasting low density lipoprotein cholesterol (LDL-C) >3 mmol/L or decreased HDL-C <1 mmol/L for males and <1.3 mmol/L for females [17].

Table 6 shows the breakdown for TC. TC as reported on iLab was elevated for 54% of the study group.

Table 6. Total Cholesterol (TC) Levels (mmol/L) of Participants.

TC (mmol/L)	$n = 112$	%
$\leq$5	47	42
5.1–6	35	31
>6	26	23
Not done	4	4
Mean (SD)	5.3 (1.04)	-

When laboratory TC levels and diagnoses recorded were compared, it was found that some patients with elevated TC levels did not have a diagnosis documented in their medical notes, nor were they prescribed lipid lowering agents. In total 41% ($n = 46$) patients had elevated cholesterol levels on iLab and were undiagnosed/untreated. A total of 36 patients had a documented diagnosis of dyslipidaemia and/or were prescribed lipid lowering agents. Of those, 58% ($n = 21$) were treated to target. Despite a diagnosis of dyslipidaemia and/or taking lipid lowering treatment, 42% ($n = 15$) had elevated TC levels.

The prevalence of T2DM, based on documentation in the medical notes, or associated drug treatment is 19% ($n = 21$). The laboratory marker used by the clozapine clinic for T2DM is HbA$_{1c}$ (Table 7).

Table 7. HbA1c Values for the study participants.

HbA$_{1c}$ (mmol/mol)	$n = 112$	%
$\leq$42 *	79	71
43–47	12	11
48–53 *	7	6
>53	9	8
Not done	5	4
Mean (SD)	40 ($\pm$10.7)	

* Levels < 42 mmol/mol are normal [18]. Those >48 mmol/mol confirm T2DM [18,19].

There were nine patients with elevated laboratory HbA_{1C} levels, indicative of pre-diabetes, not prescribed anti-diabetic treatment [20] and a further patient whereby a level >48 mmol/mol was measured but neither diagnosis nor treatment were in place.

In the case of those for whom T2DM was documented in the medical notes and/or patients were prescribed anti-hyperglycaemic agents (n = 21); six patients were well controlled with HbA_{1c} < 48 mmol/mol, six had elevated levels between 48–53 mmol/mol and nine had levels >53 mmol/mol.

Hypertension was documented in the medical notes for sixteen patients. Based on readings taken in the clozapine clinic, eight patients had readings >140/90 mmHg. Three of these patients had documented hypertension, whereas five patients were not diagnosed with hypertension and were not prescribed anti-hypertensive treatment. Constipation; a well-known adverse effect of clozapine, was documented for 21% (n = 24) of patients. Five of these patients were not prescribed treatment.

4. Discussion

In this study, the population of patients was a similar size to clozapine-related studies reported in the literature. In addition, this study group had similar characteristics to those in other related studies [2,5,10,21–23]. There were more males than females, with a mean age of 44 years, taking a mean dose of 350 ($\pm$136) mg of clozapine per day. The average BMI was 30 kg/m^2 and the percentage of patients smoking was at the lower end of figures reported in the literature at 39%, although this was a self-reported figure. There is evidence showing that in comparison to patients with schizophrenia in general; patients prescribed clozapine have a lower frequency of tobacco use [24]. The majority of patients were stabilised on treatment and residing in the community. All outpatients were self-medicating, including those in supported living arrangements, except for one older patient with Parkinson's disease, who was living in a nursing home. Nearly 90% of patients reported taking other co-prescribed medicines which are dispensed from community pharmacies. Patients were co-prescribed on average five additional medicines, similar to the figure reported by Murphy et al. [5].

4.1. Community Pharmacy Awareness

Two-thirds of community pharmacists were unaware of co-prescribed clozapine. This is greater than the figure (40%) reported by Murphy et al. [5] in a 'shared care' system in Australia. As expected, this provides evidence that shared care improves the sharing of information in relation to clozapine with community pharmacists. These results showed that most patients did not communicate directly with their community pharmacist about clozapine, or were unaware that they could consult their community pharmacist for healthcare advice. This lack of communication between patients and community pharmacists may have been due to associated mental health stigma as reported in the literature [25,26]. There may be a lack of awareness on the services pharmacists can provide, including checking for interactions or the suitability of co-prescribed medicines. Our results are in agreement with the literature as Bell et al. [8], Heald et al. [10] and Murphy et al. [5] reported a lack of communication with community pharmacists on concomitant clozapine use dispensed from secondary care.

One third of community pharmacists who were aware of concomitant clozapine therapy did not reflect this by documenting clozapine use in the patients' PMR. This showed ambiguity in their role in relation to clozapine as part of the patients' PMR. This means when a locum pharmacist, or a pharmacist unfamiliar with the patient, is dispensing medications, they will not have this information available to screen for clozapine-related DDIs and adverse effects. Additionally, when clozapine is not recorded in a patient's PMR, the software will not include clozapine when alerting the pharmacist to interaction risks. Therefore, a community pharmacist who is aware of concomitant clozapine therapy should document this in the PMR to minimise risk and enhance transfer of information for these patients. More education is required for community pharmacists on how to manage this information and the clinical relevance of this. This was an issue that had to be addressed in Australia when clozapine dispensing transferred from hospital to community pharmacy for stable patients in

2015 [6]. A lack of education and inadequate resources were identified as barriers to implementing this service change.

For more than one in ten patients, the community pharmacist reported seeing clozapine on prescriptions from the patients' GP. In some cases, pharmacists said clozapine was listed on the prescription [endorsed as "hospital only"]. Pharmacists reported that this was good practice by GPs. GPs also have a role to play in ensuring medicines prescribed in primary care are safe with clozapine. Both Murphy et al. [5] and Parker and Somasunderam [7] showed GPs omitted clozapine from their records in up to 50% of cases; however when GPs were more involved in clozapine services this figure reduces to 5%.

4.2. Drug-Drug Interactions

'Stockley's Drug Interactions' is a commonly used reference in Ireland and in the UK. Lexicomp® is a US-based resource. In practice SIC would be used first-line in CUH. The categorised severity of an interaction may differ between the grading systems in both sources, but the underlying mechanisms are the same. For patients co-prescribed other medicines ($n = 97$), DDIs with clozapine occurred in all but three patients. This was in keeping with the figure reported by Leung et al. [1]; in a similar sized population DDIs were found in all but 10 patients. There was an average of 2.9 DDI/patient. Guo et al. [27] reported that nearly a quarter of patients with schizophrenia prescribed an antipsychotic were exposed to a major or moderate DDI. Guo et al.'s [27] figures are not specific to clozapine and include all antipsychotics. In this study, which specifically focused on clozapine, the figures were much higher, with 53.5% of patients exposed to a major or moderate interaction as per Lexicomp®and 58% exposure as per Stockley (category 1&2) [13,14].

Guo et al. [27] reported on medicines that interacted with clozapine and found similar results to this study. The most frequent interacting drugs were SSRIs via CYP 2D6 pathways, phenytoin and carbamazepine via CYP3A4 induction and ciprofloxacin via CYP1A2 mechanisms [27]. Many of the interactions reported in this study group involved a risk of QT prolongation and TdP, additive bone marrow suppression and changes to clozapine serum levels. In a review of clozapine DDIs by Markowitz et al. [28], clinical significance was assessed for each interaction. Interactions between clozapine and benzodiazepines, lithium, some SSRIs, carbamazepine and phenytoin were deemed clinically significant [28]. All of these drugs, deemed by Markowitz et al. to have clinically significant interactions with clozapine, were also prescribed for patients attending the CUH clinic. These patients, who were not reviewed by clinical pharmacists, were also not fully reviewed by community pharmacists as, in at least two thirds of cases, they were uninformed of clozapine as part of a patient's PMR.

Patients in this cohort, who were living in the community, appeared to be functioning, despite interacting medicines. The clinical relevance of these interactions often becomes more prominent at the point of change i.e., drug initiation, dose change or discontinuation. Pharmacists have the knowledge, expertise and skill mix to process complex interactions and decide upon their clinical relevance at the time of dispensing new/changed medicines. They can recommend an alternative agent and/or provide counselling and rationalise drug therapy. The advice for many clozapine related DDIs is to monitor therapy and give guidance. This was not possible for this patient group without clinical or community pharmacist input. For example, four patients were taking regular domperidone despite multiple warnings on the risk of serious cardiac adverse drug reactions [29]. It is CI for those taking QT-prolonging drugs, i.e., including clozapine [29]. Without knowledge of concomitant clozapine, it was not possible to make any recommendation. One patient was found to have taken a course of the antibiotic ciprofloxacin; this has been reported in the literature to increase clozapine levels by up to 500% [1]. Monitoring of smoking status is assigned to the CCNS.

4.3. Medical Complications/Adverse Effects

Poor monitoring of the physical health of patients with schizophrenia is well documented [2,9]. Even so, there is little evidence of communication of this information to other healthcare professionals, who can act upon abnormal results [2,30,31]. Of the second generation antipsychotics, clozapine has the greatest potential to cause metabolic syndrome, thus predisposing patients to weight gain, hyperlipidaemia and hyperglycaemia [3]. In this study, three quarters of patients were overweight or obese, and 70% had laboratory results indicative of dyslipidaemia. Similarly, Bolton et al. report that 88% of their group had dyslipidaemia [21]. Over 40% of this study group had an elevated TC level and were not prescribed lipid lowering therapy. In Crawford et al.'s study, 80% of patients with dyslipidaemia were left untreated [2]. In contrast to Crawford, monitoring was better in this study group as nearly all patients had the recommended parameters measured [2]. The results demonstrated that the treatment of out-of-range parameters was not adequately managed. The results of this study support recommending measurement of waist circumference and fasting glucose for patients attending the clozapine clinic. This would ensure early prevention/prediction of metabolic syndrome onset. Interestingly, Bolton et al. [21] showed that half of their patients had metabolic syndrome, this is in agreement with other literature [3]. With more than three quarters of patients with an elevated BMI, and indications of poor glucose control with elevated HbA_{1c} levels found for both non-diabetic patients and those with T2DM, monitoring for metabolic syndrome is advised.

A fifth of patients in this study had a diagnosis of T2DM. This is in keeping with other studies with patients prescribed clozapine [21]. HbA_{1c} was >53 mmol/mol in over 40% of those with documented T2DM. This signifies poorly controlled T2DM and adds to an already increased CVD risk burden [20]. HbA_{1c} was elevated in 9% of patients not formally diagnosed with T2DM. There is an opportunity to intervene with dietary and lifestyle advice for these patients before overt T2DM manifests. More needs to be done to improve the management of T2DM in this patient group and when doing so, to incorporate the additive effect of clozapine therapy on diabetes management. Pharmacists can provide individual advice and ensure adherence to medication and blood glucose monitoring, while being cognisant of concomitant clozapine therapy.

Whilst clozapine-induced agranulocytosis is the main fear with treatment, and is the main reason for intensive monitoring, recent evidence from pharmacovigilance databases suggests that GI complications (constipation, intestinal obstruction and paralytic ileus) are the leading cause of clozapine-related deaths [32]. Clozapine-induced constipation ranges from 14% to 60% [23,33]. In this study, over a fifth of the population suffered with constipation (21.4%). This may be under-reported as it is self-managed in many cases, and documentation in the medical notes was not up to date for all patients. Leung et al. [1] reported that gastrointestinal hypo-motility can lead to hospitalisation and death. Community pharmacists play an active role in the pharmaceutical management of bowel problems on a daily basis; therefore, they would be a valuable HCP in the ongoing management of these patients. They are also vendors of codeine-based analgesia (OTC), which can contribute to constipation and hence are in a position to caution against the use of codeine-containing products in this cohort.

It is recognised that more needs to be done to improve the physical health of patients with mental health problems. The National Health Service (NHS) in the UK is committed to merging mental and physical health, and has launched 'The mental health workforce plan for England' [34]. This follows in the steps of Australia and New Zealand where provision of mental healthcare is community based where possible [12,35], and clozapine therapy is not excluded from this. As stated by Knowles et al., community access arrangements "provide community pharmacists with an opportunity to support clozapine users within the context of their overall medicine regimen, thus promoting holistic care which is an integral part of patient-centred care" [35].

Patients need education and counselling, and often clozapine counselling is done early in therapy when the patient is too unwell to retain the information provided [36]. There is evidence to show that interventions involving clinical pharmacist counselling can improve patient knowledge and this empowers patients in the management of their treatment [36].

5. Limitations

This is a single site study which limits the generalisability of the findings. We have reported on co-prescribed medicines, however additional medicines, (both those which can be bought without prescriptions and complementary and alternative therapy/products) are not included and these may contribute to additional DDIs. As patients can attend any pharmacy; there is a possibility that patients may have received other medications in pharmacies other than the ones given in the study, which may underestimate the extent of co-prescribing.

6. Conclusions

Patients prescribed clozapine are currently not receiving a seamless service, caught as they are, at the interface of primary and secondary care. Community pharmacists were not aware of prescribed clozapine in two thirds of cases. Patients in this study were exposed to clozapine-related drug-drug interactions and hence potential adverse effects. This study supports previous work on the sub-optimal management of the physical health of this patient group. There is international evidence to show clozapine can be safely dispensed from community pharmacies, exclusively, or as part of shared care settings. Ireland could follow this approach and make changes to support community dispensing of clozapine for stable patients. The remuneration model for pharmacy services needs consideration; one that would reimburse pharmacist services, including medication reconciliation and discharge summaries. This would serve as a driver to change the current, non-integrated, clozapine practice. Current pharmacy services provided to patients prescribed clozapine in secondary care need reform. There is an opportunity for pharmacist involvement in the management of all clozapine-related effects, in addition to their traditional role in haematological monitoring. This study supports the need for a clinical pharmacist to review inpatients commenced on clozapine, monitor for DDIs and provide counselling. Hospital pharmacists, with the patient's permission, could liaise with their colleagues in community pharmacies, to ensure continuity of care once patients are discharged. Resources and educational material for community pharmacists will need to be developed. Policies to provide for this change in practice will also need consideration. These patients are community based and current evidence supports empowering patients to remain in the community, whilst providing more integrated care.

Acknowledgments: The authors would like to thank all of the participants within this study.

Author Contributions: Marita Barrett and Laura J Sahm conceived and designed the study. Marita Barrett, Geraldine Scanlon, Mary Kigathi and Fidelma Corcoran were involved in patient recruitment. Marita Barrett undertook data collection. Laura J Sahm analyzed the data. Marita Barrett, Anna Keating, Deirdre Lynch, Geraldine Scanlon, Mary Kigathi, Fidelma Corcoran and Laura J Sahm were involved in drafting the manuscript and all authors reviewed and agreed upon the final draft.

References

1.   Leung, J.G.; Hasassri, M.E.; Barreto, J.N.; Nelson, S.; Morgan, R.J. Characterization of Admission Types in Medically Hospitalized Patients Prescribed Clozapine. *J. Consul. Liaison Psychiatry* **2017**, *58*, 164–172. [CrossRef] [PubMed]

2.   Crawford, M.J.; Jayakumar, S.; Lemmey, S.J.; Zalewska, K.; Patel, M.X.; Cooper, S.J.; Shiers, D. Assessment and Treatment of Physical Health Problems Among People with Schizophrenia: National Cross-sectional Study. *Br. J. Psychiatry* **2014**, *205*, 473–477. [CrossRef] [PubMed]

3.   Lambert, T. Managing the Metabolic Adverse Effects of Antipsychotic Drugs in Patients with Psychosis. *Aust. Presc.* **2011**, *34*, 97–98. [CrossRef]

4.   Knowles, S.A.; McMillan, S.S.; Wheeler, A.J. Consumer Access to Clozapine in Australia: How Does This Compare to New Zealand and the United Kingdom? *Pharm. Pract.* **2016**, *14*. [CrossRef] [PubMed]

5.   Murphy, K.; Coombes, I.; Moudgil, V.; Patterson, S.; Wheeler, A. Clozapine and Concomitant Medications: Assessing the Completeness and Accuracy of Medication Records for People Prescribed Clozapine Under Shared Care Arrangements. *J. Eval. Clin. Pract.* **2017**. [CrossRef] [PubMed]

6.   Winckel, K.; Siskindm, D.; Hollingworth, S.; Robinson, G.; Mitchell, S.; Varghese, D.; Smith, L.; Wheeler, A.J. Clozapine in the community: Improved Access or Risky Free-for-all? *Aust. N. Z. J. Psychiatry* **2015**, *49*, 863–865. [CrossRef] [PubMed]

7.   Parker, C.; Somasunderam, P. Audit of GP Practice Records of Patients Prescribed Clozapine. *Prog. Neurol. Psychiatry* **2010**, *14*, 11–16. [CrossRef]

8.   Bell, J.S.; Rosen, A.; Aslani, P.; Whitehead, P.; Chen, T.F. Developing the Role of Pharmacists as Members of Community Mental Health Teams: Perspectives of Pharmacists and Mental Health Professionals. *Res. Soc. Adm. Pharm.* **2007**, *3*, 392–409. [CrossRef] [PubMed]

9.   Van Hasselt, F.M.; Schorr, S.G.; Mookhoek, E.J.; Brouwers, J.R.; Loonen, A.J.; Taxis, K. Gaps in Health Care for the Somatic Health of Outpatients with Severe Mental Illness. *Int. J. Ment. Health Nurs.* **2013**, *22*, 249–255. [CrossRef] [PubMed]

10. Heald, A.; Livingston, M.; Yung, A.; De Hert, M.A. Prescribing in Schizophrenia and Psychosis: Increasing Polypharmacy Over Time. *Hum. Psychopharmacol.* **2017**, *32*. [CrossRef] [PubMed]

11. Taylor, D.; Sutton, J.; Family, H.E. *Evaluating the Pharmacist Provision of Clozapine Services*; University of Bath: Bath, UK, 2011.

12. Crump, K.; Boo, G.; Liew, F.S.; Olivier, T.; So, C.; Sung, J.Y.; Wong, C.H.; Shaw, J.; Wheeler, A. New Zealand Community Pharmacists' views of Their Roles in Meeting Medicine-related Needs for People with Mental Illness. *Res. Soc. Adm. Pharm.* **2011**, *7*, 122–133. [CrossRef] [PubMed]

13. WoltersKluwer. Lexicomp®Drug Interactions. Available online: sit.ucc.ieUpToDate (accessed on 7 August 2017).

14. Preston, C.L. Stockley's Drug Interactions. 2016. Available online: sit.ucc.iemedicinescomplete (accessed on 7 August 2017).

15. Kheshti, R.; Aalipour, M.; Namazi, S. A Comparison of Five Common Drug-drug Interaction Software Programs Regarding Accuracy and Comprehensiveness. *J. Res. Pharm. Pract.* **2016**, *5*, 257–263. [PubMed]

16. Summary of Product Characteristics Clozaril Ireland: Mylan. 2016. Available online: https://www.hpra.ie/img/uploaded/swedocuments/LicenseSPC_PA0013-046-002_04112016145050.pdf (accessed on 22 January 2017).

17. Catapano, A.L.; Graham, I.; De Backer, G.; Wiklund, O.; Chapman, M.J.; Drexel, H.; Hoes, A.W.; Jennings, S.S.; Landmesser, U.; Pedersen, T.R.; Reiner, Z.; et al. 2016 ESC/EAS Guidelines for the Management of Dyslipidaemia. *Eur. Heart J.* **2016**, *37*, 2999–3058. [CrossRef] [PubMed]

18. Information for Healthcare Professionals Regarding Diabetes, 2010. Health Service Executive 2010. Available online: http://www.hse.ie/eng/services/Publications/topics/Diabetes/HbA1c_Information_for_Health_Care_Professionals_regarding_Diabetes.pdf. (accessed on 18 August 2017).

19. Type 2 Diabetes in Adults: Management. Available online: https://www.nice.org.uk/guidance/ng28/chapter/1-Recommendations (accessed on 18 August 2017).

20. Harkins, V. *A Practical Guide to Integrated Type 2 Diabetes Care*; Irish College of General Practitioners: Dublin, Ireland, 2016; p. 7.

21. Bolton, P.J. Improving Physical Health Monitoring in Secondary Care for Patients on Clozapine. *Psychiatrist* **2011**, *35*, 49–55. [CrossRef]

22. Filia, S.; Lee, S.; Sinclair, K.; Wheelhouse, A.; Wilkins, S.; de Castella, A.; Kulkarni, J. Demonstrating the Effectiveness of Less Restrictive Care Pathways for the Management of Patients Treated with Clozapine. Australasian Psychiatry. *R. Aust. N. Z. Coll. Psychiatr.* **2013**, *21*, 449–455. [CrossRef] [PubMed]

23. Takeuchi, I.; Hanya, M.; Uno, J.; Amano, Y.; Fukai, K.; Fujita, K.; Kamei, H. A Questionnaire-based Study of the Views of Schizophrenia Patients and Psychiatric Healthcare Professionals in Japan about the Side Effects of Clozapine. *Clin. Psychopharmacol. Neurosci.* **2016**, *14*, 286–294. [CrossRef] [PubMed]

24. Mallet, J.; Le Strat, Y.; Schurhoff, F.; Mazer, N.; Portalier, C.; Andrianarisoa, M.; Aouizerate, B.; Brunel, L.; Capdevielle, D.; Chereau, I.; et al. Cigarette Smoking and Schizophrenia: A Specific Clinical and Therapeutic Profile? Results from the FACE-Schizophrenia Cohort. *Prog. Neuro Psychopharmac. Boil. Psychiatry* **2017**, *79*, 332–339. [CrossRef] [PubMed]

25. Calogero, S.; Caley, C.F. Supporting Patients with Mental Illness: Deconstructing Barriers to Community Pharmacist Access. *J. Am. Pharm. Assoc.* **2017**, *57*, 248–255. [CrossRef] [PubMed]

26. O'Reilly, C.L.; Bell, J.S.; Kelly, P.J.; Chen, T.F. Exploring the Relationship Between Mental Health Stigma, Knowledge and Provision of Pharmacy Services for Consumers with Schizophrenia. *Res. Soc. Adm. Pharm.* **2015**, *11*, e101–e109. [CrossRef] [PubMed]

27. Guo, J.J.; Wu, J.; Kelton, C.M.; Jing, Y.; Fan, H.; Keck, P.E.; Patel, N.C. Exposure to Potentially Dangerous Drug-drug Interactions Involving Antipsychotics. *Psychiatr. Serv.* **2012**, *63*, 1080–1088. [CrossRef] [PubMed]

28. Edge, S.C.; Markowitz, J.S.; Devane, C.L. Clozapine Drug-Drug Interactions: A Review of the Literature. *Hum. Psychopharmacol. Clin. Exp.* **1997**, *12*, 5–20. [CrossRef]

29. McNeilHealthcare(Ireland)Ltd.   Domperidone-Important   Safety   Information   from   McNeil Healthcare (Ireland) Ltd. as Approved by the Irish Medicines Board 2014.   Available online: http://www.hpra.ie/homepage/medicines/safety-notices/item?t=/domperidone---important-safety-information-from-mcneil-healthcare-(ireland)-ltd.-as-approved-by-the-irish-medicines-board&id= c3d0f925-9782-6eee-9b55-ff00008c97d0 (accessed on 7 August 2017).

30. Arif, N. Monitoring of Physical Health of Patients on Clozapine and Communication of Results with the Psychiatric Team. *Int. J. Pharm. Pract.* **2013**, *21*, 135–136.

31. Schembri, K.; Azzopardi, L.M. Clozapine Treatment in Patients Living in the Community. *J. EuroMed Pharm.* **2015**, *5*, 8–11.

32. Shirazi, A.; Stubbs, B.; Gomez, L.; Moore, S.; Gaughran, F.; Flanagan, R.J.; MacCabe, J.H.; Lally, J. Prevalence and Predictors of Clozapine-Associated Constipation: A Systematic Review and Meta-Analysis. *Int. J. Mol. Sci.* **2016**, *17*, 863. [CrossRef] [PubMed]

33. Bishara, D.; Taylor, D. Adverse Effects of Clozapine in Older Patients: Epidemiology, Prevention and Management. *Drugs Aging* **2014**, *31*, 11–20. [CrossRef] [PubMed]

34. NHS. Stepping forward to 2020/21: The Mental Health Workforce Plan for England 2017. Available online: https://www.rcpsych.ac.uk/pdf/FYFV%20Mental%20health%20workforce%20plan% 20for%20England%20FINAL.pdf (accessed on 2 August 2017).

35. Knowles, S.-A. Providing Clozapine in community pharmacy. *Aust. Pharm.* **2016**, *35*, 56–60.

36. Ni Dhubhlaing, C.; Young, A.; Sahm, L.J. Impact of Pharmacist Counselling on Clozapine Knowledge. *Schizophr. Res. Treat.* **2017**, *2017*. [CrossRef] [PubMed]

9

The Role of Pharmacists in Travel Medicine

Lee Baker

Amayeza Info Services, Johannesburg 1709, South Africa; lee@amayeza-info.co.za

Abstract: Worldwide, pharmacists, who are the most accessible health-care providers, are playing an ever increasing role in travel medicine, assisting travelers in taking the necessary precautions to ensure safe and healthy travel. This article looks at the situation in South Africa, and how pharmacists are performing these functions within the legal constraints of the Medicines and Related Substances Act 101 of 1965, which prevents pharmacists from prescribing many of the travel vaccines and medications. The scope of practice in community pharmacies increased since the successful down-scheduling of some of the antimalarials, allowing pharmacists to supply the many travelers who frequently travel to neighboring countries. As in many other countries, travel medicine in South Africa is currently thwart with products that are out of stock, and a number of temporary guidelines were put in place to deal with these. Ways to facilitate expanding the role of pharmacists in travel medicine in South Africa need to be further explored.

Keywords: pharmacists; travel medicine; malaria; malaria prophylaxis; South Africa; schedules

---

1. Pharmacist Prescribing in South Africa

There are 3370 community pharmacists in South Africa [1], and they potentially have a very important role to play in travel medicine in South Africa, especially with regards to malaria, as there are many malaria-stricken areas within a couple of hours' travel from people's homes, which are often visited on weekends. There is also a significant migrant population from neighboring countries that come to South Africa seeking work, and who go home in December (the height of malaria season). Pharmacists are the most accessible health-care professionals, and are, therefore, frequently consulted regarding malaria prophylaxis and other travel health matters. In spite of this, the formal role of pharmacists in travel medicine is in its infancy when compared to some countries such as Canada [2]. This is mainly due to legislature which prevents pharmacists from prescribing or dispensing (without a prescription) any medicine above schedule 2. Medicines in South Africa are scheduled from 0–8, which determines the rules relating to the sale thereof, with schedule 0 (S0) sold in supermarkets, and S3 and up on prescription only. Most travel vaccines are schedule 4 [3].

In addition to the scope of practice of a pharmacist, a pharmacist with the Primary Care Drug Therapy (PCDT) qualification and a Section 22A (15) permit issued by the Director General of Health is permitted to diagnose, treat, and supply medicines following the Primary Health Care Standard Treatment Guidelines and the list of approved medicines, as an authorized prescriber [4].

Section 22A(15) of the Medicines and Related Substances Act (Act 101 of 1965) states that the Director General issues Section 22A(15) permits after consultation with the South African Pharmacy Council (SAPC). Primary Care Drug Therapy (PCDT) permits are issued with a list of conditions and medications that the pharmacist in possession of the permit may prescribe and dispense. This list is in line with the Department of Health's latest Essential Medicines List. This section reads as follows: "Notwithstanding anything to the contrary contained in this section, the Director General may, after consultation with the Interim Pharmacy Council of South Africa as referred to in Section 2 of the

Pharmacy Act, 1974 (Act 53 of 1974), issue a permit to any person or organization performing a health service, authorizing such person or organization to acquire, possess, use, or supply any specified schedule 1, schedule 2, schedule 3, schedule 4, or schedule 5 substance, and such permit shall be subject to such conditions as the Director General may determine [3]." Any application for the scheduling of medicines for this purpose, or for access in terms of Section 22A(15) of the Act should, therefore, use the most recent set of Standard Treatment Guidelines/Essential Medicines List (STG/EML) for Primary Health Care (PHC) issued by the National Department of Health as a starting point, wherever appropriate. The PHC STG/EML is intended to guide the practice of medical practitioners and nurses at PHC facilities in the public sector. Pediatric vaccines against polio, tuberculosis, diphtheria, tetanus, pertussis, hepatitis B, *haemophilus influenzae* type b, measles, pneumococcal, and rotavirus infections are on the Primary Health Care Essential Medicines List, and pharmacists with this Section 22A(15) permit can administer them. The human papillomavirus (HPV) vaccine and the influenza vaccines are also on this list [5]. However, none of the travel vaccines are on this list, and the pharmacist cannot, therefore, prescribe and administer them.

2. Pharmacist Activity in Travel Medicine

Currently, 10 pharmacists are members of the South African Society of Travel Medicine (SASTM), and they have all completed the Travel Medicine Course offered once a year by the SASTM, and accredited by the Witwatersrand University. Pharmacists and nurses may only apply to do this course if they have a medical practitioner overseeing them who has either done the course or will do the course with them [6]. This is a very comprehensive course, which equips them with the knowledge they need to be able to offer travel health of the highest standard. This entitles them to apply for a yellow fever license, which allows them to administer these vaccines if they are prescribed by a doctor. Although they cannot prescribe and dispense the necessary vaccines and medicines, they usually work closely with doctors or travel clinics, and play an important role in counseling [3,6]. Most community pharmacists actively counsel travelers on a daily basis, particularly with respect to malaria prophylaxis. Topics that they give advice on, and where possible, products to minimize risks include, traveler's diarrhea, jetlag, motion sickness, altitude sickness, and prophylaxis of venous thromboembolism [7].

Very few pharmacists currently run their own travel clinics because of the constraints; however, many of the bigger pharmacy groups have started clinics that administer childhood vaccines, and they would be in a good position to open up travel clinics. A few community pharmacists completed the SASTM course and worked under the supervision of a doctor. They are in small rural towns, and they play a very important role.

Two pharmacists, who did the course, worked in a medicine information center, the only privately run one in South Africa. Only one is still employed by the center. Various services are offered, with two of them being a malaria information line and a vaccine information line. Both these services are utilized by health-care professionals, as well as by members of the public. The medicine information center is the Amayeza Info Centre www.amayeza-info.co.za.

Pharmacists have access to a number of resources to assist them with travel health. Those that are members of the SASTM have access to Travax www.travax.nhs.uk and anyone can access the Centers for Disease Control and Prevention (CDC) website for travel health https://wwwnc.cdc.gov/travel, and the World Health Organization (WHO) website for travel and health www.who.int/topics/travel/en/. South African information is available from the National Institute of Communicable Diseases www.nicd.ac.za and the South African National Travel Health Network www.santhnet.co.za.

The current president of the SASTM is a pharmacist, and, in her private capacity, she also sits on the South African Malaria Elimination Committee (SAMEC), which is a committee, made up of experts in the field of malaria, that advises the National Department of Health on malaria. This committee is involved in drawing up the Guidelines for the Treatment of Malaria in South Africa 2018 [8] and the South African Guidelines for the Prevention of Malaria 2017 [9], as well as being instrumental in getting intravenous (IV) artesunate registered in South Africa, and some of the chemoprophylaxis products down-scheduled.

3. Antimalarials through Pharmacies

For a medicine to be rescheduled in South Africa, the manufacturer is required to make a submission to the scheduling committee of the Medicines Control Council (MCC), which is now the South African Health Products Regulatory Authority (SAHPRA). In order to make antimalarials more accessible to the public, in the hopes that this would reduce the number of imported malaria cases in South Africa as the country moves toward malaria elimination, the SAMEC approached both the manufacturers and the scheduling committee with a motivation to down-schedule some of the antimalarials. After a number of years of trying to get them down-scheduled to enable a pharmacist to dispense them without a prescription, this was recently achieved. Two years ago, in March 2016, doxycycline [10], and in November 2017, atovaquone-proguanil [11] were cleared to be given out by pharmacists without a prescription. This has enormous benefit for the many travelers who only became aware of the need to obtain antimalarials close to the time of the planned trip, and who did not have sufficient time to arrange for a prescription. In order to ensure that pharmacists are adequately knowledgeable to recommend and dispense these antimalarials, a number of continuing professional development (CPD) talks were given, as well as articles being published in pharmacy and medical journals [12,13].

In the last two years, both South Africa and its neighboring countries have experienced a surge in malaria cases [14]. Namibia experienced four times more cases in 2017 compared to 2015, and incidence rates in Zambia, Mozambique, and Malawi were between 286 and 381 per 1000 people in 2016. Mozambique, which is a popular destination for South Africans, and is also one of the countries from where many of South Africa's migrant workers come, has between six and eight million cases a year. South Africa's cases increased from about 5000 cases in 2016 to more than 30,000 cases in 2017 [15]. It is hoped that improving accessibility to antimalarials will result in more travelers taking them, and in a reduction in the number of cases.

4. Future Developments

In terms of the Regulations relating to the registration of the Specialities of Pharmacists, Council recognizes Master's Programs for registration as specialists. There are two specialities currently registrable with Council, i.e., Radio-pharmacy and Clinical Pharmacokinetics [16]. The way forward would be to have travel medicine registered as a speciality. It will then be possible to design a course that will allow pharmacists to prescribe vaccines and medicines appropriate for travel (as the PCDT course only allows them to prescribe for primary care).

5. Current Challenges

Travel medicine in general, not specific to pharmacists, saw many challenges in the last year. Many of the travel vaccines and antimalarials were out of stock for months at a time; there is only one manufacturer of pediatric atovaquone-proguanil, and they were out of stock, as was the case with mefloquine, whereas doxycycline cannot be given to children under the age of eight, resulting in no antimalarials available for young children. Vaccine shortages are a worldwide problem; many parts of the world have a yellow-fever vaccine shortage, which South Africa fortunately does not. Both hepatitis A and B vaccines are in short supply, which led to the development of guidelines to deal with these [17,18].

Despite these challenges, travel medicine is alive and well in South Africa, and it is hoped that pharmacists will play an even bigger role in the near future. In a study published earlier this year, clinical outcomes and traveler satisfaction with a pharmacy-based travel clinic was evaluated in Alberta, Canada. Traveler satisfaction was reported as very high with infrequent health issues during travel, and the majority of those who did experience health problems felt that they were adequately prepared to cope with them [2]. These results support an earlier study done in Scotland [19]. Such evidence is important to promote continued expansion of pharmacists' scope in this area, and it is hoped that similar results will be seen in South Africa in the not-too-distant future.

Funding: This research received no external funding.

Acknowledgments: I would like to acknowledge Prof Larry Goodyer for assisting me with the format of this article.

References

1. Statistics of Registered Persons and Organisations. 2018. Available online: https://www.pharmcouncil.co.za/B_Statistics.asp (accessed on 22 May 2018).

2. Houle, S.K.D.; Bascom, C.S.; Rosenthal, M.M. Clinical outcomes and satisfaction with a pharmacist-managed travel clinic in Alberta, Canada. *Travel Med. Infect. Dis.* **2018**, *23*, 21–26. [CrossRef] [PubMed]

3. SAHPRA. Acts, Regulations and Government Notices. 101 Medicines and Related Substances Act 101. 1965. Available online: http://www.mccza.com/Publications (accessed on 22 May 2018).

4. SAHPRA. Scheduling of Substances for Prescribing by Authorised Prescribers. Available online: http://www.mccza.com/documents/fb489cf12.37_Scheduling_for_Prescribing_by_Authorised_Prescribers_Mar14_v1.pdf (accessed on 18 July 2018).

5. Standard Treatment Guidelines and Essential Medicines List for South Africa Primary Health Care Level 2014. Available online: http://www.health.gov.za/index.php/component/phocadownload/category/285-phc (accessed on 22 May 2018).

6. Travel Medicine Course. The South African Society of Travel Medicine. Available online: www.sastm.org.za (accessed on 15 June 2018).

7. Meyer, J.C.; Nkonde, K.; Schellack, N. Travel medicine: An overview. *S. Afr. Pharm. J.* **2017**, *84*, 19–28.

8. Guidelines for the Treatment of Malaria in South Africa. 2018. Available online: www.Santhnet.co.za (accessed on 14 June 2018).

9. South African Guidelines for the Prevention of Malaria. Available online: https://www.google.com/url?sa=t&rct=j&q=&esrc=s&source=web&cd=1&ved=0ahUKEwiLr83_lKrcAhVU_GEKHUp0AicQFggwMAA&url=http%3A%2F%2Fwww.nicd.ac.za%2Fwp-content%2Fuploads%2F2017%2F09%2FGuidelines-South-African-Guidelines-for-the-Prevention-of-Malaria-2017-final.pdf&usg=AOvVaw2JINqVj7gggDq4uz3FVVQv (accessed on 14 June 2018).

10. Government Gazette. 15 March 2016. Volume 609, No. 39815. Available online: www.gpwonline.co.za (accessed on 13 February 2018).

11. Gouws, J.C. Registrar of Medicines. Communication to Industry. Medicine Control Council. Department of Health. Available online: www.mccza.com/Publications/DownloadDoc/5587 (accessed on 13 July 2018).

12. Baker, L. Malaria prophylaxis—Can we conquer the 'mighty' parasite? *S. Afr. Pharm. J.* **2018**, *85*, 48–54.

13. Parker, S. Malaria drug: Rescheduling treatment adherence. *Med. Chron.* **2018**, *3*, 2–3.

14. Blumberg, L.; Frean, J. Malaria reduces globally but rebounds across southern Africa. *S. Afr. J. Infect. Dis.* **2017**, *32*, 3–4.

15. SADC Malaria Report 2017. Available online: https://www.google.com/url?sa=t&rct=j&q=&esrc=s&source=web&cd=1&ved=0ahUKEwiv_rXphqrcAhXVdt4KHeg9AsEQFggrMAA&url=http%3A%2F%2Fwww.health.gov.za%2Findex.php%2Fcomponent%2Fphocadownload%2Fcategory%2F422-malaria-2017%3Fdownload%3D2529%3Asadc-malaria-report-2017&usg=AOvVaw0Dwli79m7Ik4jj88aZkT7R (accessed on 18 July 2018).

16. Specialities in Pharmacy. Available online: https://www.pharmcouncil.co.za/B_Edu_AccOfCourses.asp (accessed on 22 May 2018).

17. Hepatitis A Vaccination in Adults—Temporary Recommendations. Published July 2017 PHE Publications Gateway Number: 2017175. Available online: https://www.gov.uk/government/publications/hepatitis-a-infection-prevention-and-control-guidance (accessed on 15 June 2018).

18. Hepatitis B Vaccination in Adults and Children: Temporary Recommendations from 21 August 2017. Published 21 August 2017 PHE Publications Gateway Number: 2017256. Available online: https://assets.publishing.service.gov.uk/government/uploads/system/uploads/attachment_data/file/639145/Hepatitis_B_vaccine_recommendations_during_supply_constraints.pdf (accessed on 15 June 2018).

19. Hind, C.; Bond, C.; Lee, A.J.; van Teijlingen, E. Travel medicine services from community pharmacy: Evaluation of a pilot service. *Pharm. J.* **2018**, *281*, 625–632.

10

Development and Implementation of a Global Health Elective with a Drug Discovery Game for Pharmacy Students

Jordan R. Covvey † ⓘ, Anthony J. Guarascio, Lauren A. O'Donnell ⓘ and Kevin J. Tidgewell *,† ⓘ

Duquesne University School of Pharmacy, 600 Forbes Ave, Pittsburgh, PA 15282, USA; covveyj@duq.edu (J.R.C.); guarascioa@duq.edu (A.J.G.); odonnel6@duq.edu (L.A.O.)
* Correspondence: tidgewellk@duq.edu
† These authors contributed equally to this work.

Abstract: Interest in global health education within the pharmacy curriculum has increased significantly in recent years. However, discussion of different models and methods to evaluate course structures are limited. The overall objective was to (1) describe the structure of our global health elective for pharmacy students, and (2) assess educational outcomes related to perceived/formal knowledge and attitudes associated with global health. Our elective was designed using a competency-centered approach to global health education, incorporating reflection, projects, service and game-learning. In addition to course assessments, a pre-post survey questionnaire assessing attitudes, knowledge perception, formalized knowledge and opinions was utilized. Overall, students demonstrated appropriate performance on course assessments, temporally improving throughout longitudinal projects. The survey demonstrated significant increases in knowledge perception as a result of the course; however, no change in formalized knowledge was evident through the survey assessment. Additionally, the incorporation of game-learning into the course was well received by students. Future iterations of the course will focus on utilization of different assessment methods to meet learning outcomes.

Keywords: pharmacy education; global health; active learning; curriculum; elective course

---

1. Introduction

1.1. Background

Global health is increasingly being featured within curricula in pharmacy education, primarily the result of growing interest and recognition of a wider role of pharmacists in the global environment [1,2]. Global health is widely defined as "an area for study, research, and practice that places a priority on improving health for all people worldwide ... [it] emphasizes transnational health issues, determinants, and solutions; involves many disciplines within and beyond the health sciences and promotes interdisciplinary collaboration; and is a synthesis of population based prevention with individual-level clinical care" [3]. This definition is wide-reaching, including both clinical activities as well as science, focused abroad as well as in local communities, and serves both macro- and micro-levels of public health. Accordingly, introductory course offerings for health sciences students in this area are charged to provide broad curricular exposure, focused on development first as a 'global citizen', and secondarily, to build desired skill sets that contribute in a variety of settings. In this manuscript, we detail our creation of a global health elective for pharmacy students and our initial assessment of outcomes toward serving these goals.

1.2. *Course Description*

In our school, *Perspectives in Global Health* was created as an elective course offering in the third professional year of the PharmD curriculum, with the goal of providing a global view of pharmacy and understanding of healthcare, science and the role of the pharmacist within the world. The course is team-taught by four School of Pharmacy faculty members in different disciplines, including health outcomes research, clinical specialty in infectious diseases, basic science of infectious diseases, and basic science of drug discovery. The course follows a weekly seminar format with discussion led by a faculty member, supplemented with pre-readings. Students are engaged by in-class activities to promote thinking about the topics and increase student engagement. Major topic areas covered in the course were global health status and statistics, infectious and neglected tropical diseases, global health organizational infrastructure, culture/ethics, drug discovery, international science collaborations and immigration/poverty. Learning outcomes for students by the end of the course were to: (1) demonstrate a comprehensive understanding of global health issues pertinent to pharmacy and pharmaceutical science in the past, present and future, and (2) develop an enhanced awareness and ability to work with patients, healthcare and science within a widened world view. Learning outcomes were designed to emphasize student growth and recognition regarding their personal and professional roles, as well as awareness and willingness to engage in future activities to affect global health outcomes. To meet course objectives (Appendix A) and specific learning outcomes, students are engaged in several individual and group projects across the semester, which are described in the following sections and related back to course learning objectives.

1.2.1. Neglected Tropical Diseases Eradication Plan

Students in teams are assigned an emerging and/or neglected disease and asked to submit a written proposal on the disease and how they could potentially eradicate it (learning objectives 1, 3, 4). In the class session prior to the assignment, examples of completed pathogen eradication programs (e.g., smallpox) and current pathogen eradication programs (e.g., poliovirus, Guinea worms) are discussed with emphasis on factors that made each disease amenable to eradication. Students must utilize basic science and clinical knowledge to present the causative organism, disease progression, points of intervention, risk factors, and barriers to treatment that might exist. Students are asked to develop a detailed, step-wise approach for an eradication plan, and to describe whether or not they believe eradication is feasible given current global resources available.

1.2.2. Culture/Ethics Case Study Development

Students are individually provided two of eight patient-oriented case studies regarding ethical/cultural topics in global health (learning objectives 2 and 6). Students are asked to submit a written response that details the cultural/ethical issues at hand in the described scenarios, different approaches to approaching the scenarios, and final recommendations on how they would address the issue at hand.

1.2.3. Country Health System Project

Students are asked to individually choose a country from a determined list and develop a short presentation detailing the country and a specific international health issue related to that country (learning objectives 1, 3, 5). Potential countries included Cuba, Ghana, Tanzania, India, Guyana, China, Brazil, Syria and Iran. The presentation was required to tie together the multiple topic areas covered by the course, including epidemiology of the health issue, healthcare structure of the country, culture/ethical issues to consider, potential drug utilization/development and role of organizational support for the issue. The project includes both an interim submission for faculty feedback, as well as final presentation to the class at the end of the semester.

1.2.4. Volunteer Impact for a Local Global Health Organization

All students in the course are required to attend at least one volunteer session with a local organization, Global Links, a "medical relief and development organization dedicated to supporting health improvement initiatives in resource-poor communities and promoting environmental stewardship in the US healthcare system" [4] (learning objective 3). The volunteer session involves an introduction to the organization and the services they provide, and then an activity chosen by Global Links to meet whatever current needs they have, often including sorting and categorization of medical supply donations. This activity was developed to get students engaged with an opportunity in global health at the local level and to further understanding that actions in the local community can work to aid people around the world. This activity underpins longitudinal reinforcement of the idea throughout the course that global health does not necessarily require travel abroad, but rather, focuses on serving inequities in health across the globe.

1.2.5. Patient Education Project for a Global Partner

Students additionally complete a group project partnered with another local organization focused on global health, namely the Espwa Foundation [5] (learning objectives 1, 3, 5, 6). This organization works in concert with other local partners in and around Cap-Haitien, Haiti with a goal to "identify needs and develop projects that empower and inspire hope". Two of the faculty traveled with the organization to Haiti in 2016 to help identify potential ways to make a lasting impact on the community through medical relief and related activities. A Haitian physician partnering with the Espwa Foundation was opening a hospital for the underserved area and was in the process of arranging required resources for the facility. From this, a project was created in our course for students help create patient education materials on relevant medical topics that could be used in the new hospital setting for outreach. The assignment occurs longitudinally across the course as a multi-stage assignment to assist student progress. At the beginning of the semester, students choose small groups and are offered topic areas for their project focus; examples of topics in the past have included hygiene, maternal health, cholera, malaria, Zika, mental health, nutrition/malnutrition, and chronic disease. A collaborator with the Espwa Foundation provides a guest lecture discussing the organization and their work. Students are subsequently asked to research Haitian culture, healthcare system and available resources for their project for their first assignment. Next, they create a plan for information delivery and what they plan to communicate to patients on their topic. This is followed by a brief in-class presentation of their idea for feedback from the class and course instructors. The project concludes with creation and submission of their education project materials.

1.2.6. Game of International Drug Discovery

Following a didactic session on drug discovery chemistry relevant to the global community, students are given two readings about international partnerships in drug discovery (learning objectives 7 and 8). To demonstrate how drug discovery is influenced by science, investment, biodiversity and country-specific priorities and development goals, students spend a class period playing the Game of International Drug Discovery, an investigator-designed learning activity. A full description of the game and rules is found in Appendix B. In short, students are placed into teams that represent fictitious countries with differing amounts of money, science capability and biodiversity at the start. Countries are asked to achieve a set of confidential goals through taking turns to invest in science, license drugs or explore biodiversity. Turns proceed through drawing of "drug" and "nature" cards which change the dynamics of each turn through situations such as outbreaks, natural disasters and scientific grants. Additionally, countries may interact through making agreements with each other. After the game, a short debriefing occurs in which the class discusses country-driven motivations and how the students felt about the game. Students finalize the activity by writing a short reflection on their self-assessed learning outcomes from the game and how their country's resources and goals affected how they played the game.

1.3. Study Objective

The overall objective of this study was to (1) describe the structure of a global health elective for pharmacy students, and (2) assess educational outcomes related to knowledge and attitudes associated with global health. Outcomes were evaluated through course assessments as well as a survey questionnaire regarding knowledge (perceived and formal) and attitudes regarding the course activities and topic areas.

2. Methods

2.1. Course Assessments

The tropical disease eradication plan and culture/ethics case studies were issued as individual written assignments with a single grade for each. The country health system project was split into two major components: interim submission of the presentation draft (30%) and final presentation in class, as scored by faculty (50%) and student peers (20%). The patient education project included four stages: initial country assessment (20%), plan for project (20%), presentation of idea in class (30%) and final submission of the project (30%). The Game of International Drug Discovery was followed by a reflection post-game.

2.2. Survey Questionnaire

In the second year offering of the course, an investigator-designed questionnaire was delivered as a pre-/post-survey at the beginning and end of the semester. Survey items were compiled based on a literature review performed by the investigators; with no validated tool available that met the needs of the study, the investigators worked through multiple iterations of discussion to achieve the final instrument delivered to students. The pre-survey questionnaire assessed respondent characteristics and experience relevant to global health, items on knowledge perception (8 items) and attitudes (7 items) regarding global health and formal knowledge assessment questions (16 items) in domains of global burden of disease, infectious disease, culture/ethics, drug discovery and organizational roles. Knowledge perception and attitudes were assessed using five-level Likert-type items (1 = strongly disagree, 2 = disagree, 3 = neutral, 4 = agree, 5 = strongly agree). A series of open-ended questions was also included to assess student goals for the course. For the post-survey, items on knowledge perception, attitudes and formal knowledge assessment were repeated. Additional questions on course and game outcomes (4 items each) were included for student reflection. The survey was optional to the course with no bearing on formal grade assessments. The survey questionnaire was approved by the Duquesne University institutional review board.

The survey was delivered via Qualtrics (Provo, UT, USA) and analysis was performed using SPSS Statistics 24 (IBM Corp.; Armonk, NY, USA). Descriptive analyses were conducted for each item, and internal consistency reliability for knowledge perception and attitude domains were conducted using Cronbach's alpha. Formal knowledge questions were scored as percentage correct. Paired t-tests were utilized to compare changes in pre-/post-data for knowledge perception, attitudes and formal knowledge. Statistical tests were clarified with Cohen's d effect sizes where appropriate. Qualitative data from open-ended opinion items were assessed using a content analysis strategy. Two investigators independently identified open coding categories for themes associated with each item after immersion in the data; frequency patterns for said coding were summarized quantitatively.

3. Results and Discussion

3.1. Results—Course Assessments

Across major course assessments (Table 1), overall performance was strong for the 11 students participating in the elective. For project-based assignments which included formative assessments temporally issued across the project, performance improved over time, likely based on peer and faculty feedback provided at each stage of the assessment.

Table 1. Performance on course assessments.

Course Assessment	Type	Score, Mean (SD)
Tropical disease eradication plan	Team	93.4 (1.3)
Culture/ethics case studies	Individual	89.6 (6.6)
Country health system project Interim Final	Individual	89.7 (9.2) 92.2 (4.1)
Patient education project Country assessment Plan for project Presentation Final	Team	86.4 (10.7) 90.5 (5.0) 95.5 (14.4) 96.1 (4.5)

For reflections regarding the Game of International Drug Discovery, common themes (found in more than 70% of reflections) regarding learning outcomes noted by students included; need to consider a country's motivations to accomplish goals ($n = 8$, 100%), differences between developing and developed countries ($n = 7$, 87.5%), and the ability to relate to the material better ($n = 8$, 100%). Students realized quickly that despite everyone playing the game together, there were clear differences in what goals they were seeking to accomplish. Topics mentioned in greater than half of the reflections were a better understanding of the collaborative nature of research ($n = 8$, 62.5%) and that working together made achieving goals easier ($n = 8$, 62.5%). Students also mentioned the responsibility of researchers to maintain ethics and help train developing countries ($n = 8$, 62.5%), which was something briefly mentioned in the didactic portion when discussing National Cooperative Drug Discovery Grants (NCDDGs) and International Conservation and Biodiversity Grants (ICBG), demonstrating that they were able to connect the didactic to the active learning portions of this material. Some students found the activity challenging since the topic is not something they have been exposed to regularly; however, they noted gaining first-hand knowledge and skills regarding the negotiations and various motivations encountered throughout the game.

3.2. Results—Survey Questionnaire

Out of the total of 11 students enrolled in the elective, 10 provided complete data on the pre-survey and post-survey. The cohort included seven males (63.6%), with all students having had previous community pharmacy experience, and six (54.5%) with additional experience in the hospital setting. A total of two students (18.2%) reported either previously living or studying abroad, while five (45.5%) had previously traveled abroad for vacation purposes.

Perception of knowledge regarding areas of global health was relatively low among student at the beginning of the course (Table 2), with perceived knowledge of global health systems and neglected tropical diseases rated lowest. Effect sizes for changes for all knowledge perception items were high (Cohen's d > 0.8). However, perception of knowledge for each item significantly improved at the end of the course. Among attitudes, students held very positive attitudes regarding global health both at the beginning and end of the course, rendering non-significant changes on these items.

For the formal knowledge assessment (16 items), the mean score on the pre-test was 54.2% (range: 23–69%). Highest rated items were formal knowledge of tropic disease eradication (100%), health as a human right (90.9%) and opinion status of the US healthcare system abroad (90.9%). However, scores on the post-test were similar, at 55.6% (range: 31–63%) ($p = 0.575$ for the comparison). Scores on highest rated items generally persisted for tropic disease eradication (80%), health as a human right (100%) and opinion status of the US healthcare system abroad (90%).

Table 2. Pre-post comparison of knowledge perception and attitudes regarding global health.

Statement	Pre-Score, Mean (SD) *	Post-Score, Mean (SD) *	Mean Diff	*p*-Value
Knowledge perception [†]				
I feel knowledgeable regarding the general topic and goals of global health	2.8 (0.92)	4.8 (0.42)	2.00	<0.001
I feel knowledgeable about other countries' healthcare systems	1.3 (0.48)	4.3 (0.68)	3.00	<0.001
I feel knowledgeable about neglected topical diseases	1.9 (1.1)	4.7 (0.48)	2.80	<0.001
I feel knowledgeable regarding current issues in global infectious disease	2.4 (0.70)	4.7 (0.48)	2.30	<0.001
I feel knowledgeable regarding cultural influences on health	2.9 (1.1)	4.7 (0.48)	1.80	0.001
I feel knowledgeable regarding drug discovery on the global scale	2.1 (1.1)	4.4 (0.52)	2.30	<0.001
I feel knowledgeable regarding how organizations provide volunteer clinical care abroad	2.8 (1.1)	4.5 (0.53)	1.70	0.003
I feel knowledgeable about roles/opportunities for pharmacists in global health	3.3 (0.82)	4.6 (0.52)	1.30	0.004
Attitudes [‡]				
I believe that global health should be considered an important issue to all pharmacists	4.7 (0.5)	4.7 (0.5)	0	0.999
I believe that 'thinking globally' improves the quality of care I can deliver	4.6 (0.73)	4.7 (0.5)	0.11	0.681
I believe that an experience abroad improves a pharmacist's perspective of patient care	4.7 (0.5)	4.7 (0.5)	0	0.999
I believe that I can be involved in global health initiatives without traveling abroad	3.9 (1.17)	4.4 (1.01)	0.56	0.139
I believe that health issues primarily affecting people outside of the USA are still relevant	4.6 (0.73)	4.8 (0.44)	0.22	0.347
I believe that learning about a patient's culture, religion and beliefs is important to delivering care	4.8 (0.44)	5.0 (0.0)	0.22	0.169
I believe that there is much for the USA to learn about health from around the globe	4.8 (0.44)	4.8 (0.44)	0	0.999

* 1 = strongly disagree, 2 = disagree, 3 = neutral, 4 = agree, 5 = strongly agree; [†] Cronbach's alpha = 0.537 (pre), 0.799 (post); [‡] Cronbach's alpha = 0.900 (pre), 0.747 (post).

In contrast, post-survey quantitative opinion items were uniformly and similarly rated high (Table 3) for both course outcomes as well as game outcomes. Analysis of the qualitative opinion data regarding what students hoped to gain from the course (in the pre-survey) revealed a desire for increased knowledge/understanding about health globally ($n = 5$, 45.5%) as well as interest in how their role as a pharmacist would relate to global health ($n = 4$, 36.4%). On the post-survey, when asked about what they gained from the course, all students made reference to knowledge gains, most commonly on acquiring perspective ($n = 6$, 54.5%) regarding the diversity of health, healthcare and needs globally.

Table 3. Post-survey opinions regarding the course and The Game of International Drug Discovery.

Statement	Score, Mean (SD) *
About the course [†]	
This course helped me to discover new areas of health I have not previously considered	4.6 (0.52)
This course helped me to develop a widened world view of health	4.7 (0.48)
This course helped me to understand the role of a pharmacist in global health	4.7 (0.48)
This course helped me to better focus my counseling to the needs of each unique patient	4.8 (0.42)
About the Game of International Drug Discovery [‡]	
The game helped me to understand the drug discovery process better	4.6 (0.70)
The game helped me to understand international collaborations in drug discovery	4.7 (0.68)
The game helped me to understand the importance of biodiversity	4.7 (0.68)
The game helped me to understand the differing motivations of nations with respect to drug discovery	4.7 (0.68)
The game helped me to understand the drug discovery process better	4.6 (0.70)

* 1 = strongly disagree, 2 = disagree, 3 = neutral, 4 = agree, 5 = strongly agree; [†] Cronbach's alpha = 0.937; [‡] Cronbach's alpha = 0.986.

3.3. Discussion

In this initial and preliminary assessment of our global health elective course, significant gains were evident regarding the perception of knowledge students had regarding course topics, complemented by previously established positive attitudes. Success on course instructional activities was demonstrated, but formal knowledge gains as assessed by the pre-post survey did not demonstrate significant improvements.

3.3.1. Global Health Competencies

Global health education across the health disciplines has sustained rapid expansion in recent years, albeit not without growing pains. A literature review of 238 articles in global health education by Liu et al. identified lacking curricular standardization and inclusion of professionals outside of medicine as areas for improvement [6]. Recently, the Consortium of Universities of Global Health (CUGH) has provided some guidance on these issues. This group combines expertise from several professions, including medicine, nursing, pharmacy, dentistry, public health, physical/occupational therapy and psychology. In 2015, CUGH released a list of inter-professional competencies for global health, including eight domains included at the 'global citizen' competency level, defined as "competency sets required of all post-secondary students pursuing any field with bearing on global health" [7]. These domains included global burden of disease; globalization of health and health care; social and environmental determinants of health; collaboration, partnering, and communication; ethics; professional practice; health equity and social justice; and socio-cultural and political awareness [7].

Development of our elective course and choice of topics was guided by these defined competency domains. However, other areas were added as they were felt to be specifically relevant for coverage in our curriculum structure. Notably, the competency list is highly clinically focused, and our faculty felt strongly that inclusion of basic science relevant to global health would be a useful addition. Additionally, we chose to include higher domain levels within the CUGH framework, such as capacity strengthening and strategic analysis, which were integrated into our patient education project.

3.3.2. Knowledge and Attitudes

Limited published data is available on other global health course structures and their subsequent assessments within pharmacy curricula for comparison, particularly without inclusion of global field experiences. One relevant example is available from Addo-Atuah et al., who described implementation of a global health elective which utilized team-based learning, projects and online learning [8]. Pre-post surveys from the course demonstrated non-significant improvements in knowledge and attitudes about global health as well as significant improvements in perception of skills development for areas such as grant writing, project planning and management of pharmaceutical services [8]. No major formal assessments of knowledge were conducted, although team-based learning did demonstrate improvement on assessments utilized in the course. Poirer et al. described an interprofessional, online global health course with inclusion of team-based work organized across eight topic-oriented modules [9]. Significant changes were noted across most student-assessed knowledge perceptions before and after the course. No data regarding formal knowledge assessments were reported [9].

Outcomes in the current study broadly mirror those found in these previous analyses, although we additionally attempted to assess formalized knowledge changes. Prior to the course, student perceptions of knowledge and demonstration of formalized knowledge were similarly assessed as low. However, after the course as knowledge perceptions were significantly higher, demonstration of formalized knowledge failed to follow, despite gains in this area being an intended learning outcome for the course. Several aspects may have affected achievement of this outcome. First, students may have over-rated themselves on post-assessments in an effort to justify their course progress and learning [10]. Additionally, the approach used by faculty to deliver content may have focused too heavily on exploration of ideas and concepts, which may focus more heavily on attitudinal gains. Failure to demonstrate formal knowledge may also have been the result of the assessment tool itself, including its ability to comprehensively represent the multifaceted content and scope of the course, but additionally may have resulted from the type of formative assessments utilized throughout the course. Unlike curriculum in the required coursework of our PharmD program, which commonly utilizes quizzes and examinations, we chose to approach assessment in this elective course through essays, projects and presentations. Therefore, expectation of improved formal knowledge demonstrated through the post-survey (which utilized a quiz/examination format) may have not been supported through the assessment design used in the course. Additionally, most global health education, particularly in pharmacy education [11,12], is focused in the experiential realm through short-term elective or medical missions abroad. These types of experiences may allow for enhanced reinforcement and application of global health that we were unable to realize within the confines of our didactic elective.

For attitudes, our study failed to demonstrate any differences between pre- and post-assessments. This was primarily the result of high ratings across all items in the pre-survey, and therefore limited opportunity for improvement. We hypothesize the main influence on this result is the elective nature of the course, which self-selected individuals with interest and enthusiasm for this area of study. If instead the course had been a part of the required didactic curriculum, assessments of attitudes might have demonstrated more meaningful results.

3.3.3. Game Learning

A literature review regarding the use of games in pharmacy education and their overall impact on students by Aburahma and Mohamed discussed the benefits and challenges of using games in the classroom, with most game use in pharmacy curricula involving the use of trivia-type games for review of didactic material [13]. Pharmacy education involves a large use of simulation in the clinical aspects of pharmacy for pharmacist patient interaction and evaluation of student pharmacists "soft skills" and practice readiness [14]. The use of simulations can be considered "serious gaming" but has historically been relegated to the clinical aspects of pharmacy education, yet has been shown to increase student motivation and when used properly increase student retention and understanding [15].

For this course, the corresponding author designed the Game of International Drug Discovery to utilize simulation/role-play to enhance student understanding of the complex relationships and motivations involved in international drug discovery collaborations. This topic is a good fit for game learning, due to its complexity and involvement of relationships and interactions which can be simulated in a condensed format in the classroom. One of the most significant advantages of using games is the increased engagement and excitement generated by being actively involved [13]. The topic of international collaboration would be difficult to generate interest and excitement without role-playing as the students would have no frame of reference or stake in the concepts. By allowing the students to represent countries with different resources and goals, they can rise to the understanding of differential motivations and aspirations on their own, as was shown as a common theme through their post-game reflections. When used in the proper context and developed purposefully, serious games can enhance the learning and comprehension of complex topics for students.

3.3.4. Study Limitations

Several limitations are worth mentioning for the current analysis. First of all, a very small sample size was utilized, which renders the data limited in scope and not generalizable across all curricula. We additionally used an investigator-designed survey questionnaire which was non-validated. This was primarily due to limited available literature and instruments measuring the constructs we desired to assess. Due to this, we measured the internal consistency reliability for our attitude and knowledge perception items and found an adequate coefficient of consistency. Finally, we previously mentioned the potential limitation resulting from utilization of a qualitative formal knowledge assessment (multiple choice items), which was different than the assessment methods utilized during the course (essays and projects).

3.3.5. Plans for Future Course Improvements

Based on these initial assessments of the course and alongside other faculty motivations, several changes are anticipated for future offerings. At current time, the patient education project has initiated collaboration with partners in Haiti through support of educational initiatives. Faculty are actively planning to incorporate a 'spring break-away' component to the course that will allow opportunity for students to travel to Cap-Haitien for a week for implementation of their projects and to provide longitudinal support for pharmacy services in the area. A key focus of this development has been long-term investment and building a sustainable partnership. Alongside this, at our university, a movement for creation of a global health minor/concentration is gaining traction, which will significantly increase opportunity for students not only to participate in global health education within the field of pharmacy, but also through inter-professional activities.

4. Conclusions

Our initial offering of our global health elective for pharmacy students was designed to expose students to a new area of practice through inclusion of projects, multidisciplinary topics, team-based work and community involvement. Students entered the course with positive attitudes, and knowledge perceptions regarding global health increased significantly as a result of the course. However, increased focus is needed for measuring and sustaining formal knowledge gains. Notably, our use of a novel game method was effective for engagement within the area of international drug discovery.

Acknowledgments: The authors thank the students who participated in the inaugural years of this elective course, as well as the collaborative support we have received from both Global Links and the Espwa Foundation.

Author Contributions: K.T. created the Game of International Drug Discovery and J.R.C. designed the survey tool used in the course. All authors (K.T., J.R.C., L.A.O. and A.J.G.) had input into refinement of the survey tool as well as the course content and delivery. All authors helped to write the manuscript.

Appendix A. Course Learning Objectives

Appendix A.1. Learning Objectives

1.   Build upon public health principles to identify and discuss global burden of disease
2.   Discuss the implications of immigration and movement around the globe upon healthcare infrastructure and delivery
3.   Identify and describe current priorities in health affecting the world and how these are applicable to practice in the USA
4.   Describe past and present epidemics and strategies created to protect against the future
5.   Compare/contrast infrastructures of various healthcare systems and discuss the pros/cons associated with each
6.   Discuss the place of ethics and cultural competency in global health and its importance to daily pharmacy practice
7.   Identify regulations and respect for autonomy and ownership of biodiversity of different countries and people
8.   Describe drug discovery for neglected diseases with a focus on compounds found and aspects of key chemistry

Appendix B. Game of International Drug Discovery

Appendix B.1. Game Rules and Description

In this game, players will be split into six teams representing six countries that have different levels of resources and motivations for how to win the game. As a country, a team's goal is to complete the tasks assigned to you. Every country could accomplish their goals (everyone wins) or no country could accomplish their goals (everyone loses).

There are three main characteristics that each country needs to worry about: (1) money; (2) biodiversity; and (3) science. Money can be used to buy drugs that have already been discovered, explore biodiversity for new drugs, or to invest in science points. Science points determine the number of actions that you may take on your turn. Biodiversity is a natural resource that countries may choose to protect, while others may want to exploit for gains in money and science.

Throughout the game, each country will know what the other country's resources are but will not know what other country's goals to win the game are. Each country will have different goals and objectives they must meet to "win". For example: a country could be told to earn over a specific amount of money and discover at least two cancer drugs OR a country could be told to earn over a specific amount of money but must maintain a certain level of biodiversity.

On each turn, there are three actions a player may take:

- Invest in science—purchase additional science points (up to five) for use on future turns

  o   Prices: 2nd point—$25; 3rd point—$75; 4th point—$150; 5th point—$300

- License a drug—negotiate with another country to trade money or biodiversity points for one drug card
- Explore biodiversity—explore your own or another country's biodiversity

  o   Exploring your own biodiversity is free, and you will keep all profits, drugs and biodiversity points from any discovery

  o   Exploring another country's biodiversity requires you to pay them $10 and agree to how to split royalties from any discoveries, with agreements remaining in place until the end of the turn.

Agreements regarding biodiversity must include how to divide money earned, drugs discovered and biodiversity recovered. The countries may each make one counter-offer in setting up the agreement. If an agreement is not reached, then the science point is used and the turn is over. If an agreement has been made, the country exploring will roll a die.

- Rolls of 1, 3 or 5 lead to drawing of a "drug" card
- Rolls of 2, 4 or 6 lead to drawing of a "nature" card

Available drug cards include:

- No activity found—restore biodiversity (9 cards)
- Drug recall——1 drug discovered (3 cards)
- Discover an antibiotic—$50 and +1 biodiversity pt (6 cards)
- Discover an anticancer drug—+$100 (8 cards)
- Discover a neglected tropical disease (NTD) drug—+$20 and +2 biodiversity pt (6 cards)

Available nature cards include:

- National park—+1 biodiversity pt (3 cards)
- Natural disaster——1 biodiversity pt (3 cards)
- Scientific breakthrough—+1 science pt (3 cards)
- Scientific grant—×2 benefits when working with this country for next two turns (6 cards)
- Vaccine—protection from diseases outbreak (single use) (6 cards)
- Cancer epidemic—if no anticancer drug, −1 science pt (4 cards)
- Bacterial outbreak—if no antibiotic, −25% of money (4 cards)
- NTD outbreak—If no NTD drug, −1 biodiversity pt (4 cards)

The game will play for six rounds or until time has expired. A running total of resources will be kept on the board (half points for biodiversity and money are allowed, but not for science). Upon completion of the game, each team will reveal their goals and if they accomplished them.

Country Profiles

Country	Country Type	Money	Science Points	Biodiversity Points
1	Developed	$200	3	1
2	Developed	$100	3	3
3	Developing	$100	2	3
4	Developing	$50	2	5
5	Underdeveloped	$20	1	8
6	Underdeveloped	$10	1	9

Country Goals

1. End the game with >$500 and discover 5 drugs
2. End the game with >$300, 4+ biodiversity points and discover 1 of each type of drug
3. End the game with 4+ biodiversity points, 4+ science points and discover 2 antibiotics
4. End the game with >$400, 3+ science points and 6+ biodiversity points
5. End the game with 4+ science points and discover 1 NTD drug
6. End the game with >$100, 8+ biodiversity points and 3+ science points

References

1. Gleason, S.E.; Covvey, J.R.; Abrons, J.P.; Dang, Y.; Seo, S.W.; Tofade, T.; Prescott, G.M.; Peron, E.P.; Masilamani, S.; Alsharif, N.Z. Connecting Global/International Pharmacy Education to the CAPE 2013 Outcomes: A Report from the Global Pharmacy Education Special Interest Group. Available online: http://www.aacp.org/resources/education/cape/Documents/GPE_CAPE_Paper_November_2015.pdf (accessed on 13 July 2017).

2. Bailey, L.C.; DiPietro Mager, N.A. Global health education in Doctor of Pharmacy programs. *Am. J. Pharm. Educ.* **2016**, *80*, 71. [CrossRef]

3. Koplan, J.P.; Bond, T.C.; Merson, M.H.; Reddy, K.S.; Rodriguez, M.H.; Sewankambo, N.K.; Wasserheit, J.N. Towards a common definition of global health. *Lancet* **2009**, *373*, 1993–1995. [CrossRef]

4. Global Links. Available online: https://www.globallinks.org/ (accessed on 7 July 2017).

5. Espwa Foundation. Available online: http://espwa.com/ (accessed on 7 July 2017).

6. Liu, Y.; Zhang, Y.; Liu, Z.; Wang, J. Gaps in studies of global health education: An empirical literature review. *Glob. Health Action* **2015**, *8*, 25709. [CrossRef] [PubMed]

7. Jogerst, K.; Callender, B.; Adams, V.; Evert, J.; Fields, E.; Hall, T.; Olsen, J.; Rowthorn, V.; Rudy, S.; Shen, J.; et al. Identifying interprofessional global health competencies for 21st-century health professionals. *Ann. Glob. Health* **2015**, *81*, 239–247. [CrossRef] [PubMed]

8. Addo-Atuah, J.; Dutta, A.; Kovera, C. A global health elective course in a PharmD curriculum. *Am. J. Pharm. Educ.* **2014**, *78*, 187. [CrossRef] [PubMed]

9. Poirier, T.I.; Devraj, R.; Blankson, F.; Xin, H. Interprofessional online global health course. *Am. J. Pharm. Educ.* **2016**, *80*, 155. [PubMed]

10. Kruger, J.; Dunning, D. Unskilled and unaware of it: How difficulties in recognizing one's own incompetence lead to inflated self-assessments. *J. Personal. Soc. Psychol.* **1999**, *7*, 1121–1134. [CrossRef]

11. Prescott, G.M.; Vu, B.N.; Alsharif, N.Z.; Prescott, W.A. Global health education in Doctor of Pharmacy programs in the United States. *Am. J. Pharm. Educ.* **2017**, *81*, 28. [PubMed]

12. Steeb, D.R.; Overman, R.A.; Sleath, B.L.; Joyner, P.U. Global experiential and didactic education opportunities at US colleges and schools of pharmacy. *Am. J. Pharm. Educ.* **2016**, *80*, 7. [CrossRef]

13. Aburahma, M.H.; Mohamed, H.M. Educational games as a teaching tool in pharmacy curriculum. *Am. J. Pharm. Educ.* **2015**, *79*, 59. [CrossRef] [PubMed]

14. Crea, K.A. Practice skill development through the use of human patient simulation. *Am. J. Pharm. Educ.* **2011**, *75*, 188. [CrossRef] [PubMed]

15. Cain, J.; Piascik, P. Are serious games a good strategy for pharmacy education? *Am. J. Pharm. Educ.* **2015**, *79*, 47. [CrossRef] [PubMed]

11

Assessment of Knowledge of Diabetes Mellitus in the Urban Areas

Sasikala Chinnappan [1], Palanisamy Sivanandy [2,*], Rajenthina Sagaran [3] and Nagashekhara Molugulu [4]

[1] Department of Life Sciences, International Medical University, Kuala Lumpur 57000, Malaysia; SasikalaChinnappan@imu.edu.my
[2] Department of Pharmacy Practice, International Medical University, Kuala Lumpur 57000, Malaysia
[3] School of Pharmacy, La Trobe University, Bendigo 3552, Australia; thina_1515@hotmail.com
[4] Department of Pharmaceutical Technology, International Medical University, Kuala Lumpur 57000, Malaysia; NagashekharaMolugulu@imu.edu.my
* Correspondence: PalanisamySivanandy@imu.edu.my

Academic Editor: Jeffrey Atkinson

Abstract: Diabetes is the most common cause of non-traumatic lower limb amputations and cardiovascular diseases. However, only a negligible percentage of the patients and subjects knew that the feet are affected in diabetes and diabetes affects the heart. Hence, a cross-sectional study was carried out to evaluate the knowledge of diabetes mellitus among the public of different age group, gender, ethnicity, and education level. A sample of 400 participants was randomly selected and data was collected using a structured questionnaire under non-contrived setting. The results showed that there is a statistically significant difference in knowledge on diabetes mellitus among different age groups and different ethnic origin but there is no significant difference in the knowledge among different gender and education level. Out of 400 respondents, 284 respondents (71%) knew that diabetes mellitus is actually a condition characterized by raised blood sugar. Age and education level of respondents were found to be the predominant predictive factors on diabetes knowledge, whereas the gender of respondents did not affect the findings of this study. An improved and well-structured educational programme that tackles the areas of weaknesses should be recommended to increase the level of knowledge on diabetes among Malaysians.

Keywords: diabetes mellitus; knowledge; cardiovascular disease; amputations

1. Introduction

Diabetes mellitus is a group of metabolic diseases whose common feature is an increase in the blood glucose level [1]. It is one of the most common diseases, causing significant mortality and morbidity worldwide. The development of complications in diabetes is not related to hyperglycaemia alone. Studies suggest that the genesis of complications is related not only to glycaemic control but also to blood pressure and lipid control [2].

It is a disease with serious complications that has now reached epidemic proportions and the prevalence rates are expected to go even higher in the future [3]. If the current trend continues, more than 170 million people worldwide will have this disease and this burden is projected to more than double by the year 2030. In Malaysia, diabetes mellitus is a very big growing concern. Significant changes in the lifestyles of Malaysians have contributed to the increased incidence of diabetes. Malaysia, a multiethnic nation consisting of three major races, Malays, Chinese and Indians with a population of about 30 million includes 0.86 million in the Klang district, which has a high epidemic of diabetes mellitus. The World Health Organization (WHO) has estimated that in 2030, Malaysia would have a total number of 2.48 million diabetics compared to 0.94 million in 2000 which is a 164% increase [3,4]. This rising trend is mainly due to some factors such as growing population, aging, urbanization and increasing prevalence of obesity and physical inactivity among Malaysians [5].

Diabetes Mellitus is also associated with long-term consequences that include severe complications. Knowledge is essential for adequate diabetes management and self-management education is the cornerstone of treatment for all people with diabetes. Patients need the knowledge and skills to make informed choices and to facilitate self-directed changes in behaviour and ultimately to reduce the risk of the associated complications [6]. Behaviour and lifestyle changes are the keys to successful self-management of diabetes [7]. Several studies report that the knowledge of diabetes is poor in developing and under-developed countries [8–10], and the knowledge should be improved through continuous education by health care professionals like pharmacists, nurses and physicians. Knowledge of diseases are of utmost importance to meet the challenge of increasing healthcare costs. Language is one of the main barriers in Malaysia as the majority of the population are Malay and are mostly educated in Malay language. Even though the literacy rate is higher in Malaysia compared to neighbouring countries in this region, language seems to be a barrier for getting adequate knowledge on any disease [11,12].

Having considered the above factors, it is evident that there is a need to study the knowledge of diabetes mellitus among Malaysians. Hence, in this study an attempt was made to evaluate the knowledge of diabetes mellitus among the public of different age groups, gender, ethnicity, and education level. A pretested and predesigned questionnaire was used to analyse the knowledge of diabetes and the questionnaire was revalidated by the faculties and experts in our institution.

2. Materials and Methods

A cross-sectional community-based study was conducted for a period of 4 months. Taman Sri Andalas, Taman Klang Jaya, Bandar Bukit Tinggi and Bandar Botanic of Klang district, Selangor were the study areas for this study. Regardless of ethnicity, a total of 400 participants aged 12 and above were randomly selected by using convenient sampling technique and were asked to participate in this study. Subjects of both genders with no hearing or visual impairment were included. Individuals with significant cognitive impairment and/or psychiatric comorbidity were excluded from the study.

A structured validated questionnaire prepared in American English language was employed to analyse the knowledge on diabetes [13]. The questionnaire consists of socio demographic characteristics of the respondents and an 11 items related to general awareness, symptoms, complications, prevention and control on diabetes mellitus. A study information sheet and written consent form were also included in the survey instrument.

A pilot study was carried out to find out the reliability and validity of the questionnaire. The structured questionnaire was pretested on a sample of 50 Malaysians to find out difficulties in understanding the meaning of the questions and to estimate the amount of time to answer all the questions. The feedback revealed that the questionnaires were easy to understand and quite convenient for the public as they just need to tick the correct options.

Data was collected using convenient sampling methods among the residents of Taman Sri Andalas, Taman Klang Jaya, Bandar Bukit Tinggi and Bandar Botanic. Before data collection, each participant was given a full explanation of the research project and its purpose and was then given to sign an informed consent form. A face-to-face interview was carried out for data collection. Each interview took approximately 10–15 min and was conducted at places comfortable for the participant. When it was necessary, appropriate probing questions were asked. To draw out more complete ideas from the participants, they were given freedom to express additional views on the topic at the end of the interview session.

The collected data were analysed using SPSS version 21.0. Descriptive studies were used to analyse the demographic data obtained whereas Student's t test and one-way analysis of variance were applied as appropriate. The Student's t test was used to compare two groups and one-way analysis of variance (ANOVA) test was used to compare between more than two groups. This study was approved by Ethics committee of AMU (ID: 01BP200904-00068/12/12/), Malaysia. All participants signed the informed consent form.

3. Results

In this study, the majority of respondents (49%, $n = 196$) lay within the range of 12–24 years old and only a few respondents (2%, $n = 8$) lay within the range of 64 years old and above. On the other hand, around 32% ($n = 130$) of the respondents fall between 25–44 years old and 16.5% ($n = 66$) of the respondents fall between 45 and 64 years old. The largest percentage of respondents was Indians (50.75%, $n = 203$) and the smallest percent of respondents were others consisting of the Punjabis and Serani (3%, $n = 12$). The Malays and Chinese were 18.5% ($n = 74$) and 27.75% ($n = 111$) respectively. The largest number of respondents received education from college/university ($n = 236$, 59%) and only 7.25% ($n = 29$) of respondents received education from graduate schools. On the other hand, 25% ($n = 100$) of respondents completed high school and 8.75% ($n = 35$) of respondents completed primary school education. Among the respondents in this study, around 58.5% ($n = 234$) were female and the rest 41.5% ($n = 166$) were male. In our study, there are more females in the age group of 12–24 years ($n = 117$) and 25–44 years ($n = 84$), and more males in the age range of 45–64 years ($n = 36$) and >64 years ($n = 5$). As for race, there were more female respondents in all races than males. For the education level there were more female respondents for all except for primary education level. The detailed demographic data are presented in Tables 1 and 2.

Eleven different structured questions were used to analyse the respondent's knowledge on causes, symptoms, associated complications, prevention and treatment of diabetes. The analysis revealed that out of 400 respondents, a majority (394; 98.50%) of the respondents knew about diabetes and heard about diabetes mellitus, among this, 233 were female and 161 were male. Around 67.52% ($n = 158$) female and 56.02% ($n = 93$) male participants said any one of their family members had suffered from diabetes.

In terms of their knowledge on what causes diabetes, the majority ($n = 181$; 45.25%) of the respondents agreed that eating more sugar may lead to diabetes, a similar percentage of males (46.39%) and females (44.44%) agreed with the statement. One hundred and forty one respondents (35.25%) agreed that a lack or defect of insulin may cause diabetes, among the respondents who agreed with the statement more were female (37.61%) than male (31.93%).

Table 1. Demographic characteristics of respondents ($N = 400$).

Demographic Characteristics	Number of Respondents (N)	Percentage (%)
Age in years		
12–24	196	49.00
25–44	130	32.50
45–64	66	16.50
>64	8	2.00
Sex		
Female	234	58.50
Male	166	41.50
Race		
Malay	74	18.50
Chinese	111	27.75
Indian	203	50.75
Others (Punjabi, Serani)	12	3.00
Education Level		
Primary	35	8.75
High School	100	25.00
College/University	236	59.00
Graduate School	29	7.25

Table 2. Gender-wise distribution of respondents ($N = 400$).

Demographic Characteristics	Female ($n = 234$)		Male ($n = 166$)		Total	
	N	%	N	%	N	%
Age in years						
12–24	117	50.00	79	47.60	196	49.00
25–44	84	35.90	46	27.70	130	32.50
45–64	30	12.82	36	21.70	66	16.50
>64	3	1.28	5	3.00	8	2.00
Race						
Malay	50	21.37	24	14.46	74	18.50
Chinese	67	28.63	44	26.50	111	27.75
Indian	108	46.15	95	57.23	203	50.75
Others(Punjabi, Serani)	9	3.85	3	1.81	12	3.00
Education Level						
Primary	17	7.26	18	10.84	35	8.75
High School	54	23.08	46	27.71	100	25.00
College/University	142	60.69	94	56.63	236	59.00
Graduate School	21	8.97	8	4.82	29	7.25

A total of 197 (84.19%) females and 129 (77.71%) males answered that middle age and elderly people were most commonly affected by diabetes. However, an equal number of female (7.69%) and male (10.85%) said young adults and middle age groups were commonly affected by diabetes.

The majority ($n = 356$; 89%) of the respondents reported that both sex were commonly affected by diabetes, among this 91% were female and 86.1% were male respondents. In terms of the course of this disease, around 82% of female and 80% of male respondents mentioned that diabetes will be lifelong and can be controlled with treatment.

Two hundred and eighty four (71%) respondents consisting of 170 (72.65%) females and 114 (68.68%) males stated that high blood sugar level was the main characteristics of diabetes. However, 27 (11.53%) females and 28 (16.87%) males believed that high urine sugar was the best characteristics of diabetes. The majority of the female and male respondents agreed frequent urination, hunger and thirst are the most common symptoms of diabetes.

The majority of the respondents ($n = 245$; 61.25%) mentioned that a foot problem was the most common complications of diabetes. However, Heart disease ($n = 111$; 27.75%), Kidney disease ($n = 153$; 38.25%), Eye disease ($n = 130$; 32.50%), and Stroke ($n = 80$; 20%) also reported as common complications of diabetes by the respondents. The majority of the respondents agreed healthy diet ($n = 358$; 89.5%), regular exercise ($n = 294$; 73.5%), weight control ($n = 236$; 59%) and stopping smoking ($n = 133$; 33.25%) were the best measures to prevent diabetes. However, 5 (1.25%) respondents said diabetes cannot be prevented.

In terms of the different methods of treatment for diabetes, the majority of the respondents declared drugs ($n = 351$; 87.75%) are the ideal choice of treatment, followed by Insulin ($n = 346$; 86.50%), Healthy diet ($n = 303$; 75.75%), regular exercise ($n = 256$; 64.00%) and weight control ($n = 206$; 51.50%). The data are depicted in Table 3.

The mean scores for both males and females were almost the same, implying that there was no significance difference in knowledge between the females and males ($p > 0.991$). The data are shown in Table 4. ANOVA results shows that the knowledge of respondents with different age groups and ethnicity have significant difference ($p < 0.001$). The respondents aged 12–24 have the highest mean value of 58.92 with standard deviation of 7.81 and the respondents aged 45–64 have the lowest mean value of 54.21 with standard deviation of 7.04 ($p < 0.001$). As for the ethnicity, the Chinese respondents have the highest mean value of 61.42 with standard deviation of 8.75 and the respondents from the other categories consisting of the Serani's and Punjabi's have the lowest mean value of 55.26 with standard deviation of 5.91 with a significant value of $p < 0.001$. The data are presented in Table 5.

Table 3. Assessment of knowledge on diabetes and participants' response ($N = 400$).

Question (s)	Response	Female ($n = 234$)	Male ($n = 166$)	Total ($n = 400$)
Have you heard about Diabetes Mellitus?	Yes	233 (99.57%)	161 (96.99%)	394 (98.50%)
	No	1 (0.43%)	5 (3.01%)	6 (1.50%)
Do any of your family members or relative have/had diabetes?	Yes	158 (67.52%)	93 (56.02%)	251 (62.75%)
	No	76 (32.48%)	73 (43.98%)	149 (37.25%)
As per your knowledge what causes diabetes?	Contact with another diabetic	7 (3.00%)	7 (4.22%)	14 (3.50%)
	Eating more sugar	104 (44.44%)	77 (46.39%)	181 (45.25%)
	Lack/defect of insulin	88 (37.61%)	53 (31.93%)	141 (35.25%)
	Destiny	6 (2.56%)	10 (6.02%)	16 (4.00%)
	Others (Specify)	11 (4.70%)	6 (3.61%)	17 (4.25%)
	Don't know	18 (7.69%)	13 (7.83%)	31 (7.75%)
Which age groups are most commonly affected by diabetes?	Children and adolescents	4 (1.71%)	5 (3.01%)	9 (2.25%)
	Young adults and middle aged	18 (7.69%)	18 (10.85%)	36 (9.00%)
	Middle aged and elderly	197 (84.19%)	129 (77.71%)	326 (81.50%)
	Others (specify)	2 (0.85%)	1 (0.60%)	3 (0.75%)
	Don't know	13 (5.56%)	13 (7.83%)	26 (6.50%)
Which sexes are affected by diabetes?	Males only	5 (2.14%)	6 (3.61%)	11 (2.75%)
	Females only	6 (2.56%)	8 (4.82%)	14 (3.50%)
	Both	213 (91.03%)	143 (86.15%)	356 (89.00%)
	Don't know	10 (4.27%)	9 (5.42%)	19 (4.75%)
What is the course of this disease?	Cures by itself	8 (3.42%)	4 (2.41%)	12 (3.00%)
	Short, cured with treatment	13 (5.56%)	10 (6.02%)	23 (5.75%)
	Lifelong, controlled with treatment	192 (82.05%)	134 (80.73%)	326 (81.50%)
	Others (specify)	1 (0.43%)	0 (0.00%)	1 (0.25%)
	Don't know	20 (8.54%)	18 (10.84%)	38 (9.50%)
Which of the following best characterizes the disease condition?	High blood sugar	170 (72.65%)	114 (68.68%)	284 (71.00%)
	High urine sugar	27 (11.53%)	28 (16.87%)	55 (13.75%)
	Low blood sugar	7 (3.0%)	5 (3.01%)	12 (3.00%)
	Low urine sugar	0 (0.0%)	1 (0.60%)	1 (0.25%)
	Don't know	30 (12.82)	18 (10.84%)	48 (12.00%)
What do you think are the most common symptoms of diabetes mellitus? (multiple responses possible)	Frequent urination	145 (61.96%)	86 (51.81%)	231 (57.75%)
	Frequent hunger	65 (27.78%)	67 (40.36%)	132 (33.00%)
	Frequent thirst	108 (46.15%)	73 (43.98%)	181 (45.25%)
	Asymptomatic	10 (4.27%)	3 (1.81%)	13 (3.25%)
	Others (specify)	4 (1.71%)	1 (0.60%)	5 (1.25%)
	Don't know	30 (12.82%)	43 (25.90%)	73 (18.25%)
What are the common complications resulting from diabetes mellitus? (multiple responses possible)	Heart disease	79 (33.76%)	32 (19.28%)	111 (27.75%)
	Kidney disease	110 (47.01%)	43 (25.90%)	153 (38.25%)
	Eye disease	87 (37.18%)	43 (25.90%)	130 (32.50%)
	Stroke	59 (25.21%)	21 (12.65%)	80 (20.00%)
	Foot problems	150 (64.10%)	95 (57.23%)	245 (61.25%)
	Death	41 (17.52%)	38 (22.89%)	79 (19.75%)
	Others (specify)	5 (2.14%)	0 (0.00%)	5 (1.25%)
	Don't know	19 (8.12%)	21 (12.65%)	40 (10.00%)
What measures can prevent diabetes? (multiple responses possible)	Healthy diet	214 (91.45%)	144 (86.75%)	358 (89.50%)
	Regular exercise	166 (70.94%)	128 (77.12%)	294 (73.50%)
	Weight control	136 (58.12%)	100 (60.24%)	236 (59.00%)
	Quit smoking	65 (27.78%)	68 (40.96%)	133 (33.25%)
	Others (specify)	8 (3.42%)	1 (0.60%)	9 (2.25%)
	Don't know	8 (3.42%)	7 (4.22%)	15 (3.75%)
	Cannot prevented	4 (1.71%)	1 (0.60%)	5 (1.25%)
What are the methods of treatment in this disease? (multiple responses possible)	Drugs	209 (89.32%)	142 (85.54%)	351 (87.75%)
	Insulin	205 (87.61%)	141 (84.94%)	346 (86.50%)
	Healthy diet	177 (75.64%)	126 (75.90%)	303 (75.75%)
	Regular exercise	146 (62.39%)	110 (66.26%)	256 (64.00%)
	Weight control	117 (50.00%)	89 (53.61%)	206 (51.50%)
	Quit smoking	37 (15.81%)	38 (22.89%)	75 (18.75%)
	Others (specify)	1 (0.43%)	0 (0.00%)	1 (0.25%)
	Don't know	10 (4.30%)	17 (20.24%)	27 (6.75%)

Table 4. Independent sample test for knowledge with different genders.

Sex	N	Mean	Std. Deviation	't' Value	Sig
Female	234	57.7	7.5	0.012	0.991
Male	166	57.6	8.1		

Table 5. Results of questionnaire separated by age, ethnicity and education level.

	Number	Mean	Std. Deviation	Sig
Age in years				
12–24	196	58.92	7.81	
25–44	130	57.64	7.52	
45–64	66	54.21	7.04	0.000
>64	8	55.02	6.91	
Total	400	57.73	7.82	
Ethnicity (race) of the respondents				
Malay	74	57.23	6.83	
Chinese	111	61.42	8.75	
Indian	203	55.81	6.94	0.000
Others (Punjabi, Serani)	12	55.26	5.91	
Total	400	57.72	7.82	
Education Level				
Primary	35	60.66	6.32	
High School	100	57.32	8.23	
College/University	236	57.63	7.98	0.057
Graduate School	29	55.47	6.06	
Total	400	57.72	7.84	

4. Discussion

The study explored the knowledge of diabetes mellitus among the population of Klang Valley, Malaysia. The results showed that there was a statistically significant difference in the mean knowledge of respondents with different age groups and ethnic origin ($p = 0.000$) but there was no significant difference in the knowledge among the gender and level of education ($p = 0.057$). The current literature evaluating the relationship between age and knowledge on diabetes yielded mixed findings [14–17]. In this study, there were a statistically significant difference in the mean knowledge of respondents with different age groups and the younger respondents have higher knowledge than the older respondents with higher mean value (μ: 58.92). This result is consistent with a study carried out in Ankara, Turkey that found lower level of knowledge of diabetes in older people (18.6%) [18] and in an another study carried out in Singapore that younger respondents have more exposure such as reading more books and using the Internet as sources of information compared to the older respondents [19]. There is a literature evaluating the relationship between gender and knowledge and it was reported that gender is not a determinant of knowledge on diabetes mellitus [20,21]. In Malaysia, males and females are have equal exposure and rights to be educated. This is one of the reasons that the latest Malaysian National Health Morbidity Survey IV 2015 showed that the prevalence of diabetes mellitus is higher in females at 18.3% compared to males at 16.7% [22].

Level of education was found to be the predominant predictive factors on knowledge of diabetes mellitus [20]. This was in consistent with a study carried out in southern India that level of education influences knowledge on physical activity which is included in the practice section of this questionnaire [23]. However, in this study there were no significant differences in knowledge among respondents of different education level ($p = 0.057$). This is a sign that everyone has almost the same amount of knowledge on diabetes mellitus regardless of their education level. In this study, the comparison between respondents of different ethnicity showed a significant difference in the knowledge of diabetes mellitus. Chinese showed the highest level of knowledge (μ: 61.42) whereas Indians (μ: 55.81) and other ethnics (μ: 55.26) showed the lowest level of knowledge. However, the explanations regarding ethnicity have not been discussed clearly in most literatures.

The study emphasizes that the learning about risk factors of Diabetes Mellitus and its preventive measures are the first step in prevention, since it will enable the public to make the informed decision of adopting a healthy lifestyle [24,25]. In addition to this, health care practitioners and policy makers need consistent good quality data about the distribution and determinants of Diabetes related health issues among their population [26]. These data are essential to design, frame, implement and evaluate successful interventional programs in Malaysia. The results of the study may not entirely reflect the actual knowledge on diabetes among the population of Klang valley, Malaysia. The questionnaire may not be attempted diligently, unless the respondents are educated and advised by the health care providers. The response biases may exist in this study as the respondents may tend to give more positive answers in order to maintain the high level of knowledge; hence, there might be a slight tendency to fill in more positive or neutral responses. In addition, the sample size may not be large enough to obtain reliable and consistent results.

5. Conclusions

This study indicated that there is a difference in knowledge on diabetes mellitus among different age groups and ethnicity, whereas the gender of respondents and education level of respondents do not have significant difference. Hence, there is a need to come out with some strategies to enhance the level of understanding on diabetes mellitus. An improved and well-structured educational programme(s) that tackles the areas of weaknesses is recommended to increase the level of public knowledge on diabetes mellitus. Moreover, promotion of implementing healthy lifestyle along with the information about risk factors, diet, exercise, and screening should be encouraged through health campaigns. This can be started as early as in school. This study has major implications to design future educational programmes to control diabetes mellitus. Apart from educating the public, these programmes can be designed in such a way to train and upgrade the health care professions, mainly the physicians and pharmacists, to produce competent diabetes educators who would be able to educate the public on the control of diabetes mellitus.

Acknowledgments: We acknowledge the help and support provided by the Management of AMU, Malaysia to carry out the study.

Author Contributions: Sasikala Chinnappan and Palanisamy Sivanandy conceived and designed the study and wrote the paper; Nagashekhara Molugulu guided the data collection procedures; Rajenthina Sagaran participated in the analysis of the data.

References

1.   Sarah, W.; Gojka, R.; Anders, G.; Richard, S.; Hilary, K. Global prevalence of diabetes: estimates for the year 2000 and projections for 2030. *Diabetes Care* **2004**, *27*, 1047–1053.
2.   ArulKumaran, K.S.G.; Palanisamy, S.; Rajasekaran, A. Development and implementation of patient information leaflets in diabetes mellitus. *J. Pharma. Health Serv. Res.* **2010**, *1*, 85–89. [CrossRef]
3.   Mafauzy, M. Diabetes mellitus in Malaysia. *Med. J. Malays.* **2006**, *61*, 397–398.
4.   Murata, G.H.; Shah, J.H.; Adam, K.D.; Wendel, C.S.; Bokhari, S.U.; Solvas, P.A.; Hoffman, R.M.; Duckworth, W.C. Factors affecting diabetes knowledge in type 2 diabetic veterans. *Diabetologia* **2003**, *46*, 1170–1178. [PubMed]
5.   Letchumanan, G.R.; Wan-Nazaimoon, W.M.; Wan-Mohamad, W.B.; Chandran, L.R.; Tee, G.H.; Jamaiyah, H.; Isa, M.R.; Zanariah, H.; Fatanah, I.; Ahmad Faudzi, Y. Prevalence of Diabetes in the Malaysian National Health Morbidity Survey III 2006. *Med. J. Malays.* **2010**, *65*, 173–179.
6.   Nehad, M.H.; Istabraq, D.A.A.; Jyothi, V.; Hussain, Y.; Umar, F.U. Assessment of knowledge and awareness of diabetic and non-diabetic population towards diabetes mellitus in Kaduna, Nigeria. *J. Adv. Sci. Res.* **2012**, *3*, 46–50.
7.   Linda, H.; Melinda, M.; Joni, B.; Carla, E.C.; Paulina, D.; Laura, E.; Hanson, L.; Kent, D.; Kolb, L.; McLaughlin, S.; et al. National standard for diabetes self-management education and support. *Diabetes Care* **2014**, *37*, S144–S153.

8. Palanisamy, S.; ArulKumaran, K.S.G.; Rajasekaran, A. Knowledge assessment in adverse drug reactions and reporting. *Arch. Pharm. Pract.* **2013**, *4*, 104–119.

9. Singh, A.; Shenoy, S.; Sandhu, J.S. Prevalence of type 2 diabetes mellitus among urban sikh population of Amritsar. *Ind. J. Commun. Med.* **2016**, *41*, 263–267. [CrossRef] [PubMed]

10. Acharya, K.G.; Shah, K.N.; Solanki, N.D.; Rana, D.A. Evaluation of antidiabetic prescriptions, cost and adherence to treatment guidelines: A prospective, cross-sectional study at a tertiary care teaching hospital. *J. Basic Clin. Pharm.* **2013**, *4*, 82–87. [PubMed]

11. Ahmad, B.; Ramadas, A.; Quek, K.F. The development and validation of diabetes knowledge questionnaire for the Indigenous population in Malaysia. *Med. J. Malays.* **2010**, *65*, 273–276.

12. Najib Mohd, N.M.; Dali, A.F.; Ahmad, A.; Sulaiman, S.; Hussin, S.N.; Mokhtar, N. Knowledge and Attitude on Diabetes Among Public In Kota Bharu Kelantan, Malaysia. *Int. J. Edu. Res.* **2014**, *2*, 1–10.

13. Prianka, M.; Bhaskar, P.; Debasis, D.; Nilanjan, S.; Rachna, M. Perceptions and practices of type 2 diabetics: A cross-sectional study in a tertiary care hospital in Kolkata. *Int. J. Diab. Ctries* **2010**, *30*, 143–149.

14. Lemes dos Santos, P.F.; Dos Santos, P.R.; Ferrari, G.S.L.; Fonseca, G.A.A.; Ferrari, C.K.B. Knowledge of Diabetes Mellitus: Does Gender Make a Difference? *Osong Public Health Res. Perspect.* **2014**, *5*, 199–203. [CrossRef] [PubMed]

15. Sivasankari, V.; Manivannan, E.; Priyadarsini, S.P. Drug utilization pattern of anti-diabetic drugs in a rural area of Tamilnadu, South India—A prospective, observational study. *Int. J. Pharm. Biol. Sci.* **2013**, *4*, 514–519.

16. Shah, V.N.; Kamdar, P.K.; Shah, N. Assessing the knowledge, attitudes and practice of type 2 diabetes among patients of Saurashtra region, Gujarat. *Int. J. Diabetes Dev. Ctries* **2009**, *29*, 118–122. [CrossRef] [PubMed]

17. Rodrigues, F.F.L.; Zanetti, M.L.; Santos, M.A. Knowledge and attitude: important components in diabetes education. *Rev. Latino-Am. Enferm.* **2009**, *17*, 468–473. [CrossRef]

18. Denis, C.; Oya, O.; Esin, O.; Aysun, I. Evaluation of awareness of diabetes mellitus and associated factors in four health center areas. *Patient Educ. Couns.* **2006**, *62*, 142–147.

19. Tham, K.Y.; Ong, J.J.Y.; Tan, D.K.L.; How, K.Y. How much do diabetic patients know about diabetes mellitus and its complications? *Ann. Acad. Med. Singap.* **2004**, *33*, 503–509. [PubMed]

20. Lai, S.Y.; Yahaya, H.; Noorizan, A.A.; Ahmed, A.; Rozina, G. A comparison of knowledge of diabetes mellitus between patients with diabetes and healthy adults: A survey from north Malaysia. *Patient Educ. Couns.* **2007**, *69*, 47–54.

21. Titaporn, P.; Shu-Chuen, L.; Hwee-Lin, W. A Survey of Knowledge on Diabetes in the Central Region of Thailand. *Int. Soc. Pharm. Outcomes Res.* **2009**, *12*, S110–S113.

22. National Health and Morbidity Survey 2015. Institute for Public Health, Ministry of Health Malaysia. Available online: http://www.iku.gov.my/images/IKU/Document/REPORT/nhmsreport2015vol2.pdf (accessed on 16 December 2016).

23. Murugesan, N.; Snehalatha, C.; Shobana, R.; Roglic, G.; Ramachandran, A. Awareness about diabetes and its complications in the general and diabetic population in a city in southern India. *Diabetes Res. Clin. Pract.* **2007**, *77*, 433–437. [CrossRef] [PubMed]

24. Bowman, B.; Gregg, E.; Williams, D.; Engelgau, M.; Jack, L. Translating the science of primary, secondary, and tertiary prevention to inform the public health response to diabetes. *J. Public Health Manag. Pract.* **2003**, *9*, S8–S14. [CrossRef]

25. Glasgow, R.E.; Wagner, E.; Kaplan, R.M.; Vinicor, F.; Smith, L.; Norman, J. If diabetes is a public health problem, why not treat it as one? A population based approach to chronic illness. *Ann. Behav. Med.* **1999**, *21*, 159–170. [CrossRef] [PubMed]

26. Garfield, S.; Malozowski, S.; Chin, M.; Venkat Narayan, K.; Glasgow, R.; Green Hiss, R.; Krumholz, H. Considerations for diabetes translation research in real-world settings. *Diabetes Care* **2003**, *26*, 2670–2674. [CrossRef] [PubMed]

12

Interprofessional Pharmacokinetics Simulation: Pharmacy and Nursing Students' Perceptions

Cheryl D. Cropp [1], Jennifer Beall [1,*] (iD), Ellen Buckner [2], Frankie Wallis [3] and Amanda Barron [2]

[1] McWhorter School of Pharmacy, Samford University, 800 Lakeshore Drive, Birmingham, AL 35229, USA; ccropp@samford.edu

[2] Ida Moffett School of Nursing, Samford University, 800 Lakeshore Drive, Birmingham, AL 35229, USA; ebuckne2@samford.edu (E.B.); abarron@samford.edu (A.B.)

[3] University of Alabama at Birmingham Hospital, NP1333, 1802 6th Avenue South, Birmingham, AL 35249-7010, USA; fwallis@uabmc.edu

* Correspondence: jwbeall@samford.edu

Abstract: Interprofessional practice between pharmacists and nurses can involve pharmacokinetic dosing of medications in a hospital setting. This study describes student perceptions of an interprofessional collaboration pharmacokinetics simulation on the Interprofessional Education Collaborative (IPEC) 2016 Core Competencies. The investigators developed a simulation activity for senior undergraduate nursing and second-year pharmacy students. Nursing and pharmacy students (n = 54, 91 respectively) participated in the simulation using medium-fidelity manikins. Each case represented a pharmacokinetic dosing consult (vancomycin, tobramycin, phenytoin, theophylline, or lidocaine). Nursing students completed head-to-toe assessment and pharmacy students gathered necessary information and calculated empiric and adjusted doses. Students communicated using SBAR (Situation, Background, Assessment, and Recommendation). Students participated in debrief sessions and completed an IRB-approved online survey. Themes from survey responses revealed meaningful perceptions in all IPEC competencies as well as themes of safety, advocacy, appreciation, and areas for improvement. Students reported learning effectively from the simulation experience. Few studies relate to this type of interprofessional education experience and this study begins to explore student perceptions of interprofessional education (IPE) in a health sciences clinical context through simulation. This real-world application of nursing and pharmacy interprofessional collaboration can positively affect patient-centered outcomes and safety.

Keywords: interprofessional education; pharmacy education; nursing education; pharmacokinetics; simulation

1. Introduction

Interprofessional education (IPE) is defined by the World Health Organization as "when students from two or more professions learn about, from, and with each other to enable effective collaboration and improve health outcomes" [1]. IPE is an important aspect in current health education and is necessary to train our students for the collaborative practice environment.

The simulation environment provides a unique opportunity for students to apply information they have learned in a traditional lecture-format environment to the setting of a patient care scenario. The 2016 Interprofessional Education Collaborative (IPEC) Core Competencies for Interprofessional Collaborative Practice serve as a guidance document for developing IPE activities [2].

1.1. Interprofessional Education at Samford University College of Health Sciences

In 2016, the College of Health Sciences (CHS) at Samford University moved to a shared facility. Since the move, the four schools (Pharmacy, Nursing, Health Professions, and Public Health) have developed several IPE experiences that include discussions and simulations. Simulations such as the one described here take place in a multifunction lab of a shared CHS simulation center. The 22,000-square-foot Experiential Learning and Simulation Center offers discipline-specific and interdisciplinary learning opportunities. Students engage at a variety of levels—from lab-based learning with low fidelity models, to simulated patient interactions, to complex high-fidelity simulations. The CHS Interprofessional workgroup was formed in 2013 and has developed a model for IPE at the CHS. We believe that our faith and calling inform and connect our work. We also incorporate quality and safety since quality improvement and patient/client/population safety are crucial, pervasive aspects of providing care. CHS graduates apply relationship-building values and the principles of team dynamics to perform effectively in different team roles. The CHS has developed a model for IPE below (Figure 1).

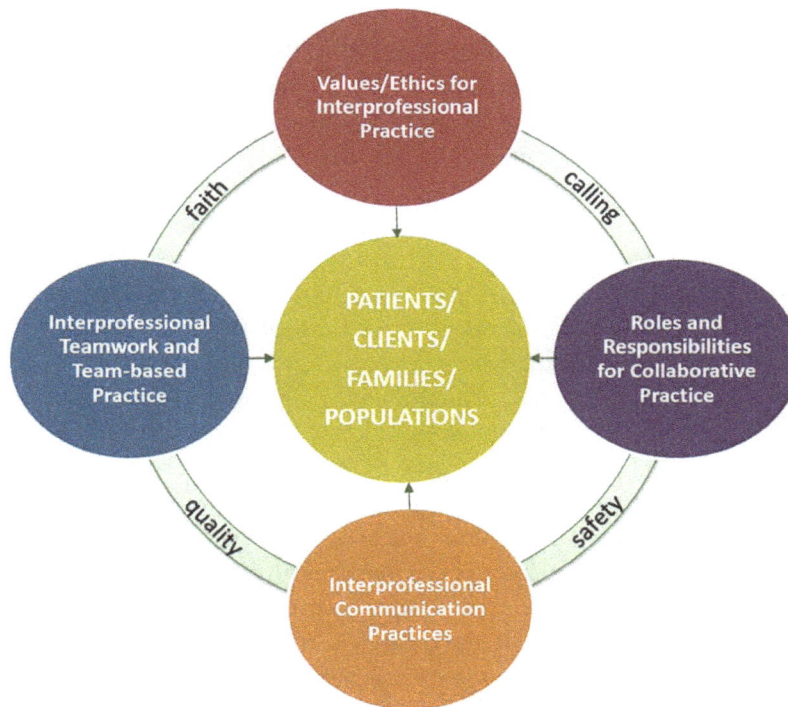

Figure 1. Samford University College of Health Sciences Model of Interprofessional Education.

In 2018, CHS colleagues proposed a staged model of IPE in which students grow in competencies across longitudinal experiences and maturing practice [3]. These stages are (a) Discuss—discuss the varied roles of IPE participants; (b) Collaborate—working together to analyze a case study and make recommendations; (c) Simulate—create a live action scenario with interprofessional team members and (d) Practice—integrate IP roles in practice settings in preceptorship and during transition to care roles. The experiences proposed here build additional strength in the third and fourth stages of Simulate and Practice transition.

1.2. Interprofessional Simulation in Literature

Simulation activities can create an opportunity for disciplines to interact and learn together prior to the completion of their degree training [4]. Smithburger and colleagues developed an elective interprofessional experience with teams that included nursing and pharmacy students. The teams were tasked with managing a complex patient case assuming their respective professional roles. Students were surveyed on their acceptance and impressions of the use of the simulation; they agreed or strongly agreed that the simulation improved their interprofessional communication and confidence in caring for a patient in a team.

In a study of nurse–physician relationships simulation was found to transform interprofessional attitudes [5]. The simulation experiences were designed to encourage open communication, shared information, and collaborative decision-making. Trust developed through the experience and reported attitudes were more positive. This study further investigated stereotype changes which was beyond the scope of the current work. In another study, five best practice components were used to structure an IPE simulation. High quality designs included debriefing practices, interprofessional education applications, validation of outcome measures, student satisfaction, and long-term information retention [6]. The current study utilizes best practices and presents initial student perceptions toward building effective IPE programs.

1.3. Nursing and Pharmacy Collaborations in Literature

Reports of effectiveness and perceptions of IPE are becoming increasingly available in the literature. Numerous articles report positive change in student attitudes, breadth of understanding, and the development of trust through interprofessional collaborative educational experiences [7]. Authors reported significant improvement in student attitudes of cultural competence, understanding of roles, interprofessional communication and teamwork.

Kostoff and colleagues incorporated SBAR (Situation, Background, Assessment, Recommendation) into their simulation to determine its impact on self-perception by pharmacy students of interprofessional competence and their reactions toward interprofessional collaboration [8]. Nursing and pharmacy students used the SBAR communication tool to share information to develop a patient care plan. Pharmacy student respondents reported that they felt it was a valuable experience, and that they planned to use SBAR in their future role as a pharmacist.

Interprofessional education simulation has shown benefits to a broad representation of disciplines and content focus. Thurston and colleagues reported specific professional stereotypes reported by nursing and pharmacy students who were naïve to IPE experiences [9]. They utilized a Student Stereotypes Rating Questionnaire and although the results were generally positive, there were significant differences noted by each profession. In a joint nursing and pharmacy IPEC job-shadowing practice experience, results showed effectiveness in increasing IPEC competencies [10]. Poirier and colleagues found differences in student self-assessment and faculty assessment of performance in a nursing–pharmacy interprofessional error disclosure in a simulation training program with recommendations to continue [11]. Both reports recommended increased IPE opportunities to include evaluative strategies.

Wilson and colleagues reported significant improvement in medication safety through an interprofessional collaboration between nurses and pharmacists in practice [12]. These authors conducted focus groups, and found that "knowing about and valuing the skills and responsibilities of other team members and respecting each person's unique contribution to the work of the team can lead to more effective communication and collaboration in the context of medication safety." Bell and colleagues described collaboration through interprofessional medication reviews in primary care [13]. In a recent report, authors described a similar positive effect for hospital-based simulation for nursing and pharmacy students [14].

Meyer and colleagues assessed the impact of a simulation with nursing and pharmacy students on their perceptions of interprofessionalism as well as the impact on knowledge of pharmacology [15]. There was a statistically significant increase in interprofessionalism, as determined by mean Attitudes Toward Health Care Teams score post-simulation compared to pre-simulation. Perceptions of the simulation were overall favorable, and over 90% of students reported that the simulation increased their knowledge of pharmacology.

Zuna and Holt investigated the use of a pharmacokinetic simulator to demonstrate one- and two-compartment drug behavior to undergraduate pharmacology students [16]. The students had received instruction in pharmacokinetic principles and calculations in a previous course. Students completed a self-assessment of their confidence and competence in working with pharmacokinetic concepts and calculations. The students self-reported a significant increase after the simulation in their competence in the math skills of pharmacokinetics, and their perceived understanding of the material compared to their perceptions before the simulation.

There have been no studies identified that investigate collaboration between nursing and pharmacy students on the topic of pharmacokinetic dosing in a simulated educational setting. Therefore, our research of this topic is groundbreaking and provides guidance on an important, useful educational activity in an effort to provide safe and effective treatment to patients.

This study describes student perceptions of an interprofessional pharmacokinetics simulation. Student perceptions of the session content, interprofessional collaboration, and the use of simulation were sought.

2. Materials and Methods

The investigators developed a simulation activity for senior undergraduate nursing and second-year pharmacy students. This was the second year for this activity. Objectives for the pharmacy students were to: (1) provide optimal drug dosing using population and patient-specific pharmacokinetic parameters; and (2) communicate effectively in the care of a patient. Objectives for nursing students were to: (3) apply principles of leadership through interprofessional collaboration, and (4) promote medication safety through interprofessional collaboration with pharmacy in patient-centered care.

2.1. Development of the Simulation and Objectives

In preparation for the simulation, we hypothesized that pharmacy and nursing students would demonstrate increased interprofessional collaboration in all the IPEC Core Competencies. We further anticipated that the competency of interprofessional communication would increase significantly with addition of shared content and best practices in medication administration and pharmacokinetic dosing. The first offering was in Spring 2017 and students' anecdotal reports were highly positive. In particular the debrief sessions included all students sharing their perceptions of the collaboration, demonstrating the collegiality that had developed among them. Based on this pilot experience, faculty chose to continue the offering and add formal qualitative measure to evaluate the simulated IPE experience.

In Spring 2018, the activity was offered to 54 nursing and 91 pharmacy students over the course of three consecutive days. The simulation took place in a five-bed flex lab using medium-fidelity manikins. Each manikin represented a different case for which the pharmacy student had been consulted to initiate or adjust pharmacokinetic dosing. The drugs for which doses were to be calculated were vancomycin, tobramycin, phenytoin, theophylline, and lidocaine. The lidocaine case was developed for the Spring 2018 activity; in Spring 2017, the fifth case was a patient receiving vancomycin and gentamicin. The cases were developed in conjunction with the instructor of record for the pharmacokinetics course, who also co-led the lab activity. Each case was designed to reinforce a pharmacokinetic principle or to provide an opportunity to practice completing a pharmacokinetic consult as would take place in an inpatient setting. Each case also had embedded in it an error or omission to provide an aspect of medication safety.

2.2. Case Studies and Core Competencies

The simulation activity was created for senior undergraduate nursing and second-year pharmacy students and was congruent with curriculum objectives for each. Nursing students had completed numerous clinical experiences and were able to integrate care expectations in the collaboration. Pharmacy students applied content on pharmacokinetics and collaborated by providing current state-of-the-science evidence-based information on nursing students' questions about medication parameters. For example, both groups were concerned with monitoring for adverse reactions or side effects and both reported they learned specific new information through the questions and answers on specific drugs. This activity takes place as part of a nursing leadership and management course, and an integrated pharmacy applications lab course. Pharmacy students completed a pharmacokinetics course the semester immediately preceding this simulation. Nursing and pharmacy students were assigned to certain days so each participated only once in the simulation. Nursing students began a head-to-toe assessment of the patient. Pharmacy students began the simulation in a classroom where they received instructions, group assignments and a worksheet to be completed. The worksheet contained a brief case vignette and space on which they could document information collected from the nursing students and the chart, as well as space for calculations. The case vignette included the pharmacokinetic consult with medical diagnosis, physical parameters, and laboratory findings. Five case studies were developed collaboratively by the pharmacy–nursing faculty team.

Case 1: Vancomycin

The patient is a 64-year old male who was hospitalized 3 days ago while on vacation in Florida for an infection in a wound on his leg. Further evaluation revealed MRSA in the wound. In addition to home meds for hypertension and ischemic heart disease, patient was placed on vancomycin with peak and trough targets.

Case 2: Theophylline

The patient is a 22-year-old female who was admitted to your hospital for an asthma exacerbation. She reports to you that she has not had her prescriptions refilled and ran out of her medications 1 week ago. Pharmacy consult included assessing adherence/compliance, determining dosage for bolus and maintenance theophylline, and discussion with patient about plans for discharge and reducing exacerbations.

Case 3: Tobramycin

The patient is a 24-year old female who resides in a long-term care facility secondary to quadriplegia. She was hospitalized for a urinary tract infection and the urine culture grew *Pseudomonas aeruginosa*. Home meds included oxybutynin, docusate sodium, and, baclofen with pharmacy to dose tobramycin.

Case 4: Phenytoin

The patient is a 30-year-old male who is admitted for a closed head trauma and has developed generalized tonic-clonic seizures. He was initially placed on lamotrigine but has not responded well to that. He was started on phenytoin a couple of days ago, but his seizure frequency increased on the second day of therapy. There are lab profiles and a consult for pharmacy to dose phenytoin.

Case 5: Vancomycin + gentamicin (Spring 2017)

The patient is a 10-year-old female admitted for osteomyelitis. Consult for pharmacy to dose vancomycin and gentamicin. Pharmacy and nursing collaboration with family to plan for discharge and monitor long-term side effects.

Case 6: Lidocaine (Spring 2018)

The patient is a 70-year-old female who resides at a local long-term care facility and is admitted for ventricular tachycardia. Consult for pharmacy to dose lidocaine to a steady-state concentration of 2 mg/L. The patient also had suspected *C. difficile* infection.

Pharmacy students then entered the simulated healthcare environment and communicated with nurses on duty. Each patient case has a team comprised of nursing and pharmacy students. They gathered the necessary information on patient status from the nursing students as well as the chart, and then conferred to calculate empiric or adjusted doses of the aforementioned medications for the patient. Once the dose was calculated, the pharmacy students communicated the planned new dosing regimen (including administration and monitoring parameters) to the nursing students using SBAR. Necessary collaborations with additional health professionals (MD, NP, or PA) were noted. Nursing and pharmacy students both participated in the debrief session including collaborative "rounds" where each discipline identified their top priority problems related to the patient case identified during the simulation. They discussed roles and responsibilities, patient-centered values, communication processes, and criticality of teamwork. Complexity in the simulation included error detection, verification of patient data, appreciation of changing status, and dosage parameters associated with age, body weight, and organ function. Both the simulation and debrief session were facilitated by nursing and pharmacy faculty, providing assistance as needed on content and the collaborative process. In the debrief, any within-profession jargon was addressed and clarified. Lack of actual patients and the absence of a physician in the consultation limited communication, however, and form the basis for our future plans.

In addition to basic case components, several cases had embedded errors or risk that students were expected to identify. For example, nursing students noted to pharmacy that potassium was still being administered even though potassium levels had reached normal range. In another example a mistake was detected when Zosyn (piperacillin/tazobactam) was substituted for Zofran (ondansetron) in the medications available for administration, even though the patient had a penicillin allergy. These safety "near misses" further strengthened the values, teamwork, and communication needed to correct medication errors by both nursing and pharmacy professions.

2.3. Surveys of Student Perceptions

A link to a 10-item survey was emailed to students (pharmacy) or available via the course learning management system (nursing). The survey was administered via SurveyMonkey. At the end of each lab session, the students were asked to complete the survey and given time in class to do so. The following questions were included in the survey (Table 1):

Table 1. Survey questions.

1.	What is your major field of study (nursing/pharmacy)?
2.	What did you learn today?
3.	What were your strengths during this activity?
4.	What were your areas for improvement during this activity?
5.	What recommendations for changing this activity do you have?
6.	What did you learn about interprofessional collaboration?
7.	What did you learn about the clinical application of kinetics in this simulation?
8.	What is the one thing you like better about lecture sessions as compared to simulation sessions?
9.	What is the one thing you like better about simulation sessions as compared to lecture sessions?
10.	Do you have any additional comments about the simulation or suggestions for improving the interprofessional education in the College of Health Sciences?

The study was conducted in accordance with the Declaration of Helsinki, and the University's Institutional Review Board approved this study as exempt since student responses were collected anonymously with no identifying information. The investigators individually gathered the results and identified themes among the responses. Student feedback was analyzed using content analysis for purposes of improving the teaching-learning environment and enhancing our knowledge of IPE and IPEC competencies. Results of the content analysis are presented below.

2.4. Significance of the Project

The safety and quality of patient care is dependent upon shared communication and understanding between health care professionals. Our project served as a template for the incorporation of interprofessional education standards into a new curriculum for the McWhorter School of Pharmacy, currently under development and scheduled for implementation in the fall of 2019. Additionally, Samford University's nursing program is exploring curriculum innovations and revisions, especially targeting opportunities for interprofessional experiences. The simulation served as a model for nursing and pharmacy interactions between each other and other health professions. This project represents a unique type of interprofessional simulation between pharmacy and nursing students related to pharmacokinetics. Interprofessional education plays an important role in both curricula, and is necessary to meet the standards for pharmacy school accreditation. Since both schools at our institution are exploring curricular revisions, this project can serve as a model for other simulations in the future.

3. Results

3.1. Sample and Response Rate

One hundred nineteen out of 145 students participated in the survey, giving a response rate of 82% (Spring 2018). Seventy-seven of the respondents (64.7%) were pharmacy students while 42 respondents (35.3%) were nursing students. Forty-two of the 54 (77.8%) nursing students and 77 of the 91 (84.6%) pharmacy students who participated in the simulation completed the survey.

3.2. Themes from Survey Responses

Themes are listed in Tables A1 and A2.

Five major areas emerged from the overall thematic analysis for the research: Interprofessional collaboration; interprofessional communication; values and ethics; roles and responsibilities; and teams and teamwork. Each of these areas relates to the Samford University College of Health Sciences IPE framework and core competencies. Other themes that arose from the data included: Safety; advocacy; appreciation for colleagues; patient-centered care; knowledge for practice; applying knowledge and evidence; professionalism; and improvements for the future. Each sample quote was selected based on a consensus of discussion of relevant themes that emerged. The data were not assessed quantitatively, therefore, frequency counts were not completed.

Interprofessional collaboration emerged as the overarching theme from the IPE event. Both pharmacy and nursing students found a common value in the collaboration efforts between the professions. They expressed the importance of working together to provide the best outcomes for the patient. The students also voiced the importance of combining discipline-specific knowledge to increase the level of care for patients.

"I learned that interprofessional collaboration can maximize the care at higher level versus working as two different units." (Pharmacy student)

"Interprofessional collaboration is vital to the health of our patients, as certain professions have more in-depth knowledge and different scopes of practice than others." (Nursing Student)

Participants also expressed an appreciation for interprofessional communication between the groups of students. The students recognized the importance of communicating with each other concerning patient status to ensure safe treatment for the patients.

"I learned the importance of communicating with nursing and other staff about monitoring labs and administering doses." (Pharmacy student)

"Pharmacy and nursing must have good communication between each other to ensure best possible care of the patient." (Nursing student)

Several students voiced interest in the different values and ethical concerns that were prioritized in the opposite profession.

"I recognized the difference between what nurses prioritize and what pharmacists generally prioritize." (Pharmacy student)

"I learned a lot about drug contraindications that I had never given thought before ... and when seeing patient allergies as well as medications ordered that a patient should not be receiving due to another medication ordered." (Nursing student)

Roles and responsibilities of both professions also emerged from the analysis. Students expressed strengths of their own profession, while also pointing out the strengths of the opposite profession throughout the scenario.

"We were the medication experts. Our strengths included correct dosing and side effects." (Pharmacy student)

"Our strengths were in assessment and specifics of care." (Nursing student)

"Nursing and Pharmacy work well together to identify patient problems. Nursing seemed to focus on the physical status of the patient while pharmacy tended to focus on the patients values. Together it made for a nice blend of patient centered care." (Pharmacy student)

"I learned that pharmacy is a good resource when you have questions about drugs and that they are very knowledgeable about the medications we were giving." (Nursing student)

"I loved to see how the pharmacy students truly focused on the medication and pharmacokinetics but I also loved showing them how the patient as a human being matters." (Nursing student)

The final major area that emerged during content analysis of the data was teams and teamwork. Participants expressed the importance of working as a team to improve patient outcomes. The students recognized the need for specialized skills set, but also the need to put the individual skills together to create a joint treatment plan.

"I learned about the complex and rewarding relationship of the nursing/pharmacy team and how our input can successfully treat a patient." (Pharmacy student)

"It really does take a team and good communication skills to improve a patient's treatment plan." (Nursing student)

In addition to the major areas that emerged during data analysis, a number of other themes were noted. Students from both professions noted an increase in knowledge for practice and expressed strength in applying knowledge and evidence from the IPE event.

"This was an excellent kinetics refresher." (Pharmacy student)

"It increased my knowledge of pharmacology, dosing, interactions, and complications of therapy." (Nursing student)

"Strength was using knowledge and applying to case studies." (Pharmacy student)

"I learned more about what pharmacy does and how much of a resource they are to our nursing practice in medication administration." (Nursing student)

Professionalism and appreciation for colleagues also emerged as themes from the IPE simulation event. Students conveyed the importance of holistically caring for individuals and using their specific skills to create the best patient outcomes. Participants also recognized the value other professions provide to the overall well-being of the patient. There was also acknowledgment of the other profession creating a different perspective of patient care.

"I need to do a better job at looking at the patient as a whole instead of basing it off of the limited numbers that I see." (Pharmacy student)

"It's important that we're knowledgeable about what other professions know and are capable of doing to maximize the outcomes of our patients." (Nursing student)

"I learned that all the different health professionals have something different to offer and it is so helpful when we put our ideas together." (Pharmacy student)

"Being able to be around pharmacy was nice concerning discussion of patient because they bring a new perspective." (Nursing student)

Themes of safety, advocacy and patient-centered care also emerged as themes from the data analysis. Participants expressed an awareness of interprofessional teams' role in the safe and effective care of patients.

"In order to make proper clinical decisions, it is important to verify the complete patient information with the nursing staff." (Pharmacy student)

"Effective communication is integral to good and safe care." (Nursing student)

"You need to treat the patient not necessarily the numbers you see. Interprofessionalism is also very important in treating the patient because the other members can tell you information that is not necessarily on the chart." (Pharmacy student)

"I learned how to properly voice patient situation and report to professionals from a different discipline." (Nursing student)

"Nursing and Pharmacy work well together to identify patient problems. Nursing seemed to focus on the physical status of the patient while pharmacy tended to focus on the patients' [lab] values. Together it made for a nice blend of patient centered care." (Pharmacy student)

Students were asked to explain what improvements could be made on the individual level and also for the simulation experience as a whole. Students expressed the need for greater communication with team members in the future, as well as increasing confidence in interacting with the other profession. In addition, both pharmacy students and nursing students conveyed the need to improve the use of the SBAR communication technique when reporting on the patient. Finally, students of both profession recognized the need for the nursing students to play a larger role in the simulation experience.

"Truly being engaged when interacting with the nursing students and members of other health professions. Not feeling uncomfortable with things I am unfamiliar with." (Pharmacy student)

"I can improve in my confidence concerning discussing patient findings with pharmacy. I want to always have it all together and there were some questions that my team did not have the answers to and that put down my confidence slightly." (Nursing student)

"Make sure that the nursing students know that what they are doing matters. Give them a bigger role in the simulation." (Pharmacy student)

"I feel like a little more planning on how to optimize the use of the nurses in the simulation would be very beneficial to the simulation experience for both professions." (Nursing student)

Participants were also asked to explain what areas of the simulation experience was preferred over a traditional lecture. Many students stated that they enjoyed the simulation experience as it allowed hands-on practice with real-life scenarios to encourage collaboration and critical thinking.

"Simulation give insight on real world situations that I see in work quite often. It is beneficial to see that we are being prepared based on real cases." (Pharmacy student)

"I learn well with hands on activities so simulations help me apply what I've read or learned in class to what I will actually be doing." (Nursing student)

"I like how it is hands-on application and gives me the ability to work with other people." (Pharmacy student)

"I like hands on learning and doing things physically helps me feel more comfortable in hospital situations because it gives me more practice." (Nursing student)

Although most students voiced preference for learning in the simulation environment, some students expressed the need for classroom lectures to set the foundational knowledge.

"Lecture sessions set the foundation for us to understand the material." (Pharmacy student)

"It gives us the appropriate information to perform well in simulation." (Nursing student)

4. Discussion

No studies were identified that investigated this collaboration between nursing and pharmacy students on the topic of pharmacokinetic dosing in a simulated educational setting, however there are numerous reports of interprofessional simulations on other topics between pharmacy and nursing students.

The five major themes from the data correlate with the CHS IPE framework. Other themes arose as well, which were investigated in other studies and allow for comparison. In the interest of highlighting one of the IPEC competencies most prominent in this study, it would likely be communication. This was one of the objectives for the pharmacy students ("communicate effectively in the care of a patient") and was an overarching theme in the students' comments. Pharmacy students had been taught the SBAR tool prior to the simulation to provide a common technique used by the nursing students. Communication was also the necessary vehicle for certain aspects of medication safety, such as the patient who was receiving potassium despite lab results indicating it was in the desired range.

This current simulation meets several of the IPEC sub-competencies for communication, such as:

- Choose effective communication tools and techniques, including information systems and communication technologies, to facilitate discussions and interactions that enhance team function.
- Communicate information with patients, families, community members, and health team members in a form that is understandable, avoiding discipline-specific terminology when possible.
- Express one's knowledge and opinions to team members involved in patient care and population health improvement with confidence, clarity, and respect, working to ensure common understanding of information, treatment, care decisions, and population health programs and policies.

Thurston and colleagues explored specific professional stereotypes reported by IPE-naive nursing and pharmacy students [9]. Pharmacy students viewed pharmacists significantly more favorably than nursing students viewed pharmacists in each area except for ability to work independently. In contrast, nursing students viewed nurses significantly less favorably than pharmacy students viewed nurses in academic ability and practical skills. The current study did not reveal more or less favorable perception of one discipline's skills or abilities. Instead students recognized their own strengths while also recognizing those of the other discipline.

Meyer and colleagues reported an overall favorable response to their interprofessional simulation to increase knowledge of pharmacology [15]. The current study reported a similar favorable response in knowledge for practice and in applying knowledge/evidence.

Effective communication was one of the objectives of this current simulation. Kostoff and colleagues reported that pharmacy students gained confidence in using SBAR and planned to incorporate it into their practice as future pharmacists [8]. The current study provided similar results. Not only did pharmacy students agree that the simulation improved their understanding of the SBAR tool, but they responded that they plan to use SBAR as a future pharmacist in healthcare communication. Nursing students had prior exposure to the SBAR format for communicating intra-professionally in patient hand-off but had not used it for interprofessional collaboration. One of the strengths of SBAR is its application to the patient's status. The giver must use critical thinking to determine the priority situation, assessment, and recommendation. The giver must select information for patient status to effectively communicate the immediate patient care issue. For nursing students it meant distilling their assessment to a focused communication to the pharmacists reflecting a medication concern. For the pharmacists their communications were strengthened by the common format and recommendations were readily understood in the context of the patient's overall care. Both groups agreed they needed more practice in use of SBAR.

Implications for Interprofessional Education

Nursing has welcomed interprofessional collaboration and IPE precisely because of its function on the frontline of patient-centered care. IPE experiences at the senior level can build on interprofessional communication approaches such as SBAR format. Nursing students at the senior level are integrating professional and clinical competencies and are well preparing to collaborate with interprofessional colleagues. In this study student perceptions specifically noted increased appreciation for their colleagues and their knowledge base in pharmacology, thus building trust and laying the groundwork for effective collaborative practice with pharmacists in the future.

Pharmacy has also welcomed interprofessional collaboration and education well in advance of its requirements in accreditation standards for schools of pharmacy. Recognizing the interactions that advanced practice pharmacy students and practicing pharmacists have with other health care providers, it is in the best interest of these students to provide them with opportunities to practice those earlier in the curriculum. The topic of pharmacokinetics provides an excellent setting for interprofessional education as this is a task where pharmacy and nursing professionals routinely interact.

Together, pharmacy and nursing students gained a higher appreciation for the others in their shared values of patient centered care, in their complementary roles, in general and applied knowledge of specific patients' needs, and in the teamwork required for effective and safe, high quality care. As educators, it is incumbent upon us to emphasize the professionalism of collaboration and importance of clear communication of within-profession jargon to the other profession in the development of collaborative IPE experiences. This simulation has provided preliminary support for further development of pharmacy–nursing simulations and collaborations in pharmacokinetics.

Future plans include incorporating standardized patient and a standardized physician provider to enhance real-world communication across all roles of medication prescribing, consulting, dispensing, and administration. Future plans also include developing evaluative measures to capture actual growth in collaborative skills and document improvements in patient safety outcomes.

Author Contributions: Conceptualization, J.B. and F.W.; Methodology, C.D.C., J.B., E.B. and F.W.; Formal Analysis, E.B. and A.B.; Investigation, C.D.C.; Data Curation, C.D.C.; Writing—Original Draft Preparation, C.D.C., J.B., E.B., F.W. and A.B.

Funding: This research received no external funding.

Acknowledgments: We wish to acknowledge Jill Hightower and Cindy Berry for their assistance with this project and Jill Pence, executive director, and faculty of the College of Health Sciences Experiential Learning and Simulation Center.

Appendix A

Table A1. Themes and pharmacy/nursing quotes on IPEC competencies and concepts.

Theme	Pharmacy	Nursing
Interprofessional collaboration	"We learned what information we needed from the nurses and what information nurses needed from us."	"Interprofessional collaboration is vital to the health of our patients, as certain professions have more in-depth knowledge and different scopes of practice than others."
	"I learned that interprofessional collaboration can maximize the care at higher level versus working as two different units."	
Interprofessional communication	"I learned the importance of communicating with nursing and other staff about monitoring labs and administering doses."	"Effective communication is integral to good and safe care."
		"Pharmacy and nursing must have good communication between each other to ensure best possible care of the patient."
Values/Ethics	"I recognized the difference between what nurses prioritize and what pharmacists generally prioritize."	"I learned a lot about drug contraindications that I had never given thought before...and when seeing patient allergies as well as medications ordered that a patient should not be receiving due to another medication ordered."
Roles/Responsibilities	"I learned about the nurse's thought processes and how we can work together for best care of the patient."	"Our strengths were in assessment and specifics of care."
	"Importance of communication with other professions and the differences in what other professions consider pertinent information versus what we as pharmacists think is the most important information."	"I loved to see how the pharmacy students truly focused on the medication and pharmacokinetics but I also loved showing them how the patient as a human being matters."
	"Nursing seemed to focus on the physical status of the patient while pharmacy tended to focus on the patients values. Together it made for a nice blend of patient centered care."	"I learned that pharmacy is a good resource when you have questions about drugs and that they are very knowledgeable about the medications we were giving."
	"Nursing and Pharmacy work well together to identify patient problems."	
	"We were the medication experts. Our strengths included correct dosing and side effects."	
Teams/Teamwork	"It takes a team to treat a patient."	"I learned how pharmacy can be consulted for med errors and medication alterations in the clinical setting."
	"I learned how to effectively work in a team with not only other pharmacy students, but also inter-professionally with the nursing students."	"It really does take a team and good communication skills to improve a patient's treatment plan."
	"I learned about the complex and rewarding relationship of the nursing/pharmacy team and how our input can successfully treat a patient."	
	"I have learned that collaborative team work is essential in developing an optimal patient care plan."	
	"Teamwork makes the dream work. Everyone's has a role to play and should be appreciated."	
Knowledge for practice	"This was an excellent kinetics refresher."	"It increased my knowledge of pharmacology, dosing, interactions, and complications of therapy."
Applying knowledge/evidence	"Strength was using knowledge and applying to case studies."	"I learned more about what pharmacy does and how much of a resource they are to our nursing practice in medication administration."
		"Being able to be around pharmacy was nice concerning discussion of patient because they bring a new perspective."

Table A1. *Cont.*

Theme	Pharmacy	Nursing
Professionalism	"I need to do a better job at looking at the patient as a whole instead of basing it off of the limited numbers that I see."	"It's important that we're knowledgeable about what other professions know and are capable of doing to maximize the outcomes of our patients."
	"I learned that it is very very important and each profession has a place to make the entire process work."	"I loved to see how the pharmacy students truly focused on the medication and pharmacokinetics but I also loved showing them how the patient as a human being matters."
Appreciation for colleagues	"I learned that all the different health professionals have something different to offer and it is so helpful when we put our ideas together."	"I learned more about what pharmacy does and how much of a resource they are to our nursing practice in med administration."
	"The patient always needs to be treated and not just the numbers."	"The patient always needs to be treated and not just the numbers."
		"Learned how to properly voice patient situation and report to professionals from a different discipline."
Patient-centered care	"Nursing and Pharmacy work well together to identify patient problems. Nursing seemed to focus on the physical status of the patient while pharmacy tended to focus on the patients' [lab] values. Together it made for a nice blend of patient centered care."	"Our strengths were in assessment and specifics of care."
	"I learned about a nurse's thought process when It comes to assessing a patient and how we can work together to get the best treatment for a patient."	"I learned about the importance I communicating with pharmacy to ensure our patient receive the best care."
Safety	"In order to make proper clinical decisions, it is important to verify the complete patient information with the nursing staff."	"Effective communication is integral to good and safe care."
Advocacy	"You need to treat the patient not necessarily the numbers you see. Interprofessionalism is also very important in treating the patient because the other members can tell you information that is not necessarily on the chart."	"We learned how to communicate and how to have a voice."
	"The patient always needs to be treated and not just the numbers."	"Learned how to properly voice patient situation and report to professionals from a different discipline."
Improvements for future	"There is still some confusion with calculating pharmacokinetic parameters differently for different drugs, and determining length of therapy for IV infusion/intermittent medications."	"I can improve in my confidence concerning discussing patient findings with pharmacy. I want to always have it all together and there were some questions that my team did not have the answers to and that put down my confidence slightly."
	"SBAR"	"SBAR"
	"I feel that I could better improve my communication skills and communicate in a more effective manner."	"I feel like a little more planning on how to optimize the use of the nurses in the simulation would be very beneficial to the simulation experience for both professions."
	"Truly being engaged when interacting with the nursing students and members of other health professions. Not feeling uncomfortable with things I am unfamiliar with."	
	"Thinking on my feet."	
	"Make sure that the nursing students know that what they are doing matters. Give them a bigger role in the simulation"	

Table A2. Students' comparisons of simulation and lecture.

	Pharmacy	Nursing
What is the one thing you like better about lecture sessions as compared to simulation sessions?	"Learning the information to be used in application sessions."	"It gives us the appropriate information to perform well in simulation."
	"Lecture sessions set the foundation for us to understand the material."	"You are given more detail and time to process information."
	"I like actually having the information directly in front of me to be able to learn from."	"Information is directly provided to us instead of us having to figure it out."
		"Lecture sessions occur at a rate in which I expect."
		"There are less expectations during lecture so I can focus 100% on the information being taught."
What is the one thing you like better about simulation sessions as compared to lecture sessions?	"I like how it is hands-on application and gives me the ability to work with other people."	"I learn well with hands on activities so simulations help me apply what I've read or learned in class to what I will actually be doing."
	"Simulation give insight on real world situations that I see in work quite often. It is beneficial to see that we are being prepared based on real cases."	"I like hands on learning and doing things physically helps me feel more comfortable in hospital situations because it gives me more practice."
	"I enjoy a change of scenery and being able to improve my skills in different settings."	"I love being hands-on. It is also easier to define my role as a nurse and the role of the pharmacist."
		"It's incredibly hands in and feels like you're working with a real patient."

References

1. World Health Organization. Framework for Action on Interprofessional Education and Collaborative Practice. 2010. Available online: http://www.who.int/hrh/resources/framework_action/en/ (accessed on 27 May 2018).
2. Interprofessional Education Collaborative (IPEC). *Core Competencies for Interprofessional Collaborative Practice: 2016 Update*; Interprofessional Education Collaborative: Washington, DC, USA, 2016.
3. Berry, C.G.; Hightower, J.; Harrison, L.; Barron, A.; Buckner, E.B. Interprofessional collaboration of nursing and pharmacy students achieved through case study examination. In Proceedings of the Alabama League for Nursing Annual Conference, Tuscaloosa, AL, USA, 2 March 2018.
4. Smithburger, P.L.; Kane-Gill, S.L.; Kloet, M.A.; Lohr, B.; Seybert, A.L. Advancing interprofessional education through the use of high fidelity human patient simulators. *Pharm. Pract. (Granada)* **2013**, *11*, 61–65. [CrossRef] [PubMed]
5. Liaw, S.Y.; Siau, C.; Zhou, W.T.; Lau, T.C. Interprofessional simulation-based education program: A promising approach for changing stereotypes and improving attitudes toward nurse-physician collaboration. *Appl. Nurs. Res.* **2014**, *27*, 258–260. [CrossRef] [PubMed]
6. Alanazi, A.A.; Nicholson, N.; Thomas, S. The Use of Simulation Training to Improve Knowledge, Skills, and Confidence Among Healthcare Students: A Systematic Review. *Internet J. Allied Health Sci. Pract.* **2017**, *15*, 1–24.
7. Costello, M.; Huddleston, J.; Atinaja-Faller, J.; Prelack, K.; Wood, A.; Barden, J.; Adly, S. Simulation as an Effective Strategy for Interprofessional Education. *Clin. Simul. Nurs.* **2017**, *13*, 624–627. [CrossRef]
8. Kostoff, M.; Burkhardt, C.; Winter, A.; Shrader, S. An interprofessional simulation using the SBAR communication tool. *Am. J. Pharm. Educ.* **2016**, *80*, 157. [CrossRef] [PubMed]
9. Thurston, M.M.; Chesson, M.M.; Harris, E.C.; Ryan, G.J. Professional stereotypes of interprofessional education naive pharmacy and nursing students. *Am. J. Pharm. Educ.* **2017**, *81*, 84. [CrossRef] [PubMed]

10. Monahan, L.; Sparbel, K.; Heinschel, J.; Rugen, K.W.; Rosenberger, K. Medical and pharmacy students shadowing advanced practice nurses to develop interprofessional competencies. *Appl. Nurs. Res.* **2017**, *39*, 103–108. [CrossRef] [PubMed]

11. Poirier, T.I.; Pailden, J.; Jhala, R.; Ronald, K.; Wilhelm, M.; Jingyang, F. Student self-assessment and faculty assessment of performance in an interprofessional error disclosure simulation training program. *Am. J. Pharm. Educ.* **2017**, *81*, 54. [CrossRef] [PubMed]

12. Wilson, A.J.; Palmer, L.; Levett-Jones, T.; Gilligan, C.; Outram, S. Interprofessional collaborative practice for medication safety: Nursing, pharmacy, and medical graduates' experiences and perspectives. *J. Interprof. Care* **2016**, *30*, 649–654. [CrossRef] [PubMed]

13. Bell, H.T.; Granas, A.G.; Enmarker, I.; Omli, R.; Steinsbekk, A. Nurses' and pharmacists' learning experiences from participating in interprofessional medication reviews for elderly in primary health care—A qualitative study. *BMC Fam. Pract.* **2017**, *18*, 30. [CrossRef] [PubMed]

14. Stehlik, P.; Frotjold, A.; Schneider, C.R. Effect of hospital simulation tutorials on nursing and pharmacy student perception of interprofessional collaboration: Findings from a pilot study. *J. Interprof. Care* **2018**, *32*, 115–117. [CrossRef] [PubMed]

15. Meyer, B.A.; Seefeldt, T.M.; Ngorsuraches, S.; Hendricks, L.D.; Lubeck, P.M.; Farver, D.K.; Heins, J.R. Interprofessional education in pharmacology using high-fidelity simulation. *Curr. Pharm. Teach. Learn.* **2017**, *9*, 1055–1062. [CrossRef] [PubMed]

16. Zuna, I.; Holt, A. ADAM, a hands-on patient simulator for teaching principles of drug disposition and compartmental pharmacokinetics. *Br. J. Clin. Pharmacol.* **2017**, *83*, 2426–2449. [CrossRef] [PubMed]

13

The Attitude of Medical and Pharmacy Students towards Research Activities: A Multicenter Approach

Akshaya Srikanth Bhagavathula [1,*] ⓘ, Deepak Kumar Bandari [2], Yonas Getaye Tefera [1], Shazia Qasim Jamshed [3] ⓘ, Asim Ahmed Elnour [4] and Abdulla Shehab [5]

[1] Department of Clinical Pharmacy, University of Gondar-College of Medicine and Health Sciences, School of Pharmacy, Gondar 196, Ethiopia; yonas1get@gmail.com

[2] Department of Clinical Pharmacy, Vaagdevi College of Pharmacy, Warangal 506001, Telangana, India; laxmideepak.pharma@gmail.com

[3] Department of Pharmacy Practice, Kulliyyah of Pharmacy, International Islamic University Malaysia, Kuantan 25200, Pahang, Malaysia; shazia_12@yahoo.com

[4] Faculty of Pharmacy, Fathima College of Health Sciences, Al Ain Campus, Al Ain 24162, UAE; asim.ahmed@fchs.ac.ae

[5] Department of Internal Medicine, College of Medicine and Health Sciences, UAE University, Al Ain 17666, UAE; A.shehab@uaeu.ac.ae

* Correspondence: akshaypharmd@gmail.com or akshaya.srikanth@uog.edu.et

Academic Editor: Jeffrey Atkinson

Abstract: Aim: To assess the attitude of medical and pharmacy students in Asian and African universities towards scholarly research activities. **Methods:** An anonymous, cross-sectional, self-reported online survey questionnaire was administered to medical and pharmacy students studying in various Asian and African universities through social media between May and July 2016. A 68-item close-ended questionnaire consisting of Likert-scale options assessed the students' research-specific experiences, and their attitudes towards scholarly research publications. **Results:** A total of 512 questionnaires were completed, with a response rate of 92% from Asia and 94% from Africa. More pharmacy students (70.8%) participated than medical students (29.2%). Overall 52.2% of the pharmacy students and 40% of medical students believed that research activities provided a means of gaining respect from their faculty members. Lack of encouragement, paucity of time, gaps in research activities and practices, and lack of research funding were some of the most common barriers acknowledged by the students. A nonparametric Mann-Whitney test showed that a statistically significant difference was observed, in that more than 80% of the pharmacy students viewed scientific writing and research activities as valuable experiences ($p = 0.001$) and would like to involve their co-students in scholarly research activities ($p = 0.002$); whereas the majority of the medical students desired to be involved more in scholarly research publications ($p = 0.033$). **Conclusion:** Pharmacy students had good attitudes towards research activities and a higher number of medical students desired to be involved more in research publications. Faculties may consider taking special research initiatives to address the barriers and improve the involvement of medical and pharmacy students in scholarly research activities.

Keywords: medical students; pharmacy students; attitude; research activities; publications

1. Introduction

Providing comprehensive patient care is an important component of all healthcare professions (HCPs). For the provision of effective care, future workers in HCPs are expected to be trained in all aspects, and to exercise proficient skills in their research-based academic education and professional practice. In order to create impact-laden critical reasoning abilities among future healthcare practitioners, research activities should be followed by seminars, conference presentations and publications as part and parcel of every healthcare discipline globally. Thus, one cannot sideline the importance of scholarly research activities as an essential component of a complete medical and health sciences curriculum in undergraduate and postgraduate education. Moreover, the initiation and incorporation of evidence-based knowledge is emphasized globally as an essential component in the modern science education. For the past few decades, a changing trend has been observed regarding the inclusion of research components in medical and pharmacy education [1–10]. These changes drive the interest among students in conducting research, and presenting and publishing their work at national and international levels. The ability of a student to carry out scholarly research is an added advantage for their academic advancement through acquisition of critical thinking and analytical skills, as well as through comprehension and analysis of the foundations of evidence-based medicine [11–13]. Several studies have shown that research experience at a student level is strongly associated with future career achievements and scholarly research initiatives [13–15]. Conducting scholarly research activities at student level is an arduous task, and in the context of this, several barriers have been reported, including lack of time, lack of support from faculties, and lack of funding sources, among others [1,11,14,16]. Despite these difficulties and predicaments, medical and pharmacy students perform their research projects across the globe.

Positive attitudes to and opportunities for research activities with adequate provision of facilities and mentorship will equip medical and other health profession students for becoming future healthcare scientists. Early identification of their passion towards research will help to discern their inclination, as well as their potential scope for professional practice in the clinical setting. Most undergraduate medicine and pharmacy programs require coursework in epidemiology, research methodology, biostatistics and literature evaluation [6,7].

However, given the demand and competing interest towards scholarly research, several studies have identified attitudinal ambivalence towards the significance of scholarly research publication [16–19]. We believe medical and pharmacy students are among the students in the major health profession discipline, who represent potential future leaders in clinical and pharmaceutical research. With this in mind, it is worth studying the attitudes of medical and pharmacy students regarding research activities. Furthermore, a better understanding of medical and pharmacy students' attitudes, of the barriers involved, and of mentors' influence, culminating in scholarly research activities and journal publication, is valuable.

The current research is an attempt in this regard, and therefore aims to investigate attitudes towards the scholarly research activities of medical and pharmacy students.

2. Methods

This was a cross-sectional survey conducted on medical and pharmacy students enrolled in various Asian (Malaysia, India, Saudi Arabia and the United Arab Emirates) and African universities (Ethiopia, Kenya and Egypt). A web-based survey through anonymous questionnaire was administered during the period May–July 2016. This online survey was designed and primarily used to gather data about students' scholarly research activities through internet and social networking sites, as well as through personal emails. The questionnaire was focused on medical and pharmacy students via an online survey instrument tool. Furthermore, e-mails carried a Uniform Resource Locator-URL link to the online survey developed and distributed through social network sites like Facebook, LinkedIn, and Twitter to encourage student participation.

Medical and pharmacy students who were enrolled at Asian and African universities were the source population. The targeted population was senior medical and pharmacy students, who were randomly selected from various universities.

An online sample size calculator—"Creative research systems" [17,19]—was used to determine the number of participants for the survey, by considering 95% confidence level with an accuracy of

50% for a student population size of 135,000 across various universities; given a confidence interval of 4.2, the recommended sample size was 542 or more. Estimating a dropout rate of 10–15%, a total of 620 students were invited to participate in the survey. Participation within these representative samples was completely voluntary, and confidentiality was maintained at all stages by not disclosing any personal information in the survey results.

The study investigators designed the survey, and the items were adopted and/or modified based on a review of the literature [1–3,6,7,13–17,19,20]. The survey questionnaire was developed in English, and tested for reliability, psychometrics, internal content and construct validity in a methodological, structured approach. A Cronbach alpha exploratory factor analysis was used as a measure of reliability. The internal consistency estimate of the reliability of the test (Cronbach's alpha) was found to be 0.76, indicating a good construct. The questionnaire was pretested in fifteen percent of the total sample size, which was not included in the study. Further, any ambiguous and unsuitable questions were modified for the final questionnaire.

The study questionnaire consisted of 68 close-ended questions subdivided into 3 categories. The first part included the socio-demographic characteristics, and contained 10 items, including age, gender, region of origin, type of studentship (medical/pharmacy), academic year, living area, type of institution, previous research grant experience, the time dedicated for research grant searching, and the number of scholarly research publications. Furthermore, the second part was comprised of 4 domains, which included a 3-point Likert scale of their priorities, which highlighted their preferences for the type of research articles that were interested in publishing (8 items), their reasons for practicing research publishing (9 items), and the important obstacles to conducting research (10 items). In addition, 12 items focused on their preferences regarding writing for publications, as well as the types of journals in which they preferred to publish their scholarly research activities (9 items). The third section contained 10 items related to their opinions towards the value of scholarly research publications, and were assessed using a 4-point Likert scale (1-strongly disagree to 4-strongly agree). The survey took an average of ten to fifteen minutes to complete.

A statistical analysis was performed using Statistical Package for Social Sciences (SPSS) version 22 for Windows. Descriptive statistics were used to describe demographics and research background experiences. For ease of reporting, differences using agreement responses of high priority (i.e., responses with "agree" and "strongly agree") were grouped together. Disagreement responses of low priority, "strongly disagree" and "disagree" of the Likert scale, were utilized. Mann-Whitney (M-W) and Chi-square tests were conducted to further analyze their opinions on possible perceptions towards scholarly research activities. Statistical significance was based on a p-value of < 0.05.

Ethical approval for conducting the study was obtained from the Institutional review board of the School of Pharmacy, University of Gondar, Ethiopia. Written informed consent was obtained from each participant prior to the administration of the study questionnaire. Confidentiality of the information of the respondents was strictly maintained.

3. Results

A total of five hundred and twelve student participants completed the survey questionnaire, with response rates of 92% from Asia and 94% from Africa. A higher percentage of pharmacy students (70.8%) participated in the survey than medical students (29.2%). The mean age of individuals sampled is 23 ± 1.42 years (range = 19–30), with 324 males (63.2%). In particular, the majority of the participants were from the fourth year of pharmacy (54.6%), studying in public universities (65.1%), and living outside their study campus (54.8%). Regarding interest towards scholarly research activities, only 19.1% (98/512) had received a research grant for conducting their research, and 48.6% of the medical and pharmacy students stated that they did not dedicate time to searching for grants. In addition, 72.5% did not publish any scholarly research (Table 1).

Table 1. Demographic characteristics of medical and pharmacy students ($N = 512$).

	Medical ($n = 150$)	Pharmacy ($n = 362$)	Total (%)
Age (years)			
<20	6	14	20 (3.9)
20–25	113	307	420 (82.0)
26–30	31	40	71 (13.8)
>30	0	1	1 (0.1)
Gender			
Male	117	207	324 (63.2)
Female	33	155	188 (36.7)
Academic year			
Fourth	80	280	360 (70.3)
Fifth	39	64	103 (20.1)
Sixth	31	18	49 (9.5)
Living area			
Outside University	44	237	281 (54.8)
Within University	106	125	231 (45.1)
Type of institution			
Public	135	198	333 (65.1)
Private	15	164	179 (34.9)
Received research grant			
Yes	26	72	98 (19.1)
No	124	290	414 (80.8)
Time dedicated for grant searching			
No hours	80	169	249 (48.6)
Daily	16	91	107 (20.8)
Weekly	27	61	88 (17.1)
Monthly	27	41	68 (13.2)
Number of scholarly research publications			
No publications	128	244	372 (72.6)
1–2	20	64	84 (16.4)
3–5	2	28	30 (5.8)
6–10	0	13	13 (2.5)
11–15	0	4	4 (0.7)
16–20	0	3	3 (0.5)
>20	0	6	6 (1.1)

Nearly 43% of both medicine and pharmacy students agreed that they were interested in focusing on original research, and 4.7% of both medical and pharmacy students were interested in systematic review studies, with a slightly higher preference by pharmacy students ($p < 0.004$). A significant number of students shared that the reasons for interest in scholarly research publications was to improve their relationships with and gain respect from faculty members (48.6%), to improve writing and research skills (44.1%), and to advance their career opportunities (42%). Nearly forty percent of the respondents from both medical and pharmacy groups felt that lack of support from their faculties, lack of time for conducting research and existence of gaps within research activities to their practice were some of the perceived barriers to conducting research. (Table 2).

Table 2. Attitude of medical and pharmacy students towards research interests ($N = 512$).

Variables	Agreement of High Priority		Percentage	p Value
	Medical ($n = 150$)	Pharmacy ($n = 362$)		
Research publications interested				
Original research	54	165	42.7	0.432
Multicenter studies	26	67	18.1	0.456
Randomized controlled trial	17	50	13.1	0.233
Meta-analysis	7	28	6.8	0.182
Systematic review	2	22	4.7	0.004
Observational studies	2	21	4.5	0.100
Comparative studies	2	18	3.9	0.854
Retrospective studies	2	12	2.7	0.105
Reasons for publications				
Advance research/share findings	32	180	41.4	<0.001 [a]
Interesting/good experience	42	116	30.8	0.041
Was encouraged by teachers	27	179	40.2	<0.001 [a]
Good achievements/goals	21	57	15.2	0.881
Compulsion from peers	34	177	41.2	<0.001 [a]
Both Job/Career advancement	45	170	41.9	<0.001 [a]
Improve writing and research skills	57	169	44.1	0.108
Better chances of to get international recognition	38	118	30.4	0.035
To have a relationship with or to gain respect from faculty members	60	189	48.6	0.010
Obstacles for conducting research				
No research course taught at faculty level	35	115	29.2	0.043
Lack of funding	37	127	32	0.006
Time-limitations	56	138	37.8	0.639
Lack of support, encouragement and rewards	70	131	39.2	0.046
The gap between research activities and practice	64	131	38	0.676
Fear of statistics and data collection	36	83	23.2	0.297
Lack of interest	34	56	17.5	<0.001 [a]
No research unit at faculty	32	88	23.4	0.643
No research in the field I am most interested in	19	68	16.9	0.734
Relationship obstacles-barriers-difficulties	19	62	15.8	0.121

[a] Mann-Whitney test was used to determine significance, defined as $p < 0.05$.

The results of the Chi-square test for difference between medical and pharmacy students in terms of their opinion on different types of research activity interests showed that there was a significant difference based on student disciplines. Interestingly, significant differences were noticed in relation to the type of research activities, except for data analysis ($p > 0.05$), the publication process ($p > 0.05$) and recognition for their research work ($p > 0.05$) (Table 3). However, the differences were significant for reviewing literature, data interpretation, writing manuscripts, collaborative research with different faculties, research learning experiences, sense of satisfaction for their research work, sharing their research ideas, and students' experiences for conducting research. Thus, the null hypothesis was accepted for three items, but rejected for these eight items. There was a difference between pharmacy and medical students for 'data interpretation' ($p > 0.001$) and 'experience for conducting research' ($p > 0.001$). Students were asked to indicate the type of journals preferred for scholarly publication using a 3-point Likert scale. The Chi-square test for differences between medical and pharmacy students' opinions on journal preferences suggests there was a statistical difference, except in their preference for open-access paid journals, paid journals with impact factors, free journals with impact factors, and Pubmed- and Scopus-indexed journals (Table 3). Therefore, the null hypothesis for journal selection was accepted for five of the nine items, but rejected in the case of open-access free journals, fast-track publishing journals, Embase indexed journals, and preferring only reputed journals for their scholarly research publications.

Table 3. Attitude of medical and pharmacy students regarding type of research activity (N = 512).

Students Interest Writing for publications		N	Chi-Square	df	p Value
Review/literature search	Medical	150	4.55	1	0.033
	Pharmacy	362			
Analyzing data	Medical	150	1.681	1	0.195
	Pharmacy	362			
Data interpretation	Medical	150	66.62	1	<0.001 [a]
	Pharmacy	362			
Writing research report, proposal or manuscript	Medical	150	8.79	1	0.003
	Pharmacy	362			
Collaboration with others or with faculty	Medical	150	7.27	1	0.007
	Pharmacy	362			
The learning experience	Medical	150	24.77	1	<0.001 [a]
	Pharmacy	362			
Sense of accomplishment/satisfaction/achievement	Medical	150	3.84	1	0.050
	Pharmacy	362			
Publication process, submission, approval and published articles appearance online	Medical	150	0.62	1	0.431
	Pharmacy	362			
Recognition	Medical	150	0.01	1	0.913
	Pharmacy	362			
Sharing ideas/adding to literature/ advancing research	Medical	150	13.53	1	<0.001 [a]
	Pharmacy	362			
A unique experience that is available to only a few students	Medical	150	24.49	1	<0.001 [a]
Type of Journals preferred for publication	Pharmacy	362			
Open access-paid journals	Medical	150	0.20	1	0.654
	Pharmacy	362			
Open access-free journals	Medical	150	8.68	1	0.003
	Pharmacy	362			
Paid journals with impact factors	Medical	150	2.75	1	0.097
	Pharmacy	362			
Free journals with impact factors	Medical	150	1.59	1	0.207
	Pharmacy	362			
Fast-track publishing journals	Medical	150	9.05	1	0.003
	Pharmacy	362			
Pubmed indexed journals	Medical	150	0.82	1	0.365
	Pharmacy	362			
Science direct/Scopus indexed journals	Medical	150	0.47	1	0.493
	Pharmacy	362			
Embase indexed journals	Medical	150	22.08	1	<0.001 [a]
	Pharmacy	362			
Only reputed journals (Lancet, Nature etc)	Medical	150	5.57	1	0.018
	Pharmacy	362			

df-differential fraction; [a] Chi-square was used to determine the significance, defined as $p < 0.05$.

Table 4 shows the result of Mann-Whitney U test for differences between medical and pharmacy students' opinions towards the value of research publications and mentor influence. Seventy-six percent of the medical and 78% of the pharmacy students felt that publishing as a student would provide them personal fulfillment. A similar percent reported that their mentors encouraged them to conduct research for publications. Interestingly, a higher proportion of pharmacy students perceived their overall writing for research publication as a good experience ($p < 0.05$), contributing to the literature during student life as a valuable experience ($p < 005$), and would likely encourage their co-students to engage in scholarly research publications ($p < 0.05$). Similarly, a high proportion of medical students perceived that they would like to publish more manuscripts for research publications, but no statistical significance was noted in this context.

Table 4. Medical and pharmacy students' attitude regarding the value of publishing and mentor influence ($N = 512$).

Statements	Agreement		p Value
	Medical Students (%)	Pharmacy Students (%)	
Publishing as a student provided me with personal fulfillment	76.6%	78.4%	0.257
Contribution to the literature as a student is a valuable experience	66.6%	82.8%	<0.001 [a]
Publishing is an excellent source of recognition for students	72.6%	78.4%	0.022
Publishing as a student provided me with formative training experience	67.3%	79.0%	<0.001 [a]
My publication will set me apart from my peers	51.3%	56.0%	0.228
I would like to publish more manuscripts	81.3%	72.6%	0.219
I encourage my co-students to publish	72.6%	81.4%	0.002
Overall, writing for publication is a good experience	70.0%	85.6%	<0.001 [a]
I received encouragement from a mentor to conduct the research for publications	71.3%	70.7%	0.282
My results with helpful for the scientific evidence	54.6%	78.7%	<0.001 [a]

Note: Responses 3 and 4 in 4-point Likert scale were grouped as "agreement" for reporting purposes; [a] Mann-Whitney test was used to determine the significance, defined as $p < 0.05$.

4. Discussion

In the current research, there are a few notable obstacles reported in terms of conducting and/or performing research. Inappropriate funding, lack of support both in kind and cash from the mentors and the institutes, and paucity of time are the hallmarks of non-accomplishment of research tasks. Aside from these, the limited number of research courses taught within medical and pharmacy curricula is one of the barriers claimed by students to conducting research. These findings mirror the conclusion derived from research in Saudi Arabia and Brazil, which showed that similar factors were predominantly cited as obstacles to conducting research [4,14,21]. Another interesting factor—'lack of same-gender research mentor'—was also outlined in recently published study by Kharraz and colleagues from Saudi Arabia [21]. Several barriers to scholarly research activities have been identified, such as lack of faculty members with appropriate expertise and sufficient time for mentoring, limited resources, and logistical difficulties [13,22].

The students have shown interest towards original article publications, and reasons for which scholarly publication was considered valuable included improving their relationships with and gaining respect from faculty members, advancing their career opportunities, and improving their writing and research skills. Research skills for pharmacy students (under- and postgraduates) are becoming more important, particularly for obtaining a decent job in a competitive market, and in order to attain scholarships for higher postgraduate studies [7,23,24]. Medical students can be potential contributors to scientific research development through participation in different clinical studies and evidence-based clinical training [8,11,25]. It is noted in the current research that slightly less than half of the respondents reported scholarly research publications as a means to improve the relationship with and gain respect from faculty members, as well as improving their writing and research skills. The motivation itself comes from research regarding whether it would be implemented as a 'core module' in future Asian and African medical and pharmacy schools. This can encompass not only research methodology aspects but can also address students' motivation for doing literature search on one's own interests, leading to critical appraisal of published studies. This literature review can serve as the backbone of one's research proposal, which itself contains minute details on executing the research and analyzing the research findings. Moreover, this concept is mirrored in a United States study in which a research elective course on dietary supplements was introduced for pharmacy students. The study findings reported enriched critical reasoning abilities and drug-literature evaluation skills among the student participants, which later contributed towards their practice readiness [24].

The medical and pharmacy schools in many developing countries are not yet offering optimum scholarly scientific writing and research opportunities [19,22,24]. To make it practically possible in Asian and African medical and pharmacy schools, sincere dedication from the faculty in terms of intellectual support and unlimited time can contribute as silently lingering motivators, culminating in the quality of the research, further motivating the student to make it publishable. Interestingly, studies from Germany and Saudi Arabia have reported that the majority of students are motivated to conduct research in order to attain and/or secure research publications [14,25]. In Saudi Arabia, one of the motivators worth mentioning is the mandatory nature of research in curricula [14]. Likewise, for nearly two decades in Germany, medical students have been required to complete a research project followed by a research thesis in order to obtain their medical degree [25]. Nykamp and associates reported that participation of pharmacy students in collaborative scholarly research opportunities with faculty members led to encouraging feedback, personal contentment, and career advancement prospects [13]. These examples can serve as models for Asian and African medical and pharmacy schools for the instituting of research modules as a core aspect in their curricula. The 'Norwegian Medical Student Research Program' is a grant scheme for all prospective and aspiring medical students to support doing research in parallel with their studies [26]. This program fortified their research environment, and helped to develop new areas of research by augmenting recruitment towards research. Nevertheless, it also instilled the inspiration to include research in the training of medical doctors [26].

The majority of the medical and pharmacy students in this study felt that publishing as a student would provide them personal fulfillment and a formative training experience, as well as regarding writing for publication to be a good experience; others claimed their mentors encouraged them to conduct research for publications. Cultivating and motivating student participation in research activities in addition to their curricular coursework should be encouraged.

Research sensitization in all undergraduate and graduate students should be advocated to enhance student participation in scholarly research activities, and to equip them with practical research experience to nurture them as future scientists.

We recommend that mindfulness towards research be addressed nationally in every Asian and African country, which could also galvanize research funding resources by means of a clear-cut expected outcome of scholarly publications and presentations in repuyearbook journals and conferences.

5. Limitations

A high response rate (>90%) is one of the strengths of the current research, and therefore contributes to the validity and usefulness of the research. Previously published studies reported response rates of not more than 75% [2,11,16,21], and we achieved a highly satisfactory response rate (>90%) [27]. Furthermore, due to the anonymous nature of the current research, the chances of bias are reduced. This does not sideline the importance of limitations, which need to be highlighted in the current research. As in any cross-sectional study, this study also adopted self-reported measures, which are generally subject to recall bias and participants' exaggerated responses; secondly, despite pilot testing of the instrument, it was not subjected to formal standardization. Due to an underpowered sample in our study, this may contribute to both false-positive and false-negative reporting by rejecting true null hypotheses [28]; therefore, caution should be taken while interpreting our findings. Furthermore, it seems that medical students are underreported in the current research, so non-responders bias is therefore a possibility not to be overlooked. We cannot generalize the findings to pharmacy and medical students on other continents, as this study only focused on those in the Asian and African region.

6. Conclusions

The present study shows pharmacy students had good attitudes towards research activities, with a higher number of medical students desiring to engage more in research publications. Faculties should implement special research initiatives to address the barriers and improve the involvement of medical and pharmacy students in scholarly research activities. The current research can serve as motivation to further explore undergraduate students' opinions towards and experiences of scholarly research activities.

Acknowledgments: We deeply express our gratefulness to the participants for giving their valuable opinions and sharing their experiences for fulfilling this research work.

Author Contributions: For research articles with several authors. ASB planned and conducted the study analysed the results and wrote the paper; DKB & YGT collected the data, entered the data into spss and anaylsed the data; ASB & AAE performed the statistical analysis, wrote and edited the paper, YGT & AS wrote and edited the paper. SQJ analysed the results, wrote and edited the paper; all the authors equally contributed in planning the study, analysed the results, wrote and edited the paper.

References

1. Amin, T.T.; Kaliyadan, F.; Al Qattan, A.E.; Al Majed, H.M.; Al Khanjaf, S.H.; Mirza, M. Knowledge, attitude and barriers related to participation of medical students in research in three Arab Universities. *Educ. Med. J.* **2012**, *4*, 43–56. [CrossRef]

2. Ismail, M.I.; Bazli, M.Y.; O'Flynn, S. Study on medical student's attitude towards research activities between University College Cork and Universiti Sains Malaysia. *Procedia Soc. Behav. Sci.* **2014**, *116*, 2645–2649. [CrossRef]

3. Reinders, J.J.; Kropmans, T.J.; Cohen-Schotanus, J. Extracurricular research experience of medical students and their scientific outputs after graduation. *Med. Educ.* **2005**, *39*, 237. [CrossRef] [PubMed]

4. Sadana, R.; D'Souza, C.; Hyder, A.A.; Chowdury, A.M. Importance of health research in South Asia. *BMJ* **2004**, *328*, 826–830. [CrossRef] [PubMed]

5. Sreedharan, J. Introduction of a research component in undergraduate medical curriculum-review of a trend. *Nepal J. Epidemiol.* **2012**, *2*, 200–204. [CrossRef]

6. Munabi, G.; Katabira, E.T.; Konde-Lule, J. Early undergraduate research experience at Makerere University Faculty of Medicine: A tool for promoting medical research. *Afr. Health Sci.* **2006**, *6*, 182–186. [PubMed]

7. Murphy, J.E.; Slack, M.K.; Boesen, K.P.; Kriking, D.M. Research-related coursework and research experience in Doctor of Pharmacy programs. *Am. J. Pharm. Educ.* **2007**, *7*, 113. [CrossRef]

8. Mark, A.L.; Kelch, R.P. Clinician scientist training program: A proposal for training medical students in clinical research. *J. Investig. Med.* **2001**, *49*, 486–490. [CrossRef] [PubMed]

9. Basnet, B.; Bhandari, A. Investing in medical student's research: Promoting future of evidence based medicine in Nepal. *Health Renaiss.* **2013**, *11*, 297–300. [CrossRef]

10. Holder, G.M.; Jones, J.; Robinson, R.A.; Krass, I. Academic literacy skills and progression rates among pharmacy students. *High. Educ. Res. Dev.* **1991**, *18*, 19–30. [CrossRef]

11. Burgoyne, L.N.; O'Flynn, S.; Boylan, G.B. Undergraduate medical research: The student perspective. *Med. Educ. Online* **2010**, *15*, 5212. [CrossRef] [PubMed]

12. Collins, J.P.; Farish, S.; McCalman, J.S.; McColl, G.J. A mandatory intercalated degree programme: Revitalising and enhancing academic and evidence-based medicine. *Med. Teach.* **2010**, *32*, e541–e546. [CrossRef] [PubMed]

13. Nykamp, D.; Murphy, J.E.; Mashall, L.L.; Bell, A. Pharmacy students' participation in a research experience culminating in journal publication. *Am. J. Pharm. Educ.* **2010**, *74*, 47. [CrossRef] [PubMed]

14. AlGhamdi, K.M.; Moussa, N.A.; AlEssa, D.S.; AlOthimeen, N.; Al-Saud, A.S. Perceptions, attitudes and practices towards research among senior medical students. *Saudi Pharm. J.* **2014**, *22*, 113–117. [CrossRef] [PubMed]

15. Dong, T.; Durning, S.J.; Gilliland, W.R.; Waechter, D.M.; Cruess, D.F.; DeZee, K.J. Exploring the relationship between self-reported experiences and performance in medical school and internship. *Mil. Med.* **2012**, *177*, 11–15. [CrossRef] [PubMed]

16. Siemens, D.R.; Punnen, S.; Wong, J.; Kanji, N. A survey on the attitude towards research in medical school. *BMC Med. Educ.* **2010**, *10*, 4. [CrossRef] [PubMed]

17. Kritikos, V.S.; Saini, B.; Carter, S.; Moles, R.J.; Krass, I. Factors influencing pharmacy students' attitudes towards pharmacy practice research and strategies for promoting research in pharmacy practice. *Pharm. Pract.* **2015**, *13*, 587. [CrossRef] [PubMed]

18. Creative Research System. Available online: http://www.surveysystem.com/sscalc.html (accessed on 14 January 2015).

19. Kritikos, V.S.; Carter, S.; Moles, R.J.; Krass, I. Undergraduate pharmacy students' perceptions of research in general and attitudes towards pharmacy practice research. *Int. J. Pharm. Pract.* **2013**, *21*, 192–201. [CrossRef] [PubMed]

20. Abu-Gharbieh, E.; Khalidi, D.A.; Baig, M.R.; Khan, S.A. Refining knowledge, attitude and practice of evidence-based medicine (EBM) among pharmacy students for professional challenges. *Saudi Pharm. J.* **2015**, *23*, 162–166. [CrossRef] [PubMed]

21. Oliveira, C.C.; de Souza, R.C.; Abe, É.H.S.; Silva Móz, L.E.; de Carvalho, L.R.; Domingues, M.A. Undergraduate research in medical education: A descriptive study of students' views. *BMC Med. Educ.* **2014**, *14*, 1–8. [CrossRef] [PubMed]

22. Kharraz, R.; Hamadah, R.; AlFawaz, D.; Attasi, J.; Obeidat, A.S.; Alkattan, W.; Abu-Zaid, A. Perceived barriers towards participation in undergraduate research activities among medical students at Alfaisal University—College of Medicine: A Saudi Arabian perspective. *Med. Teach.* **2016**, *38*, S12–S18. [CrossRef] [PubMed]

23. Wagner, J. A framework for undergraduate research in economics. *South Econ. J.* **2015**, *82*, 668–672. [CrossRef]

24. Islam, M.A.; Gunaseelan, S.; Khan, S.A. A Research Elective Course on Dietary Supplements to Engage Doctor of Pharmacy Students in Primary Literature Evaluation and Scholarly Activity. *J. Pharm. Pract.* **2015**, *28*, 577–584. [CrossRef] [PubMed]

25. Cursiefen, C.; Altunbas, A. Contribution of medical student research to the Medline TM-indexed publications of a German medical faculty. *Med. Educ.* **1998**, *32*, 439–440. [CrossRef] [PubMed]

26. Hunskaar, S.; Breivik, J.; Siebke, M.; Tømmerås, K.; Figenschau, K.; Hansen, J.-B. Evaluation of the medical student research programme in Norwegian medical schools. A survey of students and supervisors. *BMC Med. Educ.* **2009**, *9*, 1–8. [CrossRef] [PubMed]

27. Beretta, R. A critical review of the Delphi technique. *Nurse Res.* **1996**, *3*, 79–89. [CrossRef] [PubMed]

28. Button, K.S.; Ioannidis, J.P.A.; Mokrysz, C.; Nosek, B.A.; Flint, J.; Robinson, E.S.J.; Munafò, M.R. Power failure: Why small sample size undermines the reliability of neuroscience. *Nat. Rev. Neurosci.* **2013**, *14*, 365–376. [CrossRef] [PubMed]

14

Curriculum Mapping of the Master's Program in Pharmacy in Slovenia with the PHAR-QA Competency Framework

Tanja Gmeiner, Nejc Horvat, Mitja Kos, Aleš Obreza, Tomaž Vovk, Iztok Grabnar and Borut Božič *

Faculty of Pharmacy, University of Ljubljana, Aškerčeva 7, 1000 Ljubljana, Slovenia;
Tanja.Gmeiner@ffa.uni-lj.si (T.G.); Nejc.Horvat@ffa.uni-lj.si (N.H.); Mitja.Kos@ffa.uni-lj.si (M.K.);
Ales.Obreza@ffa.uni-lj.si (A.O.); Tomaz.Vovk@ffa.uni-lj.si (T.V.); Iztok.Grabnar@ffa.uni-lj.si (I.G.)
* Correspondence: borut.bozic@ffa.uni-lj.si

Academic Editor: Jeffrey Atkinson

Abstract: This article presents the results of mapping the Slovenian pharmacy curriculum to evaluate the adequacy of the recently developed and validated European Pharmacy Competences Framework (EPCF). The mapping was carried out and evaluated progressively by seven members of the teaching staff at the University of Ljubljana's Faculty of Pharmacy. Consensus was achieved by using a two-round modified Delphi technique to evaluate the coverage of competences in the current curriculum. The preliminary results of the curriculum mapping showed that all of the competences as defined by the EPCF are covered in Ljubljana's academic program. However, because most EPCF competences cover healthcare-oriented pharmacy practice, a lack of competences was observed for the drug development and production perspectives. Both of these perspectives are important because a pharmacist is (or should be) responsible for the entire process, from the development and production of medicines to pharmaceutical care in contact with patients. Nevertheless, Ljubljana's graduates are employed in both of these pharmaceutical professions in comparable proportions. The Delphi study revealed that the majority of differences in scoring arise from different perspectives on the pharmacy profession (e.g., community, hospital, industrial, etc.). Nevertheless, it can be concluded that curriculum mapping using the EPCF is very useful for evaluating and recognizing weak and strong points of the curriculum. However, the competences of the framework should address various fields of the pharmacist's profession in a more balanced way.

Keywords: pharmacy education; competences; curriculum mapping; community pharmacy; industrial pharmacy; clinical pharmacy; Delphi study; quality assurance; European framework

---

1. Introduction

Traditional universities structured programs with a defined number of courses, exams, and contact hours. It was up to the teachers to know what students needed in order to graduate from the university. The system was rather clear and worked smoothly. The majority of older pharmacists received their degrees through education structured in this way, and the pharmacy profession developed well, even excellently. Three independent factors resulted in a need to change this mindset in order to introduce competence-oriented curricula: (a) a significantly greater amount of information (not necessarily knowledge), (b) a shorter half-life of research-based knowledge, and (c) an increasing number of universities due to drastic changes in the expectations of the general population. Namely, only 2% of the population was expected to participate in higher education in the 19th century, compared to the European trend of the 21st century, in which 40% of the population is expected to participate in higher education. The change is not an issue of quantity alone, but also a question of quality. To meet the needs and expectations of society, curricula need to be reoriented from a structured mode to a competence-oriented mode [1,2].

Pharmacy education has deep roots in Slovenia. The principles of quality work in the pharmaceutical profession were introduced as early as in the 17th and 18th centuries. In 1710, a Pharmaceutical code was introduced for the Duchy of Carniola. Under the Illyrian Provinces at the beginning of the 19th century, pharmacy was taught through *materia medica* and pharmaceutical chemistry as the main subjects at the Central school in Ljubljana. Competences in pharmaceutical technology were built through traineeship at community or hospital pharmacies. University teaching of pharmacy was established in Ljubljana in the mid-20th century, with the first attempts in 1946 and 1955 as a two-year program, and starting in 1960 as a complete eight-semester program [3]. The development of undergraduate pharmacy education including clinical chemistry was based on the connection between research and practical applications in all fields of the pharmaceutical profession and science. The program was revamped several times, and it was extended to a four-and-a-half-year program in the mid-1990s. To show the integrity of the competences obtained, the curricula included awarding a diploma for individual student research work from the very beginning. After receiving their degrees, the graduates were employed as healthcare professionals (at community pharmacies, hospital pharmacies, and medical laboratories), researchers (in the public or private sector), in the pharmaceutical industry (in all four sectors: research and development, production, quality assurance, and marketing and sales), as teachers (at high schools and universities), or as professionals in pharmaceutical legislation. For employment, graduates needed to complete a probationary period and pass the final state exam. Several minor changes in the probation period based on future employers' needs were introduced before the program was harmonized according to European directives in 2004, when Slovenia entered the EU. Six months of traineeship in a pharmacy was included in the curriculum in the last semester of the five-year program [4]. Finally, the program was revamped and improved as a part of the Bologna process to a 10-semester uniform masters program: eight semesters of lectures, seminars, lab work, and other activities, one semester (6 months) of traineeship in pharmacies, and one semester of individual research work for the master's thesis. The state exam for pharmacists as healthcare professionals was integrated into the last semester, and was completed with a public defense of the master's thesis. The program was accredited by the National Agency for Quality in Higher Education in 2007 and was reaccredited in 2015 [5].

Several stakeholders were involved in the process of reform and accreditation through roundtables, workshops, meetings, written opinions, and other means. These included teachers from the university faculties involved (pharmacy, chemistry, medicine, mathematics, and physics), students (through the student counsel and the pharmacy students association), graduates, professional societies and chambers (the Slovenian Pharmaceutical Society, the Slovenian Chamber of Pharmacies, and the Slovenian Chamber of Laboratory Medicine), potential employers such as directors of community and hospital pharmacies, generic and innovative industry, and regulators (the Ministry of Health, and the Public Agency for Medicinal Products and Medical Devices). With this approach, we addressed recommendations by High Level Group on the Modernization of Higher Education, published in 2013 [1]. Namely, the program provides competences for employment in community pharmacies, hospital pharmacies, the pharmaceutical industry, medical laboratories, research laboratories, legislation, and education [6]. In some areas, an additional three or four years of specialization (as training) is necessary for special areas of the pharmacy profession, such as specializations in clinical pharmacy, medical design, medical testing, clinical chemistry, and radiopharmacy. Doctoral study is open after a degree in several fields, such as pharmacy, clinical chemistry and laboratory medicine, toxicology, biochemistry and molecular biology, and genetics [7].

The master's program in pharmacy was designed for the first-day-of-job-pharmacist; that is, for novices or beginners with limited experience [8] to be able to work autonomously. During the education process, competences are built from lower to higher levels, and therefore horizontal and vertical course linkages are very important. The primary objective of the Faculty of Pharmacy is to develop scientifically and professionally qualified, high-quality graduates familiar with ethical principles that autonomously carry out demanding tasks in community and hospital pharmacies, in all fields of the pharmaceutical industry, in clinical laboratories and laboratory medicine, laboratories for drug control and analysis, research institutions, educational organizations, state bodies, and wherever the work and presence of a pharmacist is required to increase health safety [9]. The faculty's commitment to quality teaching and research has been shown through many activities, including participation in projects initiated by EAFP [10], such as Pharmacy Education in Europe (Pharmine) and Quality Assurance in European Pharmacy Education and Training (PHAR-QA).

The European Commission has funded the international project PHAR-QA [11] to produce a consensual, harmonized framework of competences for pharmacy practice across Europe. This framework is intended to be used as a base for a QA system for evaluating university pharmacy education and training at the institutional, national, and/or European levels [12]. The second round of the PHAR-QA survey of competences for pharmacy practice in Europe was completed in 2016 [13].

The aim of this study was to evaluate the usefulness of the framework developed for pharmaceutical competences as a tool for mapping the master's pharmacy curricula by matching the existing curriculum of the master's program in pharmacy in Slovenia to the framework.

2. Materials and Methods

A team of seven members of the teaching staff in the integrated master's program in pharmacy [6] at the University of Ljubljana's Faculty of Pharmacy was involved in curriculum mapping. Two members of the team have previously been involved in the PHAR-QA project [11]; three members are responsible for coordinating the master's program, international student exchange, and traineeship as part of undergraduate study; and four members of the team are also members of the faculty management. The mapping was carried out and evaluated progressively, as indicated.

Step 1: A Microsoft Excel file was generated composing a matrix of 50 European Pharmacy Competences Framework (EPCF) competences [13] versus 60 courses in the master's curriculum. For greater transparency of the file, clusters are separated into individual worksheets and the competences within each cluster are listed in the y-axis. Courses were listed in a "drop-down" form for each year of the program in the x-axis (Figure 1).

Step 2: Primary mapping was done by a single member of the team, who copy-pasted the competences as described in the master's curriculum from each course individually based on personal assessment of the matching. In cases where competences were defined more generically (covering multiple competences), they were mapped in two or more PHAR-QA competences. For example: the competence from the program "Students acquire basic knowledge about drug action within an organism and the organism's reaction upon exposure to drug(s)" was mapped in "(29) Ability to compile and interpret a comprehensive drug history for an individual patient," "(34) Ability to identify and prioritize drug-disease interactions (e.g., NSAIDs in heart failure) and advise on appropriate changes to medication," and "(35) Knowledge of the bio-pharmaceutical, pharmacodynamic, and pharmacokinetic activity of a substance in the body."

If the description was too general, such as: "Development of competences and skills of using knowledge in a particular professional area," or not listed in the EPCF list, the faculty's competence was listed in a separate worksheet.

Step 3: The result of the primary mapping was individually evaluated and revised by the coordinator of the master's program, coordinator of the international student exchange, and coordinator of the traineeship. The revision was made based on their thorough knowledge of the course syllabuses.

Step 4: The final review of the mapping process and evaluation was made by all seven members of the team. Special attention was paid to:

- Competences absent from the curriculum;
- The number of times each competence was addressed in the curriculum;
- Building competences through teaching from lower to higher levels;
- Dedicated time and ECTS credits planned in the curriculum for teaching to build individual competences.

Step 5: Gaps and inconsistences in the curriculum and EPCF list were identified.

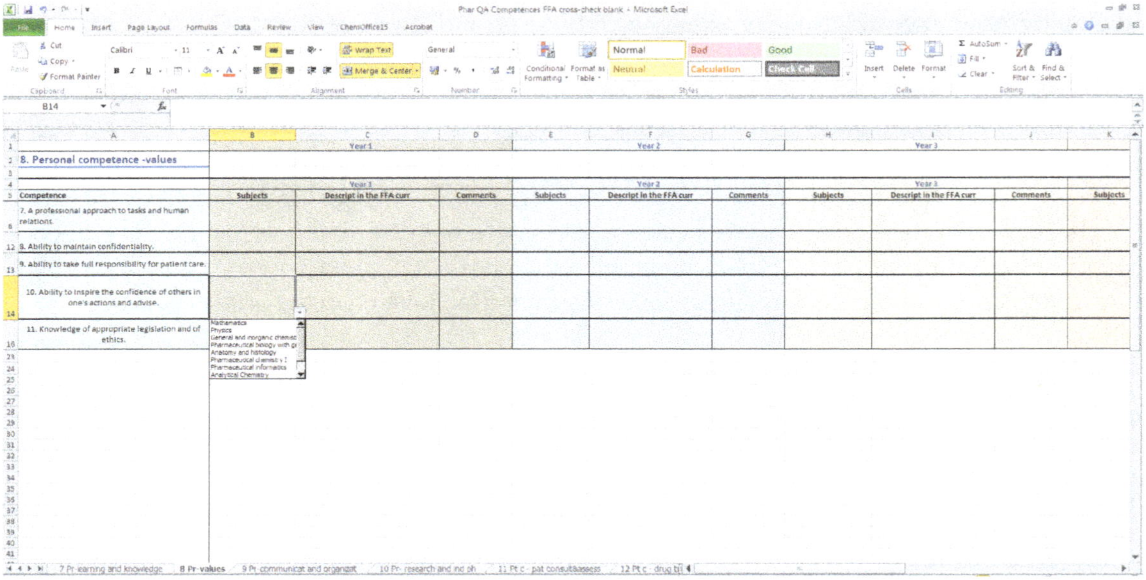

Figure 1. Screen-shot of the worksheet of a Microsoft Excel file generated for curricula mapping. Each worksheet includes one cluster of competences as defined by the Quality Assurance in European Pharmacy Education and Training (PHAR-QA) project (11). The competences within the clusters are listed in the ordinate. The courses in the master's curriculum are arranged in "drop-down" form, matching the individual year of the master's program in the abscissa.

The level of agreement of scores among individual evaluators participating in the study was assessed using the Delphi methodology [14,15]. A Delphi consensus panel was run with the aim of evaluating coverage of competences as defined by the PharQA framework in the current master's curriculum. The Delphi expert panel included four independent ratings performed by two individuals and two teams with two evaluators working together. The evaluators were six faculty professors that have insight into the pharmacy curriculum. The Delphi study consisted of two rounds. In the first round, panelists rated the coverage of the competences in the curriculum. Coverage was scored using the following five-point Likert-type scale: 0 = not covered at all, 1 = poor, 2 = fair, 3 = good, 4 = very good. Consensus on the coverage of competences was defined as the range of individual scores (Max–Min) being one or less. The panelists were also asked to provide comments on the clarity and their understanding of competences.

After the first round, the expert panel members met for a roundtable discussion. The results of the first round were presented and the panelists discussed the items for which consensus on coverage had not been attained and clarified the differences in ratings. In the second round, the panelists once again rated the coverage of competences, taking into account the roundtable discussion, the median of the panelists' answers, and the response distribution from the first round. Consensus was defined as the range being one or less.

3. Results

The starting point was the EPCF list of competences, and whether and where a particular competence is present in the curriculum was checked. The Slovenian pharmacy master's curriculum consists of 60 courses (subjects) in a 10-semester uniform program including a six-month traineeship in pharmacy, individual research work, and a master's thesis defense. The preliminary results of the competence mapping are presented in Table 1. The numbering of the competences in the table is consistent with the numbering in the PHAR-QA project [13], in which the first six questions address the profile of the respondents (age, duration of practice, country of residence, and current occupation) and were not included in the mapping process. The questions in clusters 7–16 are reflected in 60 competences for pharmacy practice across Europe: clusters 7–10 cover personal competences, and clusters 11–17 cover patient care competences.

Table 1. Results of curriculum mapping of the competences in the Slovenian master's program in pharmacy. Subjects are arranged by program years, and clusters of competences are defined by PHAR-QA. The numbers indicate how many competences from each cluster are defined in each of the subjects. Subjects are listed in alphabetical order by each year of the program.

Subject	7-Learning and Knowledge	8-Values	9-Communication and 9-Organisational 9-Skills	10-Research and Industrial Pharmacy	11-Patient Consultation and Assessment	12-Need for Drug Treatment	13-Drug Interactions	14-Drug dose and Formulation	15-Patient Education	16-Provision of Information and Service	17-Monitoring of Drug therapy	ECTS	Sum of All Competences Per Subject
	Personal Competences				Patient Care Competences								
Year 1													
Analytical Chemistry	2	0	0	0	0	0	0	0	0	0	0	8	2
Anatomy and histology	0	0	0	0	0	1	0	0	0	0	0	4	1
General and inorganic chemistry	2	0	0	0	0	0	0	0	0	0	0	8	2
Introduction to pharmacy	1	4	0	2	0	0	0	0	0	0	0	3	7
Mathematics	1	0	0	0	0	0	0	0	0	0	0	7	1
Microbiology	0	0	0	0	1	1	0	0	0	0	0	4	2
Pharmaceutical biology with genetics	5	3	3	0	0	0	0	0	0	0	0	7	11
Pharmaceutical chemistry I	2	0	0	0	0	0	0	0	0	0	0	6	2
Pharmaceutical informatics	1	0	1	1	0	0	0	0	0	0	2	5	5
Physics	1	0	0	0	0	0	0	0	0	0	0	8	1
Year 2													
Organic chemistry	0	0	1	1	0	0	0	0	0	0	0	9	2
Pharmaceutical biochemistry	2	0	0	0	0	0	0	0	0	1	0	7	3
Pharmaceutical chemistry II	1	0	0	1	0	1	1	1	0	0	0	7	5
Pharmaceutical technology I	1	1	4	4	0	0	0	1	0	1	0	20	12
Physical chemistry	1	0	0	0	0	0	0	0	0	0	0	6	1
Physical pharmacy	0	0	0	1	0	0	0	0	0	0	0	5	1
Physiology	1	0	0	0	1	0	0	0	0	0	0	6	2
Year 3													
Cosmetology	1	0	0	1	0	0	0	0	0	0	0	5	2
Hospital Pharmacy	0	1	3	1	0	1	0	1	0	0	1	5	8
Immunology	2	0	1	0	0	1	0	0	0	0	0	5	4
Instrumental Analytical Methods in Pharmacy	1	0	0	0	0	0	0	0	0	0	0	5	1
Instrumental pharmaceutical analysis	1	0	1	1	0	0	0	0	0	0	0	4	3
Nutritional Supplements	2	2	3	0	0	0	0	0	0	1	0	5	8
Pathologic physiology	2	0	0	0	0	1	0	0	0	0	0	6	3

Table 1. *Cont.*

Cluster of Competences / Subject	7-Learning and Knowledge	8-Values	9- Communication and 9-Organisational 9-Skills	10- Research and Industrial Pharmacy	11- Patient Consultation and Assessment	12- Need for Drug Treatment	13- Drug Interactions	14- Drug dose and Formulation	15- Patient Education	16- Provision of Information and Service	17- Monitoring of Drug therapy	ECTS	Sum of All Competences Per Subject
	Personal Competences				Patient Care Competences								
Year 3													
Pharmaceutical chemistry III	0	0	1	3	0	0	2	1	0	0	0	20	7
Pharmaceutical Marketing and Management	0	0	1	1	0	0	0	1	0	0	0	5	3
Pharmaceutical technology II	1	1	1	2	0	0	0	0	0	0	0	8	5
Pharmacoeconomics	0	0	2	0	0	0	0	0	0	0	1	5	3
Pharmacognosy I	2	2	3	0	0	0	0	0	0	1	0	9	8
Pharmacognosy II	2	2	3	1	0	0	0	1	0	0	0	4	9
Research methods in social Pharmacy	0	0	0	1	0	0	0	1	0	0	2	5	4
Social pharmacy	2	0	4	0	0	0	0	2	2	2	5	4	17
Year 4													
Analysis and supervision of medicinal products	2	0	0	4	0	0	0	0	0	0	0	8	6
Biochemistry of Cancer Development and Progression	1	1	0	0	0	0	0	0	0	0	0	5	2
Biopharmaceutical Evaluation of Pharmaceutical Forms	0	0	0	1	0	0	0	1	0	0	0	5	2
Biopharmaceutics with pharmacokinetics	0	0	0	2	0	1	2	2	0	0	0	9	7
Clinical chemistry	1	0	2	1	3	0	0	0	0	0	0	7	7
Clinical pharmacy	1	4	0	0	0	4	3	1	2	2	3	5	20
Design and Synthesis of Active Substances	1	0	0	1	0	0	0	1	0	0	0	5	3
Eutomers	0	0	0	2	0	0	0	1	0	0	0	5	3
Industrial pharmacy	1	0	0	4	0	0	0	0	0	0	0	5	5
Medicinal Products of alternative Medicine	3	2	2	0	0	0	0	0	0	0	0	5	7
Modified Release Pharmaceutical Forms	2	1	0	1	0	0	0	0	0	0	0	5	4
Pharmaceutical biotechnology	2	2	2	3	0	0	0	2	0	0	0	6	11
Pharmaceutical Engineering	0	0	0	1	0	0	0	0	0	0	0	5	1
Pharmacogenomics and Genetic Medicines	1	1	1	2	0	0	1	0	0	0	0	5	6
Pharmacology	1	0	0	0	0	1	2	2	0	0	0	5	6
Phytopharmaceuticals	2	2	0	0	0	0	0	0	0	1	0	5	5
Psychotropic substances and Abuse of Medicinal Products	1	0	0	0	0	2	0	0	0	0	0	5	3
Quality of Medicinal Products	0	0	0	3	0	0	0	0	0	0	0	5	3
Selected Methods of Pharmaceutical Analysis	1	0	0	0	0	0	0	0	0	0	0	5	1
Selected Topics in Clinical Biochemistry	0	0	0	0	2	0	0	0	0	0	0	5	2
Selected Topics in Pharmaceutical Biotechnology	1	2	3	2	0	0	0	1	0	0	0	5	9
Stability of medicinals	1	0	0	1	0	0	0	0	0	0	0	5	2
The Use of Genetic and Cellular Testing in Biomedicine and Pharmacy	0	1	1	0	1	0	1	0	0	0	0	5	4
Toxicological chemistry	1	0	0	1	0	1	0	0	0	0	0	5	3
Year 5													
Individual research work for master's thesis	1	1	2	0	0	0	0	0	0	0	0	25	4
Master's thesis defence	2	1	2	0	0	0	0	0	0	0	0	5	5
Traineeship	3	4	7	2	1	3	3	4	3	3	3	30	36
Sum	68	39	58	57	9	18	15	25	7	13	17	410	

Legend:

1st year of study
2nd year of study
3rd year of study
4th year of study
5th year of study

All competences as defined by the EPCF are covered in our master's curriculum, although their distribution among subjects and across program years is not balanced. During the first two years of the master's program, in which the curriculum contains typically basic subjects in the natural sciences, personal competences from clusters 7 through 11 are predominantly covered, especially those dealing with abilities to learn independently and apply logic to solve problems. Later in the program, competences from all groups are distributed more evenly. It is also evident that each subject addresses at least one EPCF competence.

The preliminary results are a rough estimate of how competences are covered in our curriculum. It was obvious that the description of competences in the curriculum was not sufficient for adequate scoring. Namely, some competences are addressed several times in a particular subject and it is not clear to what extent the competence is actually covered (i.e., mentioned, discussed, or elaborated). On the other hand, it is not possible to recognize progression in the level and sequence of student learning and performance through the program. For this reason, the evaluation was enhanced by using the Delphi approach.

Tables 2 and 3 present coverage of competence domains and individual competences in the first and second rounds of the Delphi study. Table 4 presents consensus building between the first and second rounds of the Delphi study.

Table 2. Coverage of competence domains as defined by the PHAR-QA framework in the Slovenian pharmacy curriculum. Results from both rounds of the Delphi study are presented as weighted medians of all competences in the domain. Coverage was scored using a five-point Likert-type scale: 0 = not covered at all, 1 = poor, 2 = fair, 3 = good, 4 = very good.

Domain	Coverage of the Competency Domain	
	1st Round Weighted Median	2nd Round Weighted Median
7. Personal competences: learning and knowledge.	3,4	3,4
8. Personal competences: values.	2,7	2,6
9. Personal competences: communication and organizational skills.	2,2	2,2
10. Personal competences: research and industrial pharmacy.	3,0	3,0
11. Patient care competences: patient consultation and assessment.	2,7	3,0
12. Patient care competences: need for drug treatment.	2,3	2,3
13. Patient care competences: drug interactions.	2,2	2,3
14. Patient care competences: drug dose and formulation.	3,3	3,2
15. Patient care competences: patient education.	2,0	2,0
16. Patient care competences: provision of information and service.	2,7	2,8
17. Patient care competences: monitoring of drug therapy.	2,0	2,0

Legend: An MS Excel three-color scale algorithm was used to present the results of the Delphi rounds, whereby the lowest value is presented in red, the highest in green, and the median in yellow.

Table 3. Coverage of individual competences as defined by the PHAR-QA framework in the Slovenian pharmacy curriculum. Results from both rounds of the Delphi study are presented. Coverage was scored using a five-point Likert-type scale: 0 = not covered at all, 1 = poor, 2 = fair, 3 = good, 4 = very good.

Competency Organised According to Domains	Coverage of Individual Competencies	
	1st Round Median (Min–Max)	2nd Round Median (Min–Max)
Domain: 7. Personal competences: learning and knowledge.		
1. Ability to identify learning needs and to learn independently (including continuous professional development (CPD).	3 (2–4)	3 (3–3)
2. Ability to apply logic to problem solving.	4 (4–4)	4 (4–4)
3. Ability to critically appraise relevant knowledge and to summarise the key points.	4 (3–4)	4 (3–4)
4. Ability to evaluate scientific data in line with current scientific and technological knowledge.	4 (3–4)	4 (4–4)

Table 3. *Cont.*

Competency Organised According to Domains	Coverage of Individual Competencies	
	1st Round Median (Min–Max)	2nd Round Median (Min–Max)
Domain: 7. Personal competences: learning and knowledge.		
5. Ability to apply preclinical and clinical evidence-based medical science to pharmaceutical practice.	3 (2–3)	3 (3–3)
6. Ability to apply current knowledge of relevant legislation and codes of pharmacy practice.	2,5 (2–4)	2,5 (2–3)
Domain: 8. Personal competences: values.		
1. A professional approach to tasks and human relations.	3 (2–4)	3 (3–4)
2. Ability to maintain confidentiality.	3 (2–4)	3 (3–3)
3. Ability to take full responsibility for patient care.	2 (1–2)	2 (1–2)
4. Ability to inspire the confidence of others in one's actions and advise.	2 (2–3)	2 (2–3)
5. Knowledge of appropriate legislation and of ethics.	3,5 (2–4)	3 (3–4)
Domain: 9. Personal competences: communication and organisational skills.		
1. Ability to communicate effectively—both oral and written—in the locally relevant language.	3 (3–4)	3 (3–4)
2. Ability to effectively use information technology.	2,5 (2–3)	2,5 (2–3)
3. Ability to work effectively as part of a team.	3 (2–4)	3 (3–3)
4. Ability to implement general legal requirements that impact upon the practice of pharmacy (e.g., health and safety legislation, employment law).	2,5 (2–4)	2,5 (2–3)
5. Ability to contribute to the training of staff.	1 (1–2)	1 (1–2)
6. Ability to manage risk and quality of service issues.	2 (1–2)	2 (1–2)
7. Ability to identify the need for new services.	1,5 (1–2)	1,5 (1–2)
8. Ability to understand a business environment and develop entrepreneurship.	2 (1–2)	2 (1–2)
Domain: 10. Personal competences: research and industrial pharmacy.		
1. Knowledge of design, synthesis, isolation, characterisation and biological evaluation of active substances.	4 (4–4)	4 (4–4)
2. Knowledge of good manufacturing practice and of good laboratory practice.	3 (3–4)	3 (3–4)
3. Knowledge of European directives on qualified persons.	1,5 (1–2)	1,5 (1–2)
4. Knowledge of drug registration, licensing and marketing.	3 (3–4)	3 (3–4)
5. Knowledge of the importance of research in pharmaceutical development and practice.	3,5 (2–4)	3,5 (3–4)
Domain: 11. Patient care competences: patient consultation and assessment.		
1. Ability to interpret basic medical laboratory tests.	4 (1–4)	4 (3–4)
2. Ability to perform appropriate diagnostic tests e.g., measurement of blood pressure or blood sugar.	1 (0–3)	2 (0–3)
3. Ability to recognise when referral to another member of the healthcare team is needed.	3 (2–3)	3 (2–3)
Domain: 12. Patient care competences: need for drug treatment.		
1. Ability to retrieve and interpret information on the patient's clinical background.	3 (1–3)	3 (3–3)
2. Ability to compile and interpret a comprehensive drug history for an individual patient.	2 (1–3)	2 (2–3)
3. Ability to identify non-adherence to medicine therapy and make an appropriate intervention.	2 (1–3)	2 (2–2)
4. Ability to advise to physicians on the appropriateness of prescribed medicines and—in some cases—to prescribe medication.	2 (1–3)	2 (1–2)
Domain: 13. Patient care competences: drug interactions.		
1. Ability to identify and prioritise drug-drug interactions and advise appropriate changes to medication.	3 (2–3)	3 (2–3)
2. Ability to identify and prioritise drug-patient interactions, including those that prevent or require the use of a specific drug, based on pharmaco-genetics, and advise on appropriate changes to medication.	1,5 (1–3)	2 (1–2)
3. Ability to identify and prioritise drug-disease interactions (e.g., NSAIDs in heart failure) and advise on appropriate changes to medication.	2 (1–2)	2 (1–2)
Domain: 14. Patient care competences: drug dose and formulation.		
1. Knowledge of the bio-pharmaceutical, pharmacodynamic and pharmacokinetic activity of a substance in the body.	4 (4–4)	4 (4–4)
2. Ability to recommend interchangeability of drugs based on in-depth understanding and knowledge of bioequivalence, bio-similarity and therapeutic equivalence of drugs.	3 (2–4)	3 (3–4)
3. Ability to undertake a critical evaluation of a prescription ensuring that it is clinically appropriate and legally valid.	2,5 (1–3)	2 (2–2)
4. Knowledge of the supply chain of medicines thus ensuring timely flow of quality drug products to the patient.	3 (2–3)	3 (2–3)
5. Ability to manufacture medicinal products that are not commercially available.	4 (3–4)	4 (3–4)

Table 3. *Cont.*

Competency Organised According to Domains	Coverage of Individual Competencies	
	1st Round Median (Min–Max)	2nd Round Median (Min–Max)
Domain: 15. Patient care competences: patient education.		
1. Ability to promote public health in collaboration with other professionals within the healthcare system.	2 (2–3)	2 (2–3)
2. Ability to provide appropriate lifestyle advice to improve patient outcomes (e.g., advice on smoking, obesity, etc.).	2 (2–3)	2 (2–3)
3. Ability to use pharmaceutical knowledge and provide evidence-based advice on public health issues involving medicines.	2 (2–3)	2 (2–3)
Domain: 16. Patient care competences: provision of information and service.		
1. Ability to use effective consultations to identify the patient's need for information.	2 (1–3)	2 (1–2)
2. Ability to provide accurate and appropriate information on prescription medicines.	3,5 (3–4)	3,5 (3–4)
3. Ability to provide evidence-based support for patients in selection and use of non-prescription medicines.	2,5 (2–4)	3 (3–4)
Domain: 17. Patient care competences: monitoring of drug therapy.		
1. Ability to identify and prioritise problems in the management of medicines in a timely and effective manner and so ensure patient safety.	2 (2–3)	2 (2–3)
2. Ability to monitor and report Adverse Drug Events and Adverse Drug Reactions (ADEs and ADRs) to all concerned, in a timely manner, and in accordance with current regulatory guidelines on Good Pharmacovigilance Practices (GVPs).	1,5 (1–2)	1,5 (1–2)
3. Ability to undertake a critical evaluation of prescribed medicines to confirm that current clinical guidelines are appropriately applied.	2,5 (2–3)	2,5 (2–3)
4. Ability to monitor patient care outcomes to optimise treatment in collaboration with the prescriber.	2 (1–2)	2 (1–2)
5. Ability to contribute to the cost effectiveness of treatment by collection and analysis of data on medicines use.	2 (1–3)	2 (2–3)

Legend: Results from the second round of the Delphi study that are shaded represent medians that changed from the first round of the Delphi study.

Table 4. Consensus building between the first and second rounds of the Delphi study. The frequency of ranges of individual scores (Max–Min) evaluating coverage of individual competences as defined by the PHAR-QA framework in the Slovenian pharmacy curriculum.

Range of Individual Scores (Max–Min)		2nd Round					
		0	1	2	3	4	Sum
	0	3	0	0	0	0	3
	1	2	25	0	0	0	27
1st	2	6	12	0	0	0	18
Round	3	0	1	0	1	0	2
	4	0	0	0	0	0	0
	Sum	11	38	0	1	0	50

4. Discussion

Evaluation was performed based on the curriculum [6]. The performance of the program (i.e., educational outcomes of the competences achieved) was not part of our study. The authors of this study are aware of different approaches in curriculum mapping. The final goal is to compare intended, perceived, and achieved competences as evaluated by students, graduates, teachers, and employers. Such mapping would be very useful in improving the program and its performance [16,17]. However, for preliminary mapping with the available resources, only the first step was realistic: mapping the curriculum delivered as written in the accreditation documents, expanded by evaluation of the competences present in the curricula as explained in the section Materials and Methods.

The master's program in pharmacy in Slovenia educates students for both aspects of pharmacy practice—working in health services and the pharmaceutical industry in approximately the same proportion—and most EPCF competences cover healthcare-oriented pharmacy practice; this is also reflected in the results of our evaluation. Personal competences are addressed with relatively higher frequencies due to the fact that the EPCF predominantly covers healthcare-oriented pharmacy competences. Namely, the definition of the pharmacy profession or pharmacy practice at the international level is not always clear [18]. There is no doubt that a pharmacist is a healthcare professional, but not only that. The pharmacist is "the university professional whose primary mission is the management and the exclusive responsibility for the formulation, preparation and the responsible dispensing of drugs to the population in addition to its inevitable participation in the protection of health and improvement of the quality of life" [19]. Several inconsistencies are evident regarding the pharmacist's role more broadly; that is, in the pharmaceutical industry in developing and producing medicines and in laboratory medicine. The master's program in Slovenia is designed to provide pharmacy competences within the healthcare system as well as the pharmaceutical industry, medical laboratories, research laboratories, legislation, and education. From this perspective, the PHAR-QA framework of competences does not sufficiently cover competences outside the healthcare system. Competences in drug development and production should be developed and included in greater detail.

Some definitions were found to be rather loose and/or ambiguous. For example, the competence "Knowledge of the importance of research in pharmaceutical development and practice" seems to be too general and is addressed by the majority of subjects in our curriculum. The members of the study team had difficulty understanding what the competence covers; it seems self-evident. The curriculum sets competences about research in pharmaceutical development and practice at a higher level according to Bloom's classification [20].

It was further observed that some competences are too broad, covering multiple competences. Some examples include the following: "Ability to undertake a critical evaluation of a prescription ensuring that it is clinically appropriate and legally valid" should distinguish competences of a clinical and legislative nature/origin; "Ability to advise physicians on the appropriateness of prescribed medicines and—in some cases—to prescribe medication" should distinguish counselling (i.e., advising) from taking actions (i.e., prescribing); and "Ability to identify non-adherence to medicine therapy and make an appropriate intervention" should distinguish the ability to recognize from the ability to intervene. The problem of scoring arises when two partial competences are not from the same origin and cannot be covered in the curriculum equally. For example, prescription of medicines by a pharmacist is not allowed in many EU countries, including Slovenia. Therefore it is unreasonable to include such competences in the national curriculum.

During the education process, competences are built from lower to higher levels according to Bloom's taxonomy: remember, understand, apply, analyze, evaluate, and create [21]. Not considering this, only courses at the top of the pillars are recognized as important for a particular competence whereas basic courses are overlooked. For example, the team had difficulty differentiating the following competences: "(7) Ability to apply current knowledge of relevant legislation and codes of pharmacy practice," "(8) Knowledge of appropriate legislation and of ethics," and "(9) Ability to implement general legal requirements that impact upon the practice of pharmacy"; it seems that different levels of Bloom's classification are being addressed inconsistently. To develop competences at higher levels (i.e., to be able to perform), several lower-level competences (i.e., knowledge and skills) should be adopted and included in the curriculum. Lower-level competences are usually written very generally, such as "development of skills" or "capability of practical application of knowledge," and are not linked to a specific field or competences. On the other hand, competence at the highest level, such as "Ability to use pharmaceutical knowledge and provide evidence-based advice on public health issues involving medicines," means that students have already built sufficient pharmaceutical knowledge, which should be addressed inside the curriculum as separate lower-level competences (knowledge and understanding).

The roundtable discussion of the Delphi study and further analysis of the results revealed that the majority of differences in scoring arise from different perspectives on the pharmacy profession (e.g., community, hospital, industrial, academic, laboratory medicine, or regulative); for example, "7. Personal competences: learning and knowledge. 6. Ability to apply current knowledge of relevant legislation and codes of pharmacy practice." Scoring pharmacy practice from a healthcare perspective yields different results than scoring pharmacy practice from a more general perspective, also covering industrial and regulatory aspects of the profession. Similarly, the competence "11. Patient care competences: patient consultation and assessment. 2. Ability to perform appropriate diagnostic tests, e.g., measurement of blood pressure or blood sugar" can be understood as graduates' ability to perform some basic diagnostic tests in community pharmacy, or graduates' ability to work in laboratory medicine (synonyms: clinical biochemistry, clinical biology) [22]. This is a common situation in Slovenia [23]. Different perspectives and understandings of competences as defined by PharQA were discussed in the roundtable, leading to more a balanced approach to evaluation among the panelists. This resulted in greater consensus in the second round of the Delphi evaluation process: the panelists reached consensus for 49 out of 50 competences.

Competences have to be designed to fit the first-day-of-job pharmacist [2,8]. From this perspective, it was found that some of the competences in the EPMF were rather too ambitious and require additional graduate training and/or specialization, as also discussed by Atkinson [13].

It can be concluded that curriculum mapping using EPMF is very useful for evaluating and recognizing weak and strong points of the curriculum. However, it must also be recognized that some additional improvement of the existing framework is needed. Namely, the competences of the framework should address various fields of the pharmacy profession in a more balanced way.

This study found the mapping process to be more complex than it seemed at the beginning. Not all of the pitfalls observed were addressed. For other mapping steps (e.g., perceived and achieved competences), some tuning differences in personal approaches would be necessary, and some kind of training would also be useful to support activities, which is in line with the recommendations of the European Commission [1] about teaching and learning improvement, and is also part of the Slovenian National Higher Education Program 2011–2020 [24].

Author Contributions: B.B. designed, constructed and leaded the process of curriculum mapping and analyzing. T.G. and B.B. prepared preliminary matrix courses/competences. B.B., A.O., I.G. and T.V. made preliminary mapping of the curriculum. T.G., N.H., M.K., A.O., T.V. and I.G. performed curriculum mapping. T.G., M.K., N.H. and A.O. analyzed data. B.B., M.K. and T.G. wrote the paper. All authors provided useful criticism and suggestions during paper writing.

References

1. High Level Group on the Modernisation of Higher Education. *Report to the European Commission on Improving the Quality of Teaching and Learning in Europe's Higher Education Institution*; Publications Office of the European Union: Luxembourg, 2013.

2. Božič, B. Competencies of the "first day of job" pharmacist, invited lecture. In *Abstract Book. II Congress of Pharmacists of Montenegro with the International Participation*; Potpara, Z., Ed.; UCG&FKCG: Budva, The Republic of Montenegro, 28–31 May 2015.

3. Božič, B.; Ribič, L. (Eds.) *Progress Report of the Faculty of Pharmacy for the Year 2012*; ULFFA: Ljubljana, Slovenia, 2013.

4. Directive 2005/36/EC of the European Parliament and of the Council of 7 September 2005 on the Recognition of Professional Qualifications. Available online: http://eur-lex.europa.eu/legal-content/en/TXT/?uri=CELEX%3A32005L0036 (accessed on 26 December 2016).

5. Slovenian Quality Assurance Agency for Higher Education. QA Procedures. Available online: http://www.nakvis.si/en-GB/Content/Details/78 (accessed on 26 December 2016).

6. Uniform Master's Study Programme Pharmacy, University of Ljubljana, Faculty of Pharmacy, Slovenia. Available online: http://www.ffa.uni-lj.si/fileadmin/datoteke/Dekanat/Pravilniki/PROSPECTUS_Pharmacy.pdf (accessed on 26 December 2016).

7. Interdisciplinary Doctoral Programme in Biomedicine, University of Ljubljana, Slovenia. Available online: http://www.ffa.uni-lj.si/fileadmin/datoteke/Dekanat/Studij/2013-14/Biomedicine_brochure_en_20_3_2013.pdf (accessed on 26 December 2016).

8.   Dreyfus, S.E.; Dreyfus, H.L. *A Five-Stage Model of the Mental Activities Involved in Directed Skill Acquisition*; Storming Media: Washington, DC, USA, 1980.

9.   Božič, B.; Toth, B. (Eds.) *Report on the Achievements of the Faculty of Pharmacy for 2015*. Available online: http://www.ffa.uni-lj.si/en/faculty/presentation/reports (accessed on 28 December 2016).

10. European Association of Faculties of Pharmacy. Available online: http://eafponline.eu/euprojects/ (accessed on 26 December 2016).

11. The PHAR-QA Project: Quality Assurance in European Pharmacy Education and Training. Available online: http://www.phar-qa.eu/ (accessed on 26 December 2016).

12. Atkinson, J.; Rombaut, B.; Sanchez-Pozo, A.; Rekkas, D.; Veski, P.; Hirvonen, J.; Bozic, B.; Skowron, A.; Mirciou, C. A description of the European pharmacy education and training quality assurance project. *Pharmacy* **2013**, *1*, 3–7. [CrossRef]

13. Atkinson, J.; de Paepe, K.; Sánchez Pozo, A.; Rekkas, D.; Volmer, D.; Hirvonen, J.; Bozic, B.; Skowron, A.; Mircioiu, C.; Marcincal, A.; et al. The second round of the PHAR-QA survey of competences for pharmacy practice. *Pharmacy* **2016**, *4*, 27. [CrossRef]

14. Hsu, C.C.; Sandford, B.A. The Delphi Technique: Making Sense of Consensus. *Pract. Assess. Res. Eval.* **2007**, *12*, 1–8.

15. Atkinson, J.; de Paepe, K.; Sánchez Pozo, A.; Rekkas, D.; Volmer, D.; Hirvonen, J.; Bozic, B.; Skowron, A.; Mircioiu, C.; Marcincal, A.; et al. The PHAR-QA project: Competency framework for pharmacy practice—First steps, the results of the European network Delphi round 1. *Pharmacy* **2015**, *3*, 307–329. [CrossRef]

16. Nash, R.E.; Chalmers, L.; Brown, N.; Jackson, S.; Peterson, G. An international review of the use of competency standards in undergraduate pharmacy education. *Pharm. Educ.* **2015**, *15*, 131–141.

17. Plaza, C.M.; Draugalis, J.R.; Slack, M.K.; Skrepnek, G.H.; Sauer, K.A. Curriculum mapping in program assessment and evaluation. *Am. J. Pharm. Educ.* **2007**, *71*, 20. [CrossRef] [PubMed]

18. Atkinson, J.; de Paepe, K.; Sánchez Pozo, A.; Rekkas, D.; Volmer, D.; Hirvonen, J.; Bozic, B.; Skowron, A.; Mircioiu, C.; Marcincal, A.; et al. What is a Pharmacist: Opinions of Pharmacy Department Academics and Community Pharmacists on Competences Required for Pharmacy Practice. *Pharmacy* **2016**, *4*, 12. [CrossRef]

19. Del Castillo Garcia, B. Updates to degrees in pharmacy directed to the professional development for future pharmacists as health specialists. *J. Eur. Assoc. Faculties Pharm.* **2015**. Available online: http://eafponline.eu/wp-content/uploads/2013/04/EPFN_2015_April.pdf (accessed on 27 December 2016).

20. Anderson, L.W.; Krathwohl, D.R.; Airasian, P.W.; Cruikshank, K.A.; Mayer, R.E.; Pintrich, P.R.; Raths, K.; Wittrock, M.C. *A Taxonomy for Learning, Teaching and Assessing: A Revision of Bloom's Taxonomy of Educational Objectives*; Allyn&Bacon: Boston, MA, USA, 2001.

21. Krathwohl, D.R. A revision of Bloom's taxonomy: An overview. *Theory Pract.* **2002**, *41*, 212–218. [CrossRef]

22. Dybekaer, R. Clinical laboratory work: Concept and terms. *Invited opinion. Eur. J. Clin. Chem. Clin. Biochem.* **1997**, *35*, 495–499.

23. Božič, B. Laboratory Medicine as Pharmacists' Competences. In Proceedings of the EAFP Conference 2014, Ljubljana, Slovenia, 22–24 May 2014.

24. Slovene National Higher Education Program 2011–2020, Ministry of Health. Available online: http://www.arhiv.mvzt.gov.si/nc/en/media_room/news/article/101/6960/ (accessed on 28 December 2016).

15

Uncertainty and Motivation to Seek Information from Pharmacy Automated Communications

Michelle Bones [1] and Martin Nunlee [2],*

[1] Department of Veterans Affairs, Voluntary Service, 1601 Kirkwood Highway, Wilmington, DE 19805 USA; mcnunlef@umich.edu

[2] Department of Business Administration, College of Business, Delaware State University, 1200 North Dupont Highway, Dover, DE 19901-2277, USA

* Correspondence: mnunlee@desu.edu

Abstract: Pharmacy personnel often answer telephones to respond to pharmacy customers (subjects) who received messages from automated systems. This research examines the communication process in terms of how users interact and engage with pharmacies after receiving automated messages. No study has directly addressed automated telephone calls and subjects' interactions. The purpose of this study is to test the interpersonal communication (IC) process of uncertainty in subjects in receipt of automated telephone calls ATCs from pharmacies. Subjects completed a survey of validated scales for Satisfaction (S); Relevance (R); Quality (Q); Need for Cognitive Closure (NFC). Relationships between S, R, Q, NFC, and subject preference to ATCs were analyzed to determine whether subjects contacting pharmacies display information seeking behavior. Results demonstrated that seeking information occurs if subjects: are dissatisfied with the content of the ATC; perceive that the Q of ATC is high and like receiving the ATC, or have a high NFC and do not like receiving ATCs. Other interactions presented complexities amongst uncertainty and tolerance of NFC within the IC process.

Keywords: pharmacy; patient communication; pharmacy communications; interpersonal communications; automated telemarketing telephone calls; telephone messages; automated messages; communication theory; customer relation management; CRM; pharmacy practice

---

1. Introduction

Automated messaging is a major form of patient communication for community pharmacies. Voicemails, text messages or emails serve to notify patients. These forms of communication are by their nature unidirectional, from the pharmacy to the patient. For there to be bidirectional communication, the patient must contact the pharmacy—usually this contact is by telephone. How many times have personnel in pharmacies had to respond to customers who have called concerning communications from automated systems? Automated messages—specifically automated telephone messages dates back to 1924 [1]. Accordingly, the sentiments of the intent of the sender's message, " . . . was believed . . . to save considerable expense to the companies where many "repeat" calls are necessary" [1]. The use of recorded messages blossomed in the late 20th century and exploded in the 21st century [2]. Often pharmacies send automated messages via telephone to patients, as a form of communication. The telephone, as a medium, is "cool" or one of low definition [3]. Automated telephone calls from pharmacies provide information requiring so much to be filled in by the pharmacy customer. When a pharmacy customer responds to the automated telephone call (ATC) from a pharmacy, the medium requires the individual to "actively analyze and interpret what is presented, to make sense of what they . . . hear" [4]. After receiving a message from a cool medium such as an ATC, the pharmacy customer can choose to respond to the message, thereby engaging in the interpersonal communication process. An alternative option is not to respond.

Very few studies directly addressed the role communication plays in pharmacy patients' interactions; this is one of the few studies in the pharmacy discipline that seeks to dive in-depth into the communication and interpersonal communication concepts [5,6]. By definition communication is the process of imparting or interchanging thoughts, opinions or information. Fields of study as disperse as psychology, business and engineering rely upon the same basic model of communication. A diagram of the communications process is outlined in Figure 1.

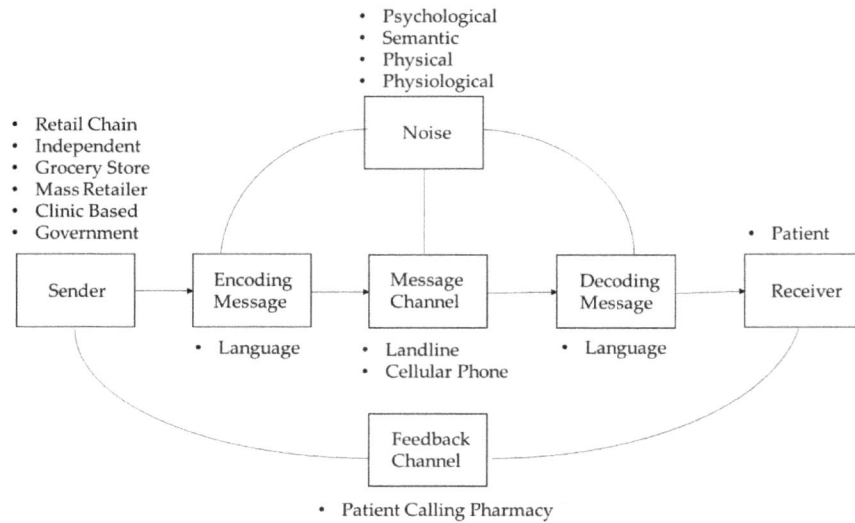

Figure 1. Diagram of communication process.

Figure 1 depicts the typical communication process. In this research we are concerned with how noise, specifically—psychological noise, influences patients' perceptions within the domain of ATCs. As indicated in the figure, noise can impact the encoding and decoding, and the message channel. Noise is anything that hinders the communication process. The four most common forms of noise are physical, physiological, semantic, and psychological. Physical noise is something that interferes with communication that is external to both the sender and receiver. Physiological noise is an internal condition of the receiver or sender that causes a distraction. Physiological noise could be caused by hunger, fatigue, malaise, medication or other factors that affect how people feel and think. In terms of oral exchanges these internal distraction, may cause senders to have problem in articulation, while receivers may have problem in hearing. Semantic noise is primarily cause by the sender. It occurs when senders encode messages in language in which the receiver is unfamiliar. Most of the work concerning the communication process in healthcare has focused on semantic noise—in the form of patient health literacy. In its most basic form, psychological noise consists of mental interference. The reader should understand that psychological noise could stem from wandering thoughts and preconceived ideas; as well as dislike of the sender, medium or receiver. To measure psychological noise, we use common constructs and in-turn scales from psychology and consumer behavior to assess patients' tendencies and attitudes and then gauge their response, by the number of feedback calls.

The motivation for why people would contact pharmacies varies. Is the ATC a channel for information seeking by pharmacy patients? Will pharmacy customers call the pharmacy seeking information pertaining to the ATC? According to Brasher et al. [6], within the health context framework, information is defined as stimuli from a person's environment that contribute to his or her knowledge or belief. Some customers will call to get clarification or confirmation, while other customers will call if they find the ATC from a pharmacy a bother or nuisance. What are the thoughts of the pharmacy patient following the receipt of an ATC from a pharmacy? If a pharmacy patient seeks information from the pharmacy, what are the contributions to the patient? Within the health context framework, "the information can be used to decrease uncertainty that is distressing, to increase certainty that allows for hope or optimism, and to invite reappraisal of uncertainty" [6]. Information seeking has been studied in the context of individuals' network of interpersonal relationships. Theories from the Social Science discipline of Interpersonal Communication will serve as the basis of analysis for the pharmacy-pharmacy patient interpersonal relationship. The selected perspective is represented by the arc of "noise" to "decoding message" outlined in Figure 1. The content of the message is not a specific focus. However, the medium of the message, via telephone, contributes to the knowledge or beliefs of the pharmacy patient. Before, discussing motivation there has to be a clear understanding of what is meant by communication.

What is communication? "A process as complex as communication is hard to summarize or define" [7]; from a business marketing perspective, "communication is the process by which we exchange or share meanings through a common set of symbols" [8]. The highest level of communication can be further delineated, from broadcasting one-way messages to interactive interpersonal communication. Focusing on interpersonal communication, it is direct, face-to-face communication between two or more people [8], and the participants receive maximum feedback [7]. A further delineation of interpersonal communication is the theory of uncertainty. Brashers [9] states that "uncertainty exist when details of situations are ambiguous, complex, unpredictable, or probabilistic; when information is unavailable or inconsistent; and when people feel insecure in their own state of knowledge or the state of knowledge in general". What factors, in an interpersonal communication relationship, can affect uncertainty? Need for Closure (NFC) is one factor. NFC is commonly defined "within the relationship exchange of information, [as] the desire for an answer on a given topic, any answer, as compared to confusion or ambiguity" [10].

Excluding pharmacy, "disciplines that have examined this depth of the uncertainty process in earnest include communications, psychology, sociology, family studies, library and information sciences, medicine, genetic counseling, business, economics and religious studies" [11]. Theories from the Social Science discipline of Interpersonal Communication serve as the basis of analysis for the pharmacy-pharmacy patient interpersonal relationship. To advance our understanding of the pharmacy-pharmacy patient communication process more empirical study is necessary. Further, socio-demographic characteristics should be examined within the framework of the information exchange process. This research focuses on the beliefs of the pharmacy patient and their motivation to contact pharmacies and directly addresses the role communication science plays in pharmacy patients' interactions in ATCs.

To examine communication processes, we will refer to pharmacy patients as "subjects". Kruglanski [10] states that subjects' desire for information or knowledge leads to NFC and is related to any particular belief properties. These properties may be content-related, structural, a novelty, desirable or formal features in given circumstances. Subjects generate theories that view their own attributes as more predictive of desirable outcomes, and they are reluctant to believe in theories relating their own attributes to undesirable events [12]. These desirable outcomes seem to be explained best by motivational ends according to Kunda [12], or otherwise stated the desire for information or knowledge is a driving motivation. The desire to seek information serves as an example of a motivational force. Motivational forces do not completely blind people to undesirable evidence or information; however, motivational forces could lead people to play down negative information. It should be noted, people's tendency to link their attributes to desirable outcomes was found only for people who cared about the outcomes. Furthermore, people threatened by undesirable evidence are reluctant to believe this evidence. The desire to seek information is tainted by self-protective motivational forces [12]. Otherwise stated, subjects are satisfied with their current state of knowledge, and do not seek information.

The framework of attribute satisfaction by consumers has been examined. Attribute satisfaction, then, is the consumer's subjective satisfaction judgment resulting from observations of attribute performance (role or event) and can be the fulfillment response consumers make when assessing performance [13]. In his research Oliver [13] looked at the role of events (e.g., attribute performance experiences) as causal agents for positive states. This analogy is extended to the summary attribute level, where the sum of positive product experiences (i.e., satisfactory attribute performances) should relate to positive affect, and negative experiences (i.e., dissatisfactory attribute performances) to negative affect [13]. If consumer's posses dissatisfactory attribute performances and negative outcomes, will they seek information to affect uncertainty?

Cosby and Stephens [14] examined stimulus influences on satisfaction decisions in a study model related to services by an entity. The communication stimuli enhanced satisfaction to services. Subjects given valid information about the services reduced search and evaluation of alternate services within the model. Henceforth in the interpersonal communication process this level of enhanced satisfaction lead to declining levels of uncertainty, with corresponding decreasing information seeking behavior [10].

In our examination, the content of the belief properties or attributes of the ATC are general satisfaction, and relevance of information. In this case, information seeking or desire for exchange of information means calling the pharmacy. Therefore, we hypothesize the following about the subjects' belief properties toward the ATC from pharmacies.

Hypothesis 1. *If subjects are dissatisfied with the content of the ATC received from a pharmacy, then they will seek information.*

Pyszczynski and Greenberg [15] conducted a study to determine causal perceptions of relevant information by subjects, including selection of information. Subjects observed an individual's behavior in a scenario. Then subjects read personality-related answers provided by the individual in the scenario. A few relevant items help explain the just-observed scenario, and the other items were irrelevant to the scenario. Next the subjects were asked something about the personality of the individual in the scenario. This study design measures the subject's motivation to voluntarily select information for use in analyzing and providing the answer to the question about the personality of the individual in the scenario. The findings revealed that when faced with disconfirming expectations subjects will seek attribution-relevant information [15]. This research demonstrated when people are confused they search for relevant information. Likewise, the relevance of the information is related to information seeking. This leads to the following hypothesis.

Hypothesis 2. *If subjects feel that the content of the ATC received from a pharmacy is relevant, then they will seek information.*

In addition, communication quality is another belief property associated with the ATC. Webster and Kruglanski [16] conducted an experiment comparing subjective certainty and susceptibility to persuasion in people with different levels of the need for closure. The experimental design was accomplished by introducing participants to differing amounts and quality of information about a situation. The investigators concluded that people with a high NFC are susceptible to the persuasion of differing quality of information, because each persuasive message gives them a chance to achieve closure [16]. This leads us to the third hypothesis, which is as follows.

Hypothesis 3a. *If a subject perceives that the quality of the ATC received from a pharmacy is high, the subject will seek information.*

Likewise, a pre-existing knowledge structure can serve as a motivating factor for search of information. If a subject has both a high affinity for receiving information, and high perception of quality, then we theorized the following:

Hypothesis 3b. *If a subject perceives that the quality of ATC received from a pharmacy is high, and like receiving the ATC, the subject will seek information.*

The extant literature on NFC, indicates the higher the need for closure, the greater the information seeking. Alternatively, a summarization of another finding by Kruglanski [8], states that if the subjects' confidence in belief properties rank high, along with a high NFC, the tendency to seek information is decreased. If the initial confidence in belief properties ranks low and NFC is high, subjects possess an increased tendency for information seeking. In examining the properties of ATC communication, we decided to test the basic premise of NFC, which leads to the following hypothesis.

Hypothesis 4a. *If subjects, NFC are high after receipt of the ATC from a pharmacy, the subjects will seek information.*

The interaction of variables surfaced from findings in an experiment [17] examining NFC effects and dependent variables to engage informational search by subjects, a multivariate analysis of variance (MANOVA) yielded a significant interaction among variables or belief properties. This unpublished study used a 2×2 factorial analysis with two independent and dependent variables to examine interactive effects of need-for-closure. The independent variables were need-for-closure and the subjects' confidence in the process. The two dependent variables were measures of the subjects' tendency to engage in information search. The analysis of data showed the two-way interactions were significant ($p < 0.01$) [17]. We chose to examine subjects' NFC based on preexisting conditions. In particular, the preexisting condition consists of whether patients receiving the ATC from pharmacies like or dislike of receiving the ATC from pharmacies. Besides generally testing NFC, we will test whether people who do not have an affinity for receiving the ATC and have a high NFC would call the pharmacy. These would most likely be the people that we mentioned earlier who call because they find ATCs a bother or nuisance. This leads us to the following sub-hypotheses.

Hypothesis 4b. *If a subject perceives that the quality of the ATC received from a pharmacy is low, and has a high NFC, the subject will seek information.*

Theses related aspects of attribute beliefs found in satisfaction, relevance, and quality along with the theory of need for closure within the theory of uncertainty as embodied in the concept of Interpersonal Communication were analyzed in a random population. We chose validated constructs scales of Satisfaction (Generalized), Information Relevance, Communication Quality and NFC to examine the pharmacy subjects' response to engaging in the interpersonal communication process. See Table 1 for a summary of the hypotheses.

Table 1. Summary of hypotheses for phenomena of behaviors of pharmacy patients in receipt of an automated telephone call (ATC).

Item	Hypothesis
1.	If subjects are dissatisfied with the content of the ATC received from a pharmacy, then they will seek information.
2.	If subjects feel that the content of the ATC received from a pharmacy is relevant, then they will seek information.
3a.	If a subject perceives that the quality of the ATC received from a pharmacy is high, the subject will seek information.
3b.	If a subject perceives that the quality of ATC received from a pharmacy is high, and like receiving the ATC, the subject will seek information.
4a.	If subjects, NFC are high after receipt of the ATC from a pharmacy, the subjects will seek information.
4b.	If a subject perceives that the quality of the ATC received from a pharmacy is low, and has a high NFC, the subject will seek information.

2. Materials and Methods

A 46-item questionnaire was compiled as a tool for the survey. Refer to Supplementary Materials for the complete survey. The questionnaire contains six validated construct scales. Validated scales have been tested with successful results many times. Validated construct scales are both reliable and reproducible. The psychometric qualities of each validated construct scales have been provided to verify the validity and reliability of each measure, giving rise to testable theories. This compilation method was utilized to collect data for analysis and inclusion in the 46-item questionnaire survey tool.

Google survey served as the platform for the survey design, and response collection. The survey was titled "Automated Telephone Calls from Pharmacies" for administration to subjects. The survey design consisted of three sections, Section 1—Pre-Interactions, Section 2—Post-interactions and Section 3—Demographics. Questions in Section 1 of the survey served to separate subjects. If subjects indicated that they have never received prescription medication or never received an ATC from a pharmacy, they were directed to Section 3 of the survey for collection of demographic data. Also, subjects were directed to Section 3 of the survey if they had never received ATCs from a pharmacy. Completion of Section 2 was limited to subjects meeting the criteria set forth in question 1 and/or 2 of Section 1. Only subjects who completed Section 2 responded to all 46-items of the survey. The completion of Section 3 of the survey was required for all subjects in fulfillment of survey completion. The estimated time for completion of the survey was 10-min. The survey was administered using Amazon Mechanical Turk (MTurk) for Social/Behavioral Research projects. MTurk is a web service that provides on-demand scalable human subjects to complete surveys. Keywords, a phrase and a short description were used to assist and guide subjects to participate in the "Automated Telephone Calls from Pharmacies" survey. The keywords are listed in Table 2.

Table 2. Keywords to recruit subjects.

Keywords (Alphabetical Order):			
Behaviors	Customers	Medicines	Prescriptions
Capsules	Healthcare	Pharmacies	Interactions
Communications	Medications	Pills	Tablets

To aid in the recruitment of subjects, potential subjects were given the following short description concerning the study:

> This is a research study that directly addresses automated pharmacy telephone calls and pharmacy customers' interactions. The purpose of this study is to examine the communication behaviors between pharmacy customers in receipt of automated telephone calls.

After subjects committed to completing the survey, they were directed to complete Section 1. Subjects who met the screening criteria were then directed to Section 2, and then they were directed to indicate their responses and preferences on the validated construct scales. Finally, subjects were directed to Section 3 to report their demographic information. The third section of the survey utilized identical socio-demographic ranges as reported in the United States census. Human subjects 18 years of age or older were eligible participants. The survey was administered using stratified sampling, in six intervals based on age to ensure representation over a continuum, see Table 3 for interval ranges. All subjects were paid for participation.

Table 3. Intervals of survey administration based on age.

Group	Age Range
1	Ages 18 years < 25 years
2	Ages 25 years < 30 years
3	Ages 30 years < 35 years
4	Ages 35 years < 45 years
5	Ages 45 years < 55 years
6	Ages 55 years or older

Sources of Validated Construct Scales

The first construct scale to be presented is the "Satisfaction (Generalized)" [18], represented by questions 6 through 10. It is a multi-item, seven-point semantic differential summated ratings scale measuring degree of satisfaction with stimuli. Scale reliability for conducted studies, as measured by Cronbach's alpha were reported as 0.96, and in other studies 0.94, 0.91, 0.90, 0.93 and 0.87. The Satisfaction scale examines a subject's degree of satisfaction after receiving automated telephone calls from a pharmacy. High scores indicate greater satisfaction with the automated telephone message, whereas low scores imply that the subjects are not pleased.

The second construct scale to be presented is Information Relevance [19], represented by questions 11 through 15. It is a five-item, seven-point summated rating scale, measuring the level of usefulness a person reports some piece of information to have. Cronbach's alpha for the Information Relevance scale were reported as 0.94, 0.94, and 0.96. The Information Relevance scale examines the level of usefulness subjects report, concerning the information provided in the automated telephone call. High scores indicate that subjects describe information related to automated telephone calls as being very relevant, whereas low scores imply that the subjects found the information less relevant.

The third construct scale to be presented is Communication Quality [20], represented by questions 16 through 20. It is a five-item, five-point semantic differential scale to assess person's perceptions of the quality of communication between them and the information provider. For reliability, Cronbach's alpha for the conducted study was 0.92. The scale examines subjects' perception of the quality of communication between themselves and the automated telephone message. This Communication Quality scale was reversed scaled. Lower scores on the scale indicate that subjects perceived that high-quality communication occurred between themselves and the automated telephone message, whereas high scores imply that the subjects perceived that low-quality communication occurred between themselves and the automated telephone message.

The forth scale to be presented is a measure of Socially Desirable Response Set (SDRS-5) [21], represented by questions 21 through 25. It is a five-item, five-point scale to evaluate susceptibility to response bias by subjects receiving automated telephone calls from pharmacies. Cronbach's alpha for the conducted study was 0.66 and 0.68. The scale evaluates a respondent's tendency to give socially-desirable response[s] [20]. This scale was used to verify that subjects were giving their true response and not giving responses that they thought were socially appropriate.

Finally, the Need for Cognitive Closure scale [22] measured subjects' tolerance or lack of tolerance for uncertainty. The Need for Cognitive Closure scale consists of 15 items, represented by questions 26 through 40. It consists of a six-point rating scale to measure a variable desire for closure along a continuum with a strong need to attain closure on one end and a high need to avoid closure at the other end [22]. Scale reliability, as measured by Cronbach's alpha was 0.79.

3. Results

There were 319 respondents who participated in the survey process. Only 294 of the 319 respondents were selected as subjects. Respondents were eliminated only as a result of the screening process or if they did not provide a response to all the questions. The demographic data collected during the survey process serves to provide characteristics of the study population. A brief overview of subject characteristics follows. The female to male ratio was approximately 2:1 respectively for all subjects. Most respondents reported having attended some college and bachelor's degree for education level. Very few respondents reported education as high school graduate or G.E.D, trade school or other post-secondary education, or associate degree. The majority of the respondents reported being married, followed by single/never married. A preponderance of respondents reported ethnicity or origin as Caucasian/White. Household income ranged from $15K to less than $150K. The interrelationships amongst the subject characteristics and responses were analyzed based on correlations and linear regression. They are not reported here, except for some comparisons, because there were no significant relationships or interaction patterns observed between survey responses and socio-demographic characteristics. None of the 294 subjects scored high on social desirability, which indicates that subjects were giving their true responses, instead of what they think is socially desirable.

To test the hypotheses, we used correlations and linear regression. The results of the analyses are shown in Table 4. The critical relationship correlations are reported in Table 4.

Table 4. Correlations of critical relationships.

	Satisfaction	Relevance	Quality	SDRS	NFC	I (Q × Like)	I (NFC × Not Like)	Contacted
Satisfaction	1							
Relevance	0.8264	1						
Quality	−0.6760	−0.6981	1					
SDRS	0.0526	0.0478	−0.0341	1				
NFC	0.1574	0.1439	−0.1997	−0.1173	1			
I (Q × Like)	0.4751	0.3631	−0.1200	−0.0420	0.0388	1		
I (NFC × not like)	−0.7663	−0.6348	0.4945	0.0089	0.0022	−0.7972	1	
Contacted	−0.0954	−0.0845	0.2210	0.0214	−0.0431	0.1082	0.0298	1

Hypothesis 1 has been confirmed. Satisfaction with the message content of automated telephone calls is negatively correlated to the number of subjects' telephone calls to the pharmacy. Although the correlation is small ($r = -0.0954$), it is significant ($p \leq 0.10$).

Hypothesis 2 has not been confirmed. Relevance of the automated telephone calls is negatively correlated to the number of subject pharmacy telephone calls to the pharmacy; however, this relationship is not significant. However, when we tested just the subjects who liked to receive ATCs, we found that the level of inverse correlation had increased ($r = -0.2030$) and significant ($p \leq 0.01$).

Quality of the automated telephone call message is positively correlated to the number of subjects' telephone calls to the pharmacy. This relationship was both positively correlated ($r = 0.221$) and significant ($p \leq 0.01$). This relationship was further tested by introducing the indicator variable of whether patients liked receiving ATCs as a moderator to quality. This means that subjects who perceive that the quality of the ATC received from a pharmacy is high will seek information. To confirm Hypothesis 3b, we need to add the interaction term and regress both the quality of the automated telephone call (Q) and the interaction of Q and liking (Like) to receive automated telephone calls—I (Q × Like)—on number of subject pharmacy telephone calls to the pharmacy—contacting pharmacies (CP). The linear model is given below.

$$CP = \beta_0 + \beta_1 \cdot Q + \beta_2 \cdot I_{Q \times Like}, \qquad (1)$$

As indicated in Table 5, although the explained variance as measured by r^2 only accounts for 26% of the explained variance, the regression coefficients were both positive and significant; with Quality remaining significant to the $p \leq 0.01$ level and interaction of liking to receive automated telephone calls and Quality significant to the $p \leq 0.05$ level. This means that Quality is positively related to the number of phone calls, and that people who like receiving ATCs play an additional role in the quality relationship. Both Hypotheses 3a and 3b have been confirmed.

Table 5. Regression results communication quality.

Variable	β_i	Std. Error	t Stat	p
Intercept	0.8473	0.0637	13.3034	$\leq$0.01
Q	0.0234	0.0056	4.1630	$\leq$0.01
I (Q $\times$ Like)	0.0138	0.0057	2.3976	$\leq$0.05

To test Hypotheses 4a and 4b, we regressed NFC, the interaction between Q and Like, and the interaction of need for closure (NFC) and not liking (NLike) to receive phone calls on to contacting the pharmacies (CP). Some of the results described in the correlation matrix (Table 4) are counter intuitive. For example, Q is negatively correlated to satisfaction. These results led us to test the interaction with Q and Like, since the interaction between NFC and NLike was significant and highly negatively correlated to satisfaction, we wanted to see if isolating people who like receiving phone calls responded differently in terms of the expected measures and whether it was significant. Said another way, we can test whether the people who were dissatisfied with receiving ATCs were driving the counter intuitive relationships. This resulted in the following linear model.

$$CP = \beta_0 + \beta_1 \cdot NFC + \beta_2 \cdot I_{Q \times Like} + \beta_3 \cdot I_{NFC \times NLike}, \tag{2}$$

The multiple coefficient of determination (r) for the regression was 0.71, r^2 was 0.50, while the adjusted-r^2 was also 0.50; with a standard error of 2.87 over 294 observations. Given a mean square error residual (MSR) of 8.23 and a mean square error regression (MSE) of 811, this yields an F(3, 293) of 98.45, meaning that the regression was significant to $p \leq 0.01$. The regression yielded the following results, Table 6:

Table 6. Regression results NFC and interaction terms.

Variable	β_i	Std. Error	t Stat	p
Intercept	6.6326	0.9998	6.6336	$\leq$0.01
NFC	−0.0795	0.0142	−5.6087	$\leq$0.01
I (Q $\times$ Like)	0.7958	0.0702	11.3405	$\leq$0.01
I (NFC $\times$ not like)	0.1636	0.0101	16.2671	$\leq$0.01

Hypothesis 4a has not been confirmed. In general NFC is negatively related to the number of subjects making telephone calls to the pharmacy. This means that people with a high need for closure are generally less likely to contact their pharmacies. This result lends credence to Kruglanski findings [10] that if the subjects' confidences in belief properties rank high, along with a high NFC, the tendency to seek information is decreased. Hypotheses 4b has been confirmed—people who have a high NFC, who do not like receiving telephone calls from their pharmacy also are likely to call their pharmacy.

By splitting the relationships using the interaction terms, we received confirmation that the negative relationship between satisfaction and communication quality was driven by NLike. Since the β_1 coefficient for NFC remained negative, it is consistent with the overall correlations described in Table 4, this indicates that the regression model is correctly specified. A correctly specified model lends credence that the relationships in the linear regression are credible, and not an artifice of multicollinearity. It is interesting that NFC only plays a role in increasing communication with subjects who do not like to receive ATCs from their pharmacy. See Table 7 for a summary of the hypotheses and results.

Table 7. Summary of hypotheses and results for phenomena of behaviors of pharmacy patients in receipt of an automated telephone call (ATC).

Item	Hypothesis	Result	Relationship	Significance
1.	If subjects are dissatisfied with the content of the ATC received from a pharmacy, then they will seek information.	Confirmed	$r = -0.0954$ negative as predicted	$p \leq 0.10$
2.	If subjects feel that the content of the ATC received from a pharmacy is relevant, then they will seek information.	Not confirmed	$r = -0.2030$ predicted positive but negative relationship	$p \leq 0.01$
3a.	If a subject perceives that the quality of the ATC received from a pharmacy is high, the subject will seek information.	Confirmed	$r = 0.221$ positive as predicted	$p \leq 0.01$
3b.	If a subject perceives that the quality of ATC received from a pharmacy is high, and like receiving the ATC, the subject will seek information.	Confirmed	$\beta = 0.0234$ positive as predicted	$p \leq 0.01$
4a.	If subjects, NFC are high after receipt of the ATC from a pharmacy, the subjects will seek information.	Not confirmed	$\beta = -0.0795$ predicted positive but negative relationship	$p \leq 0.01$
4b.	If a subject perceives that the quality of the ATC received from a pharmacy is low, and has a high NFC, the subject will seek information.	Confirmed	$\beta = 0.1636$ positive as predicted	$p \leq 0.01$

4. Discussion

We asked how many times have pharmacy personnel answered a telephone, to respond to communications from an automated system received by a subject? We were not able to answer that question, but we were able to survey subjects and determine their motivation for wishing to communicate with their pharmacy.

Some of the results revealed the situational impact of information seeking. For example, although subjects who like to receive ATCs find the information significantly relevant ($p \leq 0.01$), the relationship between contacting pharmacies and relevance was inversely correlated. This could be interpreted to mean that since the information is relevant, subjects have no reason to contact the pharmacy after receiving an ATC. This has no bearing on whether patients would contact their pharmacies if they needed information.

We found that NFC played a role only for patients who least liked receiving ATCs. Since we defined a high call volume, as being an individual who makes twelve or more calls to a pharmacy per year, this would mean that a large number of people make these calls based upon not liking to receive automated messages. Although some portion of the calls may be related to therapeutic questions, we suspect a great many are related to either patients' confusion about why they received the ATC, or a desire to express their displeasure. These incidences of communication would be less productive than addressing patient care needs.

We are less certain about the alternative—the patients who call as a result of having an affinity to receive ATCs. Since there is an interaction between liking the ATC and Quality, there is a need to address why these patients like receiving ATCs. Do these patients just like the aspect of communicating, or do they appreciate the information and seek further guidance and clarity? If it is the later condition of seeking guidance or clarity, then either the message needs to be refined or this follow-up call provided the opportunity to engage in meaningful communication that contributes to better patient care.

What we have found is consistent with other work in human communication research. Kellermann and Reynolds [23] found that while a low tolerance for uncertainty motivates greater information seeking, it is in the negative context. If there is a high level of affinity, then people find it easier to conduct communication. This affinity is a form of attractiveness. Only in the case where there is a high incentive or importance will there be communication under all conditions. This means that patients do not necessarily contact pharmacies based upon whether they are uncertain about the information. Rather, they will contact the pharmacy if they already have a positive relationship or they have a low tolerance for uncertainty. This in-turns means that information sharing will not occur; unless patients are comfortable with the pharmacy, or they have a clear understanding of the need or importance of sharing information.

Readers should notice that both interaction terms are positive and significant. In one case, subjects who like to receive ATCs from pharmacies and who have an affinity for receiving telephone calls were more likely to seek further information. In the other case, people who have a high need for closure, who do not like receiving telephone calls from their pharmacy also were likely to call their pharmacy. This is most interesting, since it indicates that communication is a complex multidimensional concept. Further these findings could possibly be explained by Webster and Kruglanski experimental situation model [18]. If the attribute of attractiveness to the task in the model decreased, subjects reflected a high NFC. We saw that the subjects who did not like receiving ATCs from pharmacies, or found ATCs from pharmacies unattractive possessed a high NFC, and called the pharmacy.

Although there needs to be further study and refinement on patient communication, one thing our study makes clear is that interpersonal communication is a complex process. The present results open new challenges for this research area. Our findings are consistent with what Kellermann and Reynolds [23] found. By extension, people are more likely to share information if they are comfortable with their provider, or if they already are aware of the importance of the message. This means that ATCs can only serve a limited role. Sending patients a reminder message to pick-up medication or get a flu vaccine via an ATC only works, if they already like the pharmacy or feel that these things are important to them. Otherwise, patients will only contact their pharmacy if they have a low tolerance for uncertainty. They do not contact their pharmacy to avoid uncertainty.

5. Conclusions

We were able to identify sub-sets within the study population where either communications and/or interpersonal communication occurred. The contributing factors differed for both groups. The less satisfied subjects—who scored high on the NFC scale—were with the ATC medium, the more likely they were to contact the pharmacy. On the other end of the spectrum, subjects that liked receiving ATCs and perceive the quality of the ATC as high were more likely to contact the pharmacy. Both of these groups of subjects sought to further engage in the interpersonal communication process.

We do not know how often subjects specifically call pharmacies after receiving ATC. We were unable to determine the degree to which subjects responded to telephone calls because of the limited response options. Question #4 of the survey asked subjects how many times they received calls from pharmacies, while question #5 asked subjects how many times subjects contacted the pharmacy. These scales were less refined. Only three response options were provided for both questions #4 and #5. We recommend refining the number of response options within these questions in future studies, specifically at the lower range. A more refined scale providing seven anchors would yield more precise results. We can only generalize how subjects with a high propensity to contact their pharmacies after receiving an ATC from pharmacies respond. No further interpretation can be made from the study design. Specifically, a more refined scale is important in the formation of a nuanced understanding of the interpersonal communication process.

We believe that by having a better understanding of patients' communication traits or beliefs and their receptivity to communication will allow senders to design better mechanisms to interact with patients. To arrive at better mechanisms, further study is needed on why some people (a) do not like receiving ATCs, or (b) what attributes of the ATC interact with some peoples' innate need for closure. Minor changes to the form or substance of the communication may make an impact on how pharmacies can better utilize forms of communication. Having an understanding of how and when patients wish to receive communication is critical to designing better communication mechanisms. Accordingly, Sileo and Kayson [24] found that the time of day can affect responsiveness to messaging. Care must be taken to insure that healthcare providers consider patients' receptivity to communication, not just the message itself. As illustrated by Xu, Bates and Schweitzer [25]—when examining telephone messaging in facilitating communications, they were unable to find a significant difference among specific message types. Extensions to this research will allow practitioners to improve the communication process, by either changing ATC messages or segmenting patients, or some combination of changing ATC messages and segmenting patients and then tailoring the message according to patient segments.

Author Contributions: M.B. and M.N. conceived and designed the study; M.B. performed the administration of the survey for the study; M.N. analyzed the data; M.B. and M.N. wrote the paper.

Acknowledgments: Funding for the survey administration was provided by Delaware State University, College of Business, Department of Business Administration, Principle Investigator Account for Martin Nunlee.

References

1. Popular Mechanics Phone Calls Are Answered by Machine. Available online: http://blog.modernmechanix.com/phone-calls-are-answered-by-machine/ (accessed on 8 October 2017).
2. Seelhorst, M. Think it's New? Think Again! After the Beep, Leave a Message. *Pop. Mech.* **1998**, *175*, 48.
3. Lapham, L.H.; Mcluhan, M. *Understanding Media (Reprint): The Extensions of Man*; MIT Press Edition; Massachusetts Institute of Technology: Cambridge, MA, USA, 1964; Volume 1, p. 365.
4. Thompson, S. What Did Marshall Mcluhan Mean by Hot and Cool Media? Available online: https://www.quora.com/What-did-Marshall-McLuhan-mean-by-hot-and-cool-media (accessed on 2 January 2018).
5. Worsely, A. Perceived reliability of sources of health information. *Health Educ. Res.* **1989**, *4*, 367–376. [CrossRef]
6. Brasher, D.E.; Goldsmith, D.J.; Hsieh, E. Information Seeking and Avoidance in Health Contexts. *Hum. Commun. Res.* **2002**, *28*, 258–271. [CrossRef]
7. Trenholm, S.; Jensen, A. *Interpersonal Communication*; International; Oxford Univ. Press: New York, NY, USA, 2009; Volume 1, p. 4.
8. Charles, W.L.; Joseph, F.H. *Carl McDaniel, Essentials of Marketing*, 4th ed.; Cengage Learning: Boston, MA, USA, 2004; p. 409.
9. Brashers, D.E. Communication and Uncertainty Management. *J. Commun.* **2001**, *51*, 477–497. [CrossRef]
10. Kruglanski, A.W. Motivation for Judging and Knowing: & nbsp; Implications for Causal Attribution. In *Handbook of Motivation and Cognition Foundations of Social Behavior*; The Guilford Press: New York, NY, USA, 1990; Volume 2, pp. 336–368.
11. Afifi, W.A.; Weiner, J.L. Toward a Theory of Motivated Information Management. *Commun. Theory* **2004**, *14*, 167–190. [CrossRef]
12. Kunda, Z. Motivated Inference: Self-serving Generation and Evaluation of Causal Theories. *J. Personal. Soc. Psychol.* **1987**, *53*, 636–647. [CrossRef]
13. Richard, L. Oliver Cognitive, Affective, and Attribute Bases of the Satisfaction Response. *J. Consum. Res.* **1993**, *20*, 418–430.
14. Crosby, L.A. Effects of Relationship Marketing on Satisfaction, Retention, and Prices in the Life Insurance Industry. *J. Mark. Res.* **1987**, *24*, 404–411. [CrossRef]
15. Pyszczynski, T.A.; Greenberg, J. Role of Disconfirmed Expectancies in the Instigation of Attributional Processing. *J. Personal. Soc. Psychol.* **1981**, *40*, 31–38. [CrossRef]
16. Webster, D.M.; Kruglanski, A.W. Individual Differences in Need for Cognitive Closure. *J. Personal. Soc. Psychol.* **1994**, *67*, 1049–1062. [CrossRef]
17. Peri, N.; Kruglanski, A.; Zakai, D. Interactive Effects of Initial Confidence and Epistemic Motivations on the Extent of Informational Search. Tel-Aviv University, Tel-Aviv, Israel, Unpublished work. 1986.

18. Crosby, L.A.; Stephens, N. Marketing Scales Handbook, A Compilation of Multi-Item Measures. In *Satisfaction (Generalized)*; Bruner, G.C., Hensel, P.J., Eds.; American Marketing Association: Chicago, IL, USA, 1998; Volume 2, pp. 550–552.

19. Mishra, S.; Umesh, U.N.; Stem, D. Marketing Scales Handbook A Compilation of Multi-Item Measures. In *Information Relevance*; Bruner, G.C., Hensel, P.J., Eds.; American Marketing Association: Chicago, IL, USA, 1998; Volume 2, pp. 337–338.

20. Mohr, J.J.; Sohi, R.S. Marketing Scales Handbook, a Compilation of Multi-Item Measures. In *Communication Quality*; Bruner, G.C., James, K.E., Hensel, P.J., Eds.; American Marketing Association: Chicago, IL, USA, 2001; Volume 3, pp. 885–886.

21. Hays, R.D.; Hayashi, T.; Stewart, A.L. A Five-item Measure of Socially Desirable Response Set. *Educ. Psychol. Meas.* **1989**, *49*, 629. [CrossRef]

22. Roets, A.; Van Hiel, A. Item Selection and Validation of a Brief, 15-item Version of the Need for Closure Scale. *Personal. Individ. Differ.* **2011**, *50*, 90–94. [CrossRef]

23. Kellermann, K.; Reynolds, R. When Ignorance Is Bliss The Role of Motivation to Reduce Uncertainty in Uncertainty Reduction Theory. *Hum. Commun. Res.* **1990**, *17*, 5–75. [CrossRef]

24. Sileo, F.J.; Kayson, W.A. When Will Annoying Phone Calls Be Listened to? Effects of Sex, Tone of Voice, and Time of Day. *Psychol. Rep.* **1988**, *62*, 351–355. [CrossRef]

25. Xu, M.; Bates, B.J.; Schweitzer, J.C. The Impact of Messages on Survey Participation in Answering Machine Households. *Public Opin. Q.* **1993**, *57*, 232–237. [CrossRef]

16

Current Status and Future Suggestions for Improving the Pharm. D Curriculum towards Clinical Pharmacy Practice

Saima Mahmood Malhi *, Hassan Raza ⓘ, Kiran Ajmal, Sumbul Shamim, Saniya Ata, Salman Farooq, Syed Muhammad Sharib and Sidrat-ul Muntaha

Faculty of Pharmaceutical Sciences, Dow College of Pharmacy, Dow University of Health Sciences, OJHA Campus, Karachi 74200, Pakistan; rph.hassan@hotmail.com (H.R.); kiran_ajmal@yahoo.com (K.A.); sumbul.shamim@gmail.com (S.S.); saniyaata@gmail.com (S.A.); alisalman_2008@yahoo.com (S.F.); sharib_syed@hotmail.com (S.M.S.); sidrarizwan5@hotmail.com (S.-u.-M.)
* Correspondence: saima.mahmood@duhs.edu.pk or smmhej@gmail.com

Abstract: Objectives & Background: Good curriculum is reflected as the backbone for standard universities to develop competitive professionals having great potential. Pharmacy education in Pakistan has gone through the same developmental stages as in other countries, but is still striving for improvement. In the present study, we want (i) to know the opinion on whether the current pharmacy curriculum requires any improvement in order to meet the training needs of pharmacy professionals regarding clinical knowledge and pharmacy practice; and (ii) to present some humble suggestions to decision-making authorities in order to improve it with respect to patient-focused programs (PFP). **Methods**: The study was conducted in two sessions. In first session, a questionnaire was distributed to pharmacy students of eight public/private sector universities of Karachi ($N = 354$) offering Pharm. D degrees. The second session dealt with the pharmacy teachers, deans, and practicing pharmacists in health care facilities (who are in any ways also related to academia), in order to take their opinions on and suggestions for the development of a better Pharm. D curriculum ($N = 135$). **Results**: Our results showed that 75.2% of respondents agree that the Pharm. D curriculum does not meet the international standards of practice, and 88.4% of respondents support the addition of more clinical aspects than industrial ones, as Pharm. D could be both clinically and industrially oriented, according to the needs of the Pakistani people. Furthermore, 80.2% of respondents are of the view that an apprenticeship should be included in last two years, while 88.4% demand a 'paid residency program' to facilitate the hospital, clinical and compounding areas of pharmacy. In addition, we also received a number of verbal suggestions for improving the Pharm. D curriculum being followed in Pakistan. **Discussion & Conclusions**: We conclude that our Pharm. D curriculum needs additions in terms of clinical practice by providing residencies and electives in health care settings. Accordingly, the need for a clinically oriented curriculum is highlighted in Pakistan, keeping in mind the continuing importance of the industrial viewpoint. Various studies have criticized the pharmacy curriculum in Pakistan in the past. Conversely, we suggest some changes in the curriculum, as change is always needed for a better tomorrow.

Keywords: Pharm. D curriculum; current pharmacy practice; patient focused program; paid residency program; questionnaire

1. Introduction

A doctor of pharmacy degree program must have a multidisciplinary curriculum that produces pharmacists with sufficient mental acuity to differentiate their position as a provider of pharmaceutical care from that simply of a dispenser of drugs [1]. The Pharm. D program in the United States is the epitome of the practice-based model, as it evolved from industrial and compounding pharmacy to a more patient-focused program [2]. The pharmacy program in Pakistan was initiated as a three-year baccalaureate program and then, in 1978–1979, it was lengthened to a four-year program. At that time, the pharmacy curriculum was directed mainly towards the production of pharmaceuticals, which helped provide the pharmaceutical industry with well-qualified and skilled human resources, but there was no consideration of the public health role of the pharmacist [3]. Hence, in Pakistan, the Pharm. D degree (a 5-year program) was introduced as the basic degree in pharmacy in 2003–2004, replacing the 4-year traditional bachelor of pharmacy (B Pharm) degree [4]. Many researchers [5] have previously criticized this program, as it is just a tool to make the pharmacy students eligible for the pharmacy entrance tests of the United States and the Gulf countries. In a paper titled "Pharm. D in Pakistan: A Tag or a Degree", the authors criticized the Pharm. D degree of being a tag, due to its lack of true clinical arrangement. Nevertheless, it is also true that the Pharm. D degree, even in United States, took years to fully develop, and it is also questionable today as to whether they have achieved their goal or not. Pakistan, being a developing country, introduced the Pharm. D degree in 2003, and a number of changes have occurred in its curriculum over the last decade. However, when this curriculum [6] was closely analyzed, it seemed that it was still in a transitional form from an industrial program to a clinical, patient-focused care program. This could be explained by the fact that the current curriculum offered to students comprises 198 credit hours in total. The yearly distribution of credit hours is as follows: first professional = 42 credit hours, second professional = 43 credit hours, third professional = 39 credit hours, fourth professional = 38 credit hours, and final professional = 36 credit hours. These are distributed across four departments; Pharmacology, Pharmaceutics, Pharmacognosy and Pharmaceutical Chemistry. Pharmacy practice has not been introduced as a fifth department at the time of this study. Clinical pharmacy courses (comprising only 6 credit hours of theory and 2 credit hours of practical work) is being taught under the supervision of department of pharmaceutics in collaboration with the department of pharmacology at this time. Thus, in order to make an effort for improvement in the curriculum, we conducted a survey to take the suggestions of 'Pharm. D teachers and students', so that these can be communicated effectively to the authorities for consideration.

2. Methodology

2.1. Study Design and Study Period

A cross-sectional study was conducted in two sessions by developing and distributing two different self-administered questionnaires between the months of August 2013 and March 2014. While developing the questionnaire, we tried to follow the roadmap provided by McLaughlin et al. (2013), i.e., guidelines for the conduct of educational research in terms of research design (defining, collecting, and analyzing educational data), ethical considerations, and the value of educational transformations in guiding curricular development [7]. As a practice, questionnaire-based studies in our university need not be evaluated by an institutional review board of university as a requirement; rather, they can be evaluated by getting verbal or written permission from sub-committees of the institutes under the umbrella of the university. Hence, we verbally informed the scientific review committee of the Dow College of Pharmacy about the study, and received permission following a discussion session with our dean. The survey was initially begun with pharmacy students studying in various institutes and universities of Karachi, and then subsequently continued with pharmacy teachers, deans and practicing pharmacists related to academia. The second questionnaire was developed on the basis of earlier study, addressing not only Karachi, but all of Pakistan, to obtain suggestions.

2.2. Study Population and Setting

The study was conducted in a total of eight universities (either from public or private sectors) of Karachi, Pakistan, that offer Pharm. D programs; namely, Dow University of Health Sciences, University of Karachi, Federal Urdu University of Science and Technology, Jinnah Sindh Medical University, Jinnah University for Women, Baqai Medical University, Ziauddin Medical University, and Hamdard Medical University.

First Session-Third to fifth professional pharmacy undergraduate Pakistani students were randomly selected as the study population for the first session. A maximum of 1000 students can be enrolled in each academic year in the selected universities in total. Verbal consent was received from each student participating in the study following an explanation of the purpose of the study. Participation in the study was voluntary, and the identity of each student remained anonymous.

Second Session-Pharmacy teachers, deans, and practicing pharmacists in Pakistan with either four years of a B. Pharmacy or five years of a Pharm. D basic degree were randomly selected as the study population for the second session. A maximum of 250 pharmacy teachers were teaching in the selected universities at the time of study. The survey was self-addressed in all institutes in Karachi that offer a Pharm. D degree, and an online form was published to take opinions from throughout Pakistan. Teachers with basic degrees other than B. Pharmacy or Pharm. D, pharmacists working in industry, students and non-practicing pharmacists were excluded in the second session of study.

2.3. Data Collection

First Session-A 14-item questionnaire on Pharm. D in Pakistan was distributed randomly among 500 students in the first session.

Second Session-In the second session, a 27-items questionnaire was distributed randomly to 221 pharmacy teachers, deans, and practicing pharmacists of Pakistan at random.

All of the participants in both sessions were asked to respond to each of the items on the questionnaires, and were evaluated using a 5-point Likert scale ranging from 1 = *Strongly Disagree* to 5 = *Strongly Agree*. Any score above 3.0 was considered as positive, and below 3.0 was considered negative.

2.4. Data Analysis

The retrieved questionnaires were then entered into Microsoft Excel, and then downloaded into the Statistical Package for Social Sciences (SPSS 16.0, Chicago, IL, USA) for analysis. Means and standard deviations for each of the items were calculated for both of the questionnaires.

3. Results

A total of 500 persons were available to respond to the questionnaire. Of these, 354 completed the questionnaire. Hence, the percentage response rate was calculated to be 70.8% for the first session. Table 1 shows the mean level of agreement of students in response to each of the 14 items in the questionnaire in the first session. Data for a total of 135 respondents were received and analyzed, out of a total of 221 professionals approached in the second session. Thus, the response rate by teachers, deans, and practicing pharmacists was estimated to be 61.1%. Table 2 shows the mean level of agreement in response to the 27-item questionnaire distributed in second session. Pharmacy deans and practicing pharmacists from all over Pakistan were included in the study population through an online survey form, and the questionnaire was self-administered in Karachi universities offering Pharm. D programs.

Table 1. 'Mean level of agreement' of students who responded to the 14-item questionnaire for the first session on a 5-point Likert scale.

Descriptive Statistics			
Questions	N	Mean	Std. Deviation
1-year paid residency should be provided in a health care sector	354	4.47	0.821
The pharmacy curriculum should place more emphasis on clinical aspects	354	4.36	0.831
The pathology course is not enough for clinical practice	354	4.24	0.936
Electives should be divided into industrial and clinical categories	354	4.24	0.870
Electives should be provided in all disciplines of clinical sciences	354	4.08	0.887
Physical assessment, neuropsychiatric therapeutics, infectious disease therapeutics, poison management & drug abuse, and cardiopulmonary therapeutics should all be included as separate disciplines	354	4.08	0.966
Current pharmacy curriculum does not meet the international standards of pharmacy practice	354	4.03	0.918
Pharmacogenetics should be included as a separate course	354	3.92	0.965
The ongoing pharmacy curriculum has too many repetitions	354	3.88	0.937
The curriculum for basic medical sciences is not sufficient	354	3.86	0.902
The medical microbiology and immunological basis for therapy should be separated from pharmaceutical microbiology as a discipline	354	3.86	1.032
The discipline of pharmacognosy can be more concise, and clinical pharmacognosy can be added	354	3.79	1.004
Clinical biochemistry should be included as a separate discipline	354	3.65	1.060
I am satisfied with the changes made in the Pharm. D curriculum	354	3.46	1.072
Valid N (list wise)	354		

Table 2. 'Mean level of agreement' of teachers, deans, and practicing pharmacists who responded to the 27-item questionnaire for the second session on a 5-point Likert scale.

Descriptive Statistics			
Questions	N	Mean	Std. Deviation
The Pharm. D degree should include a paid residency program to facilitate hospital, clinical and compounding pharmacy	135	4.37	0.826
The Pharm. D degree should be more practical and clinically oriented	135	4.33	0.938
Pharm. D degree in Pakistan should be both clinically and industrially oriented, according to the needs of the Pakistani people	135	4.32	0.869
Elective on Poison management & drug abuse must be provided	135	4.27	0.885
The Program should be run by the residency program director (RPD), residency activities coordinator, chief resident, or department chair or director	135	4.22	0.835
Elective on clinical pharmacokinetics and laboratory data interpretation must be added	135	4.16	0.948
Elective on infectious disease therapeutics (airborne/waterborne/blood borne) must be added	135	4.16	0.979
Pharm. D should include a practical apprenticeship in last two years in different wards of tertiary health care	135	4.13	1.018
Elective on pharmacovigilance must be added	135	4.06	0.944
Elective on oncology therapeutics must be added	135	4.05	0.964
Electives on Endocrine therapy & special patient population groups (such as infants, paeds, geriatrics, pregnancy, immunocompromised and renal and hepatic insufficient patients) must be provided	135	4.05	1.002

Table 2. *Cont.*

Descriptive Statistics			
Questions	N	Mean	Std. Deviation
Electives on Renal/GI/Nutrition therapy should be provided	135	4.04	0.988
Elective on cardiopulmonary therapeutics should be provided	135	4.04	0.988
Ambulatory patient care can be added as an elective	135	4.01	1.018
Electives should be provided in all the disciplines during final year.	135	3.99	1.007
Electives on pharmacogenetics and pharmacogenomics should be provided	135	3.95	0.949
Clinical pharmacy should not be included as a subject, rather it should be introduced as a discipline or department	135	3.95	1.115
The Pharm. D curriculum in Pakistan does not meet the international standards of practice	135	3.93	1.009
Elective on pharmacoeconomics should be provided	135	3.91	0.934
Clinical immunology/Hematology can be added as topics	135	3.90	0.984
Clinical microbiology can be added as topics	135	3.90	0.995
Electives on neuropsychiatric therapeutics must be provided	135	3.89	0.975
Physical assessment/Patient and family counseling can be added	135	3.85	1.062
Clinical biochemistry can be added as a subject	135	3.79	1.010
Self care and home care can also be added as subject	135	3.77	1.029
The Pre-Pharmacy includes all the basic subjects and industrial subjects necessary for a pharmacist to work in industry	135	3.33	1.112
The basic Pharm. D degree should be divided into Pre-Pharm. D and professional Pharm. D	135	3.08	1.191
Valid N (listwise)	135		

Our results showed that mean level of agreement for both sessions was 4.03 and 3.93, respectively, when we analyzed the opinion that the Pharm. D curriculum does not meet the international standards of practice. For the question that Pharm. D should be both clinically and industrially oriented according to the needs of the Pakistani people, the mean level of agreement was 4.32. Regarding having a more clinically oriented or patient-focused curriculum, rather than a curriculum focusing exclusively on industrial concerns, the mean level of agreement was 4.36 and 4.33, respectively. To improve clinical knowledge and practice further, it was suggested that electives should be provided in all of the clinical disciplines (mean level of agreement for both the sessions was 4.28 and 3.99, respectively. Moreover, the mean level of agreement for starting an apprenticeship in the last two years was found to be 4.13. Last, but not least, the study revealed that a 'paid residency program' to facilitate the hospital, clinical and compounding areas of pharmacy should be provided to undergraduate students, and that the program should be run by a residency program director (mean level of agreement for the first session was 4.47 and for the second session was 4.37). These results are summarized in Tables 1 and 2. Table 3 describes the percentage data of respondents regarding the division of the Pharm. D curriculum in two categories, such as pre-pharmacy and professional Pharm. D, along with the details of the subjects on which these should focus. Although most of the respondents (approx. 62% and 52%) rejected this division and the idea of pre-pharmacy, 70.3% of respondents still agreed with the suggestion of the inclusion of clinical pharmacy as a separate division, rather than as a mere course. In this connection, the percentages of responses that agreed with the idea of various topics being included as part of the clinical pharmacy course, or rather, in various courses within the discipline of clinical pharmacy, are illustrated in Figure 1).

Table 3. Percentage responses about Pre-Pharm. D and professional Pharm. D.

	Valid Response	Frequency	Percent	Valid Percent
The basic degree of Pharm. D should be divided into Pre-Pharm. D and Professional Pharm. D	Negative Response	49	36.3	36.2963
	Neutral	34	25.2	25.18519
	Positive Response	52	38.5	38.51852
	Total	135	100	100
	Valid Response	**Frequency**	**Percent**	**Valid Percent**
The Pre-Pharmacy Includes all the basic subjects and industrial subjects necessary for a pharmacist to work in industry	Negative Response	37	27	27.40741
	Neutral	33	24	24.44444
	Positive Response	65	48	48.14815
	Total	135	100	100
	Valid Response	**Frequency**	**Percent**	**Valid Percent**
Clinical Pharmacy should not be included as a subject rather it is introduced as a discipline or department	Negative Response	22	16.2963	16.2963
	Neutral	18	13.33333	13.33333
	Positive Response	95	70.37037	70.37037
	Total	135	100	100

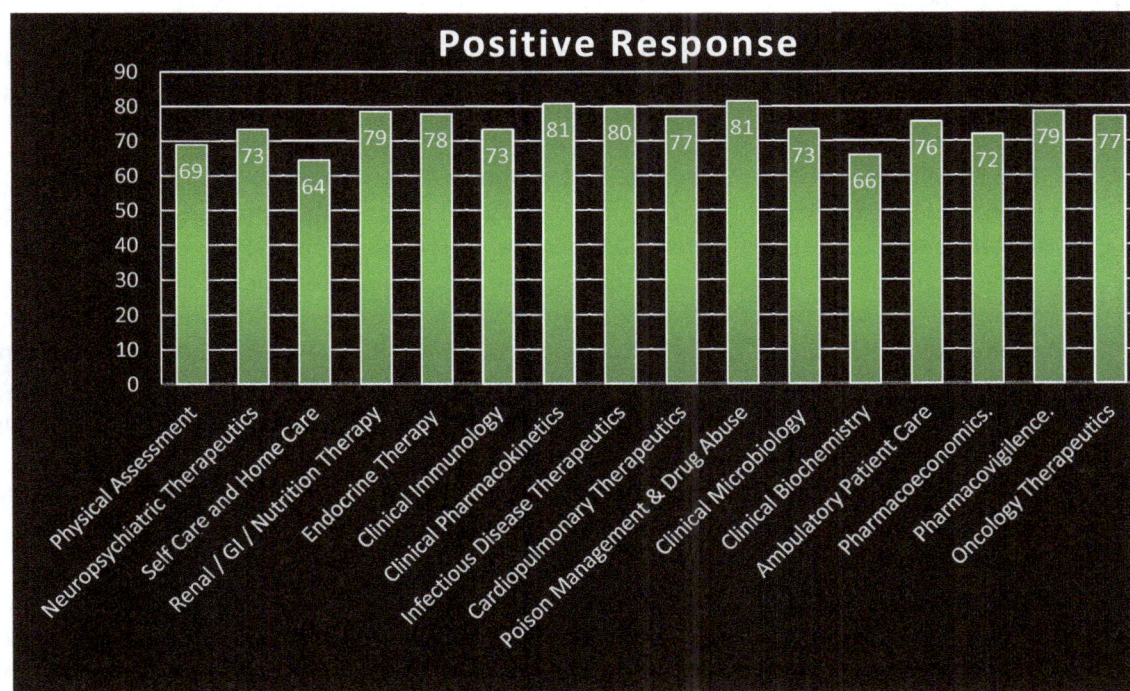

Figure 1. Percentage responses for various topics/electives as part of clinical pharmacy course/discipline.

4. Discussion

Alsharif, in 2012, found and reported that many pharmacy institutions worldwide were struggling with the same issues, whether in the United States or in other parts of the world, with the increased role that pharmacists play in the healthcare system on a local and global level [8]. According to economical facts and figures provided by Economic Adviser's Wing, Finance Division, Government of Pakistan, Islamabad, Pakistan earns 20.30% of its GDP from industrial sector [9]. Pharmaceutical industry in Pakistan is the 4th largest in the large-scale manufacturing sector of the country that contributes nearly 1 percent of the country's GDP [9,10]. According to a representative of the Pakistan Pharmaceutical Manufacturers Association, (PPMA), the pharmaceutical industry in Pakistan has experienced an impressive growth of 17 per cent during 2013, which is more than the global pharmaceutical average annual growth rate of 8 per cent [9,11].

Hence, fresh pharmacy graduates have a better future in industry, compared to other "health care settings", because clinical and community pharmacy is not truly established, even today, except in a few private hospitals. Nevertheless, current mergers of pharma industries have shifted the paradigm. Consequently, introducing a hybrid program that facilitates both of these aspects—i.e., industry and clinical/community—would be pretty good.

Previous studies related to the development of Pharm. D curricula in Pakistan have criticized it for not being productive. A few of the critical statements are as follows:

(1)   The curriculum of Pharm. D Pakistan is inadequate due the lack of experienced academics [12] and practice-based facilities, and it does not contribute to health care policy [2].

(2)   The Pharm. D degree was started without any planning [2].

(3)   "The Pharm. D degree is just a tool to help students qualify for job opportunities in Gulf countries, as well as to make the so-called "doctors" eligible to appear for the license examination in the United States or elsewhere" [13].

(4)   Whether the curriculum, without any proper clinical attachment, with just a couple of visits to hospitals, would serve the purpose is a doubtful issue [14].

(5)   In Pakistan, the hospital pharmacy/clinical pharmacy is at a preliminary level [12], etc.

Instead of echoing the criticism reported in literature, we thought about the scope of the study to be discussed, i.e., that this study should not be performed to further criticize, but rather to suggest some revisions. For example:

i.   as the "International Pharmaceutical Federation (FIP) Global Competency Framework" suggests that pharmacy professionals must be ready in terms of their professional knowledge, skills, efficiency and availability for placements at international sites [1], we suggest that our pharmacy council should encourage the provision of a "one year paid residency program" for pharmacy students, and that the residency program should be coordinated by a residency program director (RPD), residency activities coordinators, chief resident, and/or department chair or director. In addition to the enhancement of expertise, this experience could serve to increase the students' respect towards national, local and ethnic identities, increasing professional harmony, as well.

ii.   Electives should be given in all disciplines of clinical pharmacy and electives should be divided into clinical and industrial categories. This will enhance their ability to integrate knowledge towards pharmacy practice.

iii. The pharmacy degree should be divided into a two-phase degree program, i.e., Pre-Pharmacy and Pharm. D. The Pre-Pharmacy degree should be of two or three years, and should contain all the basic subjects of formulation, and the courses needed for industry. Whereas, the Pharm. D should be more practically focused towards public health, and contain electives, an apprenticeship and internship program, and have more therapeutic subjects. As a result, depending upon the aptitude of students, the choice of degrees can be varied.

iv.   The curriculum should place more emphasis on clinical aspects by adding therapeutics, clinical pharmacology, molecular pharmacology, clinical microbiology and pharmacogenetics as separate disciplines, rather than mere topics. In this way, students can compete internationally, having been equipped with the necessary applied knowledge following the standards.

5. Conclusions

Our study concludes that still, after a decade of development, our Pharm. D curriculum is facing a transition state from an industrial focus to a more patient care-oriented focus. This type of curriculum is quite beneficial for Pakistani people, and it is a necessity in this day and age. However, further improvements should be encouraged to add clinical and therapeutic courses to make this program more patient focused. For this purpose, the higher authorities should review the curriculum in the light of the suggestions of pharmacy teachers, students and, especially, practicing pharmacists given above, since our study shows more than 90% of practicing pharmacists and teachers agree to the suggested changes in the curriculum.

Acknowledgments: We acknowledge the cooperation of deans and faculty members of various universities of Karachi to complete the study. We are thankful to Salman Farooq and Saniya Ata for their untiring efforts for data entry and record keeping.

Author Contributions: Saima Mahmood Malhi and Hassan Raza are responsible for initiating and designing the study, data interpretation, and manuscript writing. Saima Mahmood Malhi is further responsible for the analysis of data, discussion questionnaire development and overall review of the manuscript. Kiran Ajmal contributed to developing the questionnaire and providing necessary information regarding the curriculum. She also reviewed the manuscript. Hassan Raza and Syed Muhammad Sharib played a part in design and development of the questionnaire, and conducting the study. Sumbul Shamim provided the permission to conduct the study and took care of legal aspects. Data collection, data interpretation and application of statistics were done by Saima Mahmood Malhi, Hassan Raza, Saniya Ata, Salman Farooq, Syed Muhammad Sharib and Sidrat-ul-Muntaha.

References and Note

1. Hawboldt, J.; Nash, R.; Patrick, B.F. How Two Small Pharmacy Schools' Competency Standards Compare with an International Competency Framework and How Well These Schools Prepare Students for International Placements. *Pharmacy* **2017**, *5*, 14. [CrossRef]

2. Jamshed, S.; Babar, Z.U.D.; Masood, I. The Pharm. D Degree in Developing Countries. *Am. J. Pharm. Educ.* **2007**, *71*, 125. [CrossRef] [PubMed]

3. Azhar, S.; Hassali, M.A.; Izham, M.; Ibrahim, M.; Ahmad, M.; Masood, I.; Shafie, A.A. The role of pharmacists in developing countries: The current scenario in Pakistan. *Hum. Resour. Health* **2009**, *7*, 54. [CrossRef] [PubMed]

4. Hadi, M.A.; Hughes, J. Broader Perspective Needed on the Pharm. D Degree in Pakistan. *Am. J. Pharm. Educ.* **2009**, *73*, 114. [CrossRef] [PubMed]

5. Anderson, C.; Futter, B. Pharm. D or Needs Based Education: Which Comes First? *Am. J. Pharm. Educ.* **2009**, *73*, 92. [CrossRef] [PubMed]

6. Pharmacy Council of Pakistan. Revised Pharm. D Curriculum Final 2013. Available online: http://www.pharmacycouncil.org.pk/ (accessed on 9 September 2013).

7. McLaughlin, J.E.; Dean, M.J.; Mumper, R.J.; Blouin, R.A.; Roth, M.T. A Roadmap for Educational Research in Pharmacy. *Am. J. Pharm. Educ.* **2013**, *77*, 218. [CrossRef] [PubMed]

8. Alsharif, N.Z. Globalization of Pharmacy Education: What is Needed? *Am. J. Pharm. Educ.* **2012**, *76*, 77. [CrossRef] [PubMed]

9. Economic Adviser's Wing, Finance Division, Government of Pakistan, Islamabad. Highlights of Pakistan Economic Survey 2014–2015. PCPPI—2551(2015) Fin.Div-2-6-2015-500.

10. Ahmed, V.; Batool, S. India-Pakistan Trade: A Case Study of the Pharmaceutical Sector. In *India-Pakistan Trade Normalisation*; Springer: Berlin, Germany, 2014.

11. Zaman, K. Review of Pakistan Pharmaceutical Industry: SWOT Analysis. Available online: http://www.ojs.excelingtech.co.uk/index.php/IJBIT/article/view/30 (accessed on 19 July 2017).

12. Khan, T.M. Challenges to pharmacy and pharmacy practice in Pakistan. *Australas. Med. J.* **2011**, *4*, 230–235. [CrossRef]

13. Jamshed, S.; Baber, Z.U.D.; Izham, M.; Ibrahim, M. Pharm. D in Pakistan: A Tag or a Degree? *Am. J. Pharm. Educ.* **2009**, *73*, 13. [PubMed]

14. Pakistan Pharmaceutical Industry analysis of Pakistan. Available online: https://www.scribd.com/doc/32476064/Pharamaceutical-Industry-Analysis-of-Pakistan (accessed on 5 March 2014).

17

Training Needs of Manitoba Pharmacists to Increase Application of Assessment and Prescribing for Minor Ailments into Practice: A Qualitative and Quantitative Survey

Brenna Shearer [1,2,*], Sheila Ng [1,*], Drena Dunford [1] and I fan Kuo [1]

1   College of Pharmacy, Faculty of Health Sciences, University of Manitoba, Winnipeg, MB R3E 0T5, Canada; drena.dunford@umanitoba.ca (D.D.); i.kuo@umanitoba.ca (I.f.K.)
2   Independent Researcher Pharmacists Manitoba, Winnipeg, MB R3C 4H1, Canada
*   Correspondence: bshearer@pharmacistsmb.ca (B.S.); sheila.ng@umanitoba.ca (S.N.)

Abstract: Current literature demonstrates the positive impact of pharmacists prescribing medication on patient outcomes and pharmacist perceptions of the practice. The aim of this study was to understand the factors affecting prescribing practices among Manitoba pharmacists and identify whether additional training methods would be beneficial for a practice behavior change. A web-based survey was developed and participation was solicited from pharmacists in Manitoba. Descriptive statistics were calculated to summarize the frequency of demographic characteristics. Chi-square tests were used to explore possible correlations between variables of interest and thematic analysis of qualitative data was completed. A total of 162 participants completed the survey. The response rate was 12.3%. Of those who had met the requirements to prescribe, none were doing so on a daily basis and 23.5% had not assessed or prescribed since being certified. Respondents identified the top barriers for providing this service as a lack of sufficient revenue and a lack of time. Qualitative analysis of responses identified additional barriers including a limiting scope and inadequate tools. Approximately half (54.4%) of respondents expressed that additional training would be of value. The themes identified from the survey data suggest that practice-based education would help pharmacists apply skills. In addition, expansion of prescribing authority and strategies addressing remuneration issues may help overcome barriers to pharmacists prescribing within Manitoba.

Keywords: pharmacists; prescribing; professional development; minor ailments; continuing education needs; survey

1. Introduction

Pharmacy practices have expanded in some regions of Canada to include the authority to prescribe medications for a variety of conditions [1]. Legislation and regulation governing the scope of pharmacy practices are a provincial/territorial jurisdiction in Canada and, therefore, varies substantially across the country. Pharmacists in the province of Manitoba were granted regulatory authority to assess and prescribe medication for ambulatory ailments due to the passing of the Pharmaceutical Act and Regulations in January 2014. The Pharmaceutical Regulations enable pharmacists to prescribe any Schedule II or III drug listed in the National Association of Pharmacy Regulatory Authorities (NAPRA) manual (non-prescription) and Health Canada approved medical devices. In addition, authorization to prescribe specific medications for select self-limiting conditions and smoking cessation (list specified in the Pharmaceutical Regulations Schedule III) can be obtained by any licensed pharmacist with successful completion of an education program approved by the provincial regulatory body known as the College of Pharmacists of Manitoba. The authorization to prescribe a drug for self-limiting conditions requires the completion of a web-based independent study program with an exam administered by the College of Pharmacists of Manitoba [2].

In the 20 months following the expansion of this scope of practice, 425 pharmacists had successfully completed the requirements of the Manitoba Certification for Authorization to Prescribe a Drug Included in the Schedule 3 to the Pharmaceutical Regulation for Self-Limiting Conditions (College of Pharmacists of Manitoba, personal email, 3 September 2015). Two hundred and twenty-five (225) pharmacists have successfully completed the Manitoba Certification to Prescribe a Drug Included in Schedule 3 to the Pharmaceutical Regulations for Smoking Cessation (College of Pharmacists of Manitoba, personal email, 3 September 2015). With more than 1501 licensed pharmacists in Manitoba, the uptake by pharmacists has been slow.

Across Canada there is variation in publicly funded and third party health insurance benefits to compensate for pharmacist initiated assessment and prescribing services [3]. While pharmacists in Manitoba have one of the most comprehensive scopes of practice, they have one of the most limited compensation models along with one of the most detailed training requirements [1,4]. Compensation frameworks may play a pivotal role in pharmacist decision-making regarding the application of these services into practice especially in Manitoba where a publicly funded framework for services has not kept pace with the rest of Canada [4]. However, a growing body of literature demonstrates the positive impact on patient outcomes of pharmacist prescribing medication, pharmacist perceptions of the practice, and practice changes [3].

Knowledge translation literature describes successful integration of knowledge into practice as a key factor to improve practitioner confidence [5]. Research on practice changes has demonstrated that significant factors for success include pharmacist's perceptions about factors influencing uptake of prescribing practices, identifying positive practice settings, confidence, and training programs incorporating both the knowledge and the ability to apply knowledge [3,6–9]. Some studies have indicated that pharmacists preferred live training programs and evaluated these as the most valuable for improving confidence [10,11]. In addition, communication and counseling skills are stated as important components for reducing practice barriers and ensuring confidence above and beyond continuing education programs [6,12]. Pharmacist prescribing education programs vary widely across the country, which may affect the consistency of application within the profession [1].

There has been no research evaluating how many Manitoba pharmacists with prescribing certifications are actively practicing this expanded scope of practice, what gaps exist between continuing professional development and application to the practice, what the training and education needs of pharmacists are to successfully apply this knowledge into practice, and what factors influence pharmacists to engage in prescribing authority education. The information gathered can inform and impact the development of effective continuing education programs that address pharmacists' needs. The aim of this research study is to understand the factors impacting prescribing authority practice among Manitoba pharmacists and identify whether additional training methods would be beneficial for practice behavior change.

2. Methods

2.1. Survey Design

An anonymous web-based survey was developed, which includes a variety of question modalities such as multi-select questions, single-select questions, dichotomous answers, rank ordering, and open-ended free text. Questions included demographic information, the status of Certification in Prescribing for Self-Limiting Conditions, factors affecting adoption of prescribing knowledge into the practice, and attitudes regarding training needs to increase the provision of prescribing drugs into clinical practice. A literature search was completed to identify previous surveys, which evaluated pharmacist's continuing education needs and preferences. Relevant resources were identified [6,7,11–17].

The research team reviewed the literature for relevant questions, themes, and modified questions to pertain specifically to pharmacist's continuing education needs and preferences for prescribing drugs for self-limiting conditions in Manitoba. Additional questions were developed to assess the demographic and status of certification specific to Manitoba.

The survey contained three question streams that filtered participants based on their status of completion of the self-study program required for prescribing drugs for self-limiting conditions. The status was broken down into four categories, which includes: (1) pharmacists that have completed the self-study program, (2) pharmacists in progress of completing the self-study program, (3) pharmacists who had not started but plan to initiate the self-study program, and (4) pharmacists with no plans to start the self-study program. All streams answered four demographic questions and one status of certification question. Participants in all categories answered a question regarding either experienced or anticipated barriers as well as four questions regarding continuing education preferences and needs. Wording was modified within the questions to reflect participants' current prescribing status. Participants who had completed the self-study program (category 1) answered three additional questions regarding the frequency of and fees charged for prescribing.

The draft survey was first piloted among eight pharmacist volunteers from the Pharmacists Manitoba Board of Directors. The pilot survey resulted in no changes. The final survey was administered through FluidSurveys™.

2.2. Recruitment and Data Collection

Recruitment of participants took place over an eight-month period from June 2016 to January 2017. The non-probability convenience sampling method was utilized. Email databases from all provincial pharmacy organizations including the Canadian Society of Hospital Pharmacists (CSHP) Manitoba Branch, the College of Pharmacists of Manitoba (CPhM), and Pharmacists Manitoba were used to distribute the survey link and information to capture all pharmacists licensed in Manitoba. The project received approval by the University of Manitoba Health Research and Ethics Board (approval number HS19741) and all participants provided informed consent prior to data collection.

2.3. Statistical Analysis

Descriptive statistics were calculated to summarize the frequency of demographic characteristics for overall survey respondents and subgroups of survey respondents. Chi-square tests were used to explore possible correlation between variables of interest (i.e., barriers, service fees, and preferences for training) and demographics for each group. Those who were in the process of completing or planning on initiating the self-study program answered the same set of survey questions and were treated as the same group in the analyses. All statistical analyses were carried out in the statistical software SAS® 9.4 (SAS Institute; Carey, NC, USA). Qualitative analysis of free text responses was also completed using FluidSurveys™. In addition, the research team completed realist thematic analysis to identify the main themes to summarize collective responses using word repetitions and key-words-in-context methods [18].

3. Results

3.1. Demographics of Survey Respondents

During the eight-month recruitment period, 185 participants consented to the research study. Of those, 162 completed the online survey (completion rate 87.6%). The survey response rate was estimated to be 12.3% based on the total number of pharmacists invited to participate in the study (185 respondents out of 1501 licensed pharmacists). The majority of the respondents practiced in the retail setting (90.7%), worked in the Winnipeg Regional Health Authority (WRHA) catchment (52.5%), and were predominantly employed in a full-time position (75.3%). Most respondents had been in practice for more than 15 years (45.7%), which was followed by those in practice for six to

15 years (32.1%), and those in practice for fewer than six years (22.2%). The characteristics of survey respondents are described in Table 1.

Table 1. Characteristics of survey respondents (*n*, %).

	Overall (*n* = 162)	Self-Study Completed (*n* = 115)	Self-Study in Progress (*n* = 9)	Self-study not Started but Plan to Initiate (*n* = 23)	No Plans to Start Self-Study (*n* = 15)
Number of years practicing as pharmacist					
<6 years	36 (22.2%)	29 (25.2%)	1 (11.1%)	5 (21.7%)	1 (6.7%)
6–15 years	52 (32.1%)	33 (28.7%)	2 (22.2%)	7 (30.4%)	10 (66.7%)
>15 years	74 (45.7%)	53 (46.1%)	6 (66.7%)	11 (47.8%)	4 (26.7%)
Employment status					
Full time	122 (75.3%)	94 (81.7%)	5 (55.6%)	14 (60.9%)	9 (60.0%)
Part time	27 (16.7%)	16 (13.9%)	3 (33.3%)	4 (17.4%)	4 (26.7%)
Casual or on leave	12 (7.4%)	4 (3.4%)	1 (11.1%)	5 (21.7%)	2 (13.3%)
Primary area of employment					
Retail/community	147 (90.7%)	111 (96.5%)	6 (66.7%)	20 (87.0%)	10 (66.7%)
Hospital	8 (4.9%)	1 (0.9%)	1 (11.1%)	1 (4.3%)	5 (33.3%)
Government or academia	3 (1.9%)	2 (1.8%)	1 (11.1%)	0	0
Other	3 (1.9%)	1 (0.9%)	1 (11.1%)	1 (4.3%)	0
Location of employment by health region					
Winnipeg (Churchill)	85 (52.5%)	55 (47.8%)	6 (66.7%)	12 (52.2%)	1 (6.7%)
Interlake Eastern	16 (9.9%)	12 (10.4%)	1 (11.1%)	3 (13.0%)	0
Northern	5 (3.1%)	3 (2.6%)	0	1 (4.3%)	1 (6.7%)
Prairie Mountain Health	25 (15.4%)	19 (16.5%)	1 (11.1%)	4 (17.4%)	1 (6.7%)
Southern Health-Sante Sud	22 (13.6%)	20 (17.4%)	0	2 (8.7%)	12 (80.0%)

Of the 162 respondents, 115 (71.0%) reported having completed the self-study program for assessments and prescribing for minor ailments. Nine individuals (5.6%) were in progress of completing the self-study program, 23 (14.2%) respondents had yet to start but were planning to initiate the program, and 15 (9.3%) pharmacists expressed having no plans to start the program. There were no significant differences in demographics between the groups with the exception of pharmacists in the hospital setting being less likely to initiate a self-study program for assessments and prescribing for minor ailments than pharmacists in the retail setting (62.5% vs. 6.8%, $p < 0.0001$).

3.2. Assessment and Prescribing Skills for Self-Limiting Conditions in the Practice Setting

Amongst the 115 respondents who have completed the self-study program, none were providing assessment and/or prescribing services for minor ailments on a daily basis and 27 (23.5%) had not assessed or prescribed for minor ailments since receiving their certification. Of the 88 pharmacists who had provided minor ailments assessment or prescribing services, 52 (59.1%) reported having done so 1 to 5 times in the past 30 days, and 48 (54.5%) described having charged a fee for their services with a median amount of $20. The employment status was found to be significantly correlated with charging service fees for minor ailments assessment and prescribing where those not in a full-time employment position were more likely to have charged a fee (84.6% vs. 51.4%, $p = 0.03$). No correlation was found between charging a clinical service fee and other demographic characteristics.

3.3. Perceived Barriers for Applying Assessment and Prescribing Skills

When asked about barriers, the majority (83.5%) of the respondents certified to assess and prescribe drugs for minor ailments reported having encountered issues in providing such a service (Table 2). The top barriers identified were 'lack of sufficient revenue attached to expanded role' (26.2%), 'lack of time at work' (23.5%), and lack of patients presenting with minor ailments (11.9%). The region of employment was found to be correlated with reporting barriers where those in the WRHA catchment were more likely to have responded to having barriers than those outside of the WRHA area (90.9% vs. 76.7%, $p = 0.04$). No correlation was found between barriers and other respondent characteristics.

Table 2. Barriers identified by respondent subgroups (*n*, %).

	Self-Study Completed (*n* = 115)	Self-Study in Progress/Plan to Initiate (*n* = 32)	No Plans to Start Self-Study (*n* = 15)
Encountered barriers in applying assessment and prescribing skills for minor ailments			
Yes	96 (83.5%)	–	–
No	19 (16.5%)	–	–
Anticipated encountering barriers in applying assessment and prescribing skills for minor ailments			
Yes	–	20 (62.5%)	–
No	–	12 (37.5%)	–
Identified barriers to taking on expanded role of applying assessment and prescribing skills for minor ailments			
Yes	–	–	14 (93.3%)
No	–	–	1 (0.06%)
Specific barriers identified (*n*, %)			
Lack of sufficient revenue attached to expanded role	68 (26.2%)	14 (29.8%)	10 (66.7%)
Lack of training in expanded role	11 (4.2%)	1 (2.1%)	–
Lack of confidence in skills	25 (9.6%)	4 (8.5%)	0
Clinical uncertainty	12 (4.6%)	0	1 (6.7%)
Lack of time at work	61 (23.5%)	15 (31.9%)	8 (53.3%)
Lack of performance feedback	2 (0.8%)	2 (4.3%)	–
Lack of motivation to take on new responsibilities	10 (3.8%)	3 (6.4%)	7 (46.7%)
Lack of support from management	14 (5.4%)	4 (8.5%)	4 (26.7%)
Lack of patients presenting with minor ailments	31 (11.9%)	2 (4.3%)	–
Lack of satisfaction with current training and certification program	–	–	2 (13.3%)
Irrelevant to practice	–	–	4 (26.7%)
Other	26 (10.0%)	2 (4.3%)	2 (13.3%)

– question not applicable and was not asked. Other: respondents were given the option of adding additional barriers in a free text format. These results are explored further in qualitative analysis.

Of the 32 respondents who were in the process of completing the self-study program or were planning to initiate the program, 20 (62.5%) reported anticipating barriers that would prevent them from applying the assessment and prescribing skills for minor ailments in their practice. The top barriers identified were similar to the group who had been certified with 'lack of sufficient revenue attached to expanded role' (29.8%) and 'lack of time at work' (31.9%) as the most common barriers. The potential obstacles identified also included a 'lack of confidence in skills' (8.5%) and a 'lack of support from management/head office' (8.5%). No correlation was found between anticipating barriers and any of the demographic characteristics.

A minority of 15 respondents expressed having no plans to start the self-study program for the assessment and drug prescribing for self-limiting conditions. When asked about specific barriers that prevented them from taking on the expanded practice role, many perceived a 'lack of sufficient revenue attached', a 'lack of time at work,' and a 'lack of motivation to take on new responsibilities' as factors deterring them from undertaking the program.

The survey also encouraged respondents to provide additional comments on their experience and their perspectives of providing assessment and drug prescribing services for self-limiting conditions. Some common themes that emerged from these open-ended questions included a lack of public and private payer remuneration for services, a limiting scope of practice and prescribing formulary, insufficient public awareness of services, and an absence of adequate documentation and decision-making tools (see Figure 1).

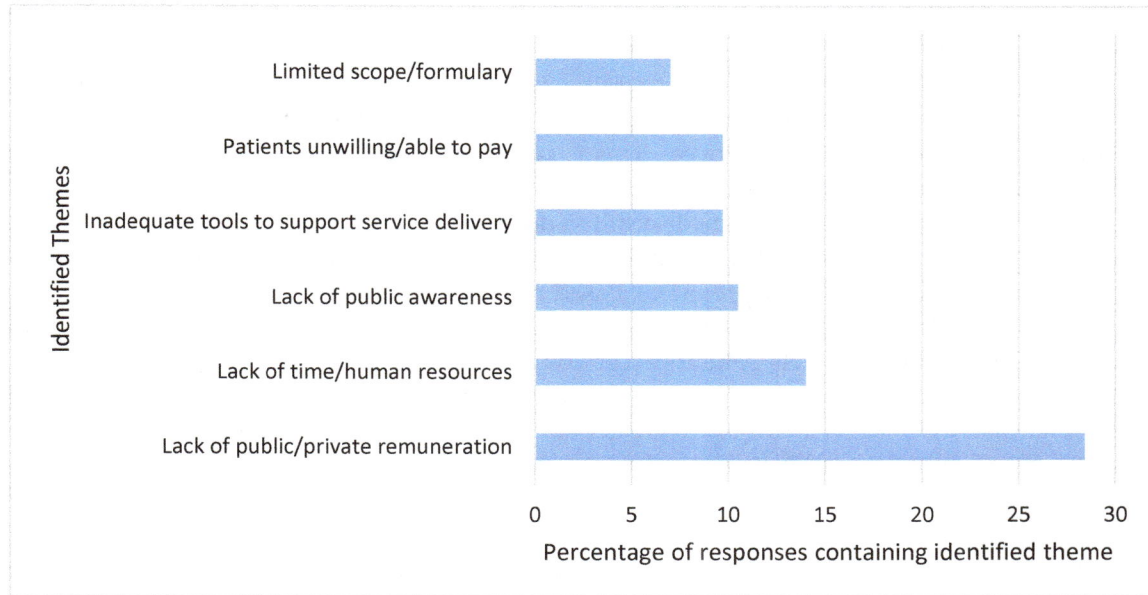

Figure 1. Themes identified from thematic analysis of open-response comments of pharmacists' experience and perspectives of providing assessment and drug prescribing services.

3.4. Preferences for Continuing Education

Respondents who have completed the self-study program, were in the process of completion, or were planning to initiate the program were also asked whether they felt additional training and continuing education would improve their application of assessment and drug prescribing services for minor ailments. Approximately half (54.4%) of the 147 respondents expressed that additional training would be of value in applying their expanded role with 29.3% and 16.3% respectively responding no or unsure for the benefit of additional training in this area. Attitudes towards additional training did not correlate with demographic characteristics. Respondents were split between the types of education opportunity with 46.2% and 53.8% preferring self-guided study and live sessions, respectively. Internet-based written materials were the preferred type of self-guided training/continuing education format while live lectures, hands-on workshops, and topic-specific short seminars were the top ranked medium for live training. There was no correlation with years of practice and type of education preferred.

4. Discussion

This is the first survey to investigate the factors affecting the prescribing authority practice among Manitoba pharmacists and identify whether an additional training method would be beneficial for practice behavior changes. While the response rate to the survey was less than desired, the information gathered provides valuable insight into pharmacist preferences and perceptions about educational needs and barriers affecting the assessment and prescribing scope of practice.

The web-based survey response rate was 12.3%. Johnson and Wislar and Dillman have identified declining response rates to surveys in the past few decades [19,20]. For this study, the sample size needed to achieve a 95% confidence level with a confidence interval of 4 would have required 433 participants (28% response rate). Research has identified lower response rates from web-based survey methodology even though there is a growing prevalence as a preferred methodology due to the ease of data collection and analysis, faster response time, and lower cost [8,21,22]. Web-based surveys with low response rates are consistent in the literature, have been identified as reliable for evaluation, and are not restrictive to the generalizability of findings [23–25]. Furthermore, web-based survey response rates of less than 10% have been reported as reliable for evaluation [22,26–28]. For survey response rates, Johnson and Wislar state that "there is no scientifically proven minimally acceptable response rate" [19] (p. 1805).

Barriers identified in this study for providing assessment and prescribing services for minor ailments included lack of sufficient revenue, lack of time, lack of support from employers, and lack of eligible patients requiring the services. This is consistent with findings of research related to medication assessment services in other Canadian settings. Isenor et al. described time, staffing, and reimbursement as barriers identified to fully adopting prescribing. Guirguis et al. described limitations in the practice environment including staffing [29,30]. While pharmacists are one of the most accessible primary care health care providers, based on the number of patient visits compared with primary care physicians, a limited range of prescribing authority combined with lack of appropriate remuneration potentially impacts patient perception of the pharmacist's role and the pharmacist's full adoption of services into practice [31]. Previous research supports these research findings that identify pharmacist's perceived barriers to greater adoption of services into practice to include a lack of support from employers, a lack of appropriate remuneration, and a need for personalized education and practice as factors affecting the application of new scopes of practice [9,10,32].

Although to a lesser extent, lack of confidence in skills was another barrier identified by some pharmacists. Previous research of allied health professionals with prescribing responsibility identified "personal anxiety undermining confidence to prescribe" as a theme affecting the continuing professional development needs of these prescribers [33]. Clinical uncertainty was not a major barrier identified in our study. Therefore, continued professional development may need to focus on strategies to increase confidence that extend beyond clinical content. Further research to explore the rationale for lack of confidence may be beneficial.

This study highlighted factors for understanding the continuing education needs of pharmacists to enhance adaptation of expanded prescribing skills into practice as an important component for understanding behavior and practice changes. Research has highlighted a strong relationship between the community pharmacy organizational culture (such as cultural values for innovation, competitiveness, and social responsibility) with a pharmacist provision of expanded scope of practice services [34].

While prior research added to the knowledge of factors affecting education participation and environmental factors impacting the adoption into practice, this study builds on that knowledge by focusing on pharmacist education preferences as an additional key element for improving the application of these skills into practice. Previous research has ascertained that pharmacists undertake continuing education based on factors including achieving licensure requirement, relevance to personal interest, and self-improvement [35].

Continuing education preferences of Manitoba pharmacists was consistent with findings from previous research studies, which indicated that training preferences of pharmacists was highest for live support programs [10,11]. While 54.4% of our respondents expressed value in additional training to support application of expanded roles, respondents were split between self-guided study and live sessions [9,11–14]. In Manitoba, a 15-hour online training module reflective of the prescribing authority range is available from the provincial regulatory body. In addition, an 8-hour continuing education in-person workshop has been jointly offered by the university and provincial advocacy body to enhance the theory-based learning with low uptake in the courses offered. Continuing education (CE) courses of self-study, distance learning, and live CE programs are most common yet less effective in improving clinical practice behavior while interactive workshops are the most favorable format to enhance the translation of CE learning into practice [13,14]. To improve the adoption of new skills into practice, Ontario pharmacists identified limitations with existing continuing education resources and identified preferences for individual practice support [9].

The findings of this study indicate that, in Manitoba, a blend of in-person education and support directly within the pharmacy along with employer education and integration may enhance opportunities for growth and adoption of new scopes of service by pharmacists and the pharmacy business. Alternative options for reimbursement beyond public funding may be required as a component of business model development for services. Since this study identified a limited prescribing scope as a barrier, increasing the pharmacist scope of prescribing authority in Manitoba may also provide additional interest by pharmacists and employers, increase visibility of the role of the pharmacist among patients and other health care providers, and open the door for constructive dialogue with government and private funders about how pharmacists can advance health care system accessibility.

Strengths & Limitation

The strengths of this research include a specific focus on perceptions of pharmacists regarding education preferences and barriers to implementing patient assessment and drug prescribing skills for minor ailments in one province of Canada. In addition, this research evaluates the differences in perceptions between pharmacists who have completed, are in the process of completing or intending to complete certification, and those with no intention to gain additional certification. Strong interest and support from the provincial regulatory body and professional associations is evident from the distribution of the survey to all licensed pharmacists in the province through their regular electronic communications. Pharmacists Manitoba in partnership with the College of Pharmacy, University of Manitoba share a common goal of advancing the pharmacist's professional practice. The survey was supported by all provincial organizations involved with licensing pharmacists and advocating for pharmacists, which increased the reach to pharmacists regardless of where they practice or the type of practice location. The information gathered in this research survey provides valuable knowledge to support the development of continuing education programs to enhance the application of practice skills in pharmacies.

A limitation of this study is the use of a web-based survey alone to capture pharmacist perceptions and a lower than desired response rate. Personalized invitations to complete the survey to stratified groups of pharmacists, those who have completed certification, and those who have not may have bolstered response rates by each group and provided more robust findings for evaluation and analysis. This study is limited to Manitoba pharmacists and, therefore, may have limited application to a national audience. However, the results confirm that perceptions of educational needs and barriers to practice application are consistent with the research literature. In spite of the specific education requirements for prescribing authority in Manitoba [12], pharmacist perceptions about barriers to the implementation of skills into practice are also consistent with the research literature.

This study lacked an evaluation of employer-specific perceptions of current and expected education requirements to support the patient assessment and drug prescribing services. A comparison of employee and employer expectations of skills post certification may provide insight as to what employers would support to advance the integration of new services.

5. Conclusions

In order to attain the optimal outcomes from pharmacists prescribing medication for minor ailments in Manitoba, continuing education that addresses the needs of pharmacists, reduces perceived barriers, and is delivered in an effective manner is required. As highlighted by the findings of this research study, pharmacists in Manitoba share similar concerns, issues, and education support needs as those in other parts of the country. The themes identified for continuing education suggest that personalized and practice-based education would help pharmacists apply these skills into practice. Educational programming, which addressed barriers identified by Manitoba pharmacists in providing prescribing services, may be beneficial. In order to address identified barriers, it could be beneficial to incorporate prescribing into a busy practice site (overcoming time management and human resource barriers) as well as include strategies to promote pharmacy services and development and implementation of fee-for-service models. In addition to education support for pharmacists, employers should direct more support for the implementation of services as well as strategies to overcome remuneration issues and mechanisms to expand prescribing authority in order to motivate the public and funders to utilize pharmacist's knowledge and skills to their full scope.

Author Contributions: Conceptualization, B.S., S.N. and D.D. Data curation, I.f.K. Formal analysis, S.N. and I.f.K. Funding acquisition, S.N. and D.D. Investigation, B.S. and S.N. Methodology, B.S., S.N., I.f.K., and D.D. Project administration, B.S. and S.N. Writing-original draft, B.S., S.N., and I.f.K. Writing-review & editing, B.S., S.N., I.f.K., and D.D.

Funding: This research was funded by the District Five National Association of Boards of Pharmacy and American Association of Colleges of Pharmacy.

Acknowledgments: The authors would like to thank Trevor Shivdatt who was a fourth-year pharmacy student at the time of the study for his assistance in building the survey. The authors thank Amani Hamad who was a PhD student at the College of Pharmacy for her assistance in study analysis. The authors also thank the Pharmacists Manitoba and The College of Pharmacists of Manitoba for survey distribution as well as our funding sponsor District V NAPRA/AACP.

References

1.   Habicht, D.; Ng, S.; Dunford, D.; Shearer, B.; Kuo, I.F. Incorporating assessment and prescribing for ambulatory ailments skills into practice: An environmental scan of continuing education for pharmacist prescribing in Canada. *Can. Pharm. J.* **2017**, *150*, 316–325. [CrossRef] [PubMed]

2.   College of Pharmacists of Manitoba. A guide to pharmacy practice in Manitoba. 2018. Available online: http://www.cphm.ca/uploaded/web/Legislation/Pharmacy-Practice-Guide/Guide-to-Pharmacy-Practice-Final.pdf (accessed on 4 August 2018).

3.   Faruquee, C.F.; Guirguis, L.M. A scoping review of research on the prescribing practice of Canadian pharmacists. *Can. Pharm. J.* **2015**, *148*, 325–348. [CrossRef] [PubMed]

4.   Canadian Pharmacists Association. A Review of Pharmacy Services in Canada and the Health Economic Evidence. 2016. Available online: https://www.pharmacists.ca/cpha-ca/assets/File/cpha-on-the-issues/Pharmacy%20Services%20Report%201.pdf (accessed on 4 August 2018).

5.   Grol, R.; Grimshaw, J. From best evidence to best practice: Effective implementation of change in patients' care. *Lancet* **2003**, *362*, 1225–1230. [CrossRef]

6.   George, J.; Pfleger, D.; McCaig, D.; Bond, C.; Stewart, D. Independent prescribing by pharmacists: A study of the awareness, views and attitudes of Scottish community pharmacists. *Pharm. World Sci.* **2006**, *28*, 45–53. [CrossRef] [PubMed]

7.   Pfleger, D.E.; McHattie, L.W.; Diack, H.L.; McCaig, D.J.; Stewart, D.C. Views, attitudes and self-assessed training needs of Scottish community pharmacists to public health practice and competence. *Pharm. World Sci.* **2008**, *30*, 801–809. [CrossRef] [PubMed]

8.   Partin, M.R.; Powell, A.A.; Burgess, D.J.; Haggstrom, D.A.; Gravely, A.A.; Halek, K.; Bangerter, A.; Shaukat, A.; Nelson, D.B. Adding Postal Follow-Up to a Web-Based Survey of Primary Care and Gastroenterology Clinic Physician Chiefs Improved Response Rates but not Response Quality or Representativeness. *Eval. Health Prof.* **2015**, *38*, 382–403. [CrossRef] [PubMed]

9.   Gregory, P.A.M.; Teixeira, B.; Austin, Z. What does it take to change practice? Perspectives of pharmacists in Ontario. *Can. Pharm. J.* **2018**, *151*, 43–50. [CrossRef] [PubMed]

10.   Houle, S.K.D.; Grindrod, K.A.; Chatterley, T.; Tsuyuki, R.T. Paying pharmacists for patient care: A systematic review of remunerated pharmacy clinical care services. *Can. Pharm. J.* **2014**, *147*, 209–232. [CrossRef] [PubMed]

11.   McCullough, K.B.; Formea, C.M.; Berg, K.D.; Burzynski, J.A.; Cunningham, J.L.; Ou, N.N.; Rudis, M.I.; Stollings, J.L.; Nicholson, W.T. Assessment of the pharmacogenomics educational needs of pharmacists. *Am. J. Pharm. Educ.* **2011**, *75*, 51. [CrossRef] [PubMed]

12.   Kibicho, J.; Pinkerton, S.D.; Owczarzak, J. Community-Based Pharmacists' Needs for HIV-Related Training and Experience. *J. Pharm. Pract.* **2014**, *27*, 369–378. [CrossRef] [PubMed]

13. Maio, V.; Belazi, D.; Goldfarb, N.I.; Phillips, A.L.; Crawford, A.G. Use and effectiveness of pharmacy continuing-education materials. *Am. J. Health Syst. Pharm.* **2003**, *60*, 1644–1649. [PubMed]

14. Hasan, S. Continuing education needs assessment of pharmacists in the United Arab Emirates. *Pharm. World Sci.* **2009**, *31*, 670–676. [CrossRef] [PubMed]

15. Bascom, C.S.; Rosenthal, M.M.; Houle, S.K.D. Are pharmacists ready for a greater role in travel health? An evaluation of the knowledge and confidence in providing travel health advice of pharmacists practicing in a community pharmacy chain in Alberta, Canada. *J. Travel Med.* **2015**, *22*, 99–104. [CrossRef] [PubMed]

16. Amery, J.; Lapwood, S. A study into the educational needs of children's hospice doctors: A descriptive quantitative and qualitative survey. *Palliat. Med.* **2004**, *18*, 727–733. [CrossRef] [PubMed]

17. Awad, N.I.; Bridgeman, M.B. Continuing-education program planning: Tips for assessing staff educational needs. *Am. J. Health Syst. Pharm.* **2014**, *71*, 1616–1619. [CrossRef] [PubMed]

18. Braun, V.; Clarke, V. Using thematic analysis in psychology. *Qual. Res. Psychol.* **2006**, *3*, 77–101. [CrossRef]

19. Johnson, T.P.; Wislar, J.S. Response rates and nonresponse errors in surveys. *JAMA* **2012**, *307*, 1805–1806. [CrossRef] [PubMed]

20. Dillman, D. *Mail and Internet Surverys: The Tailored Design Method*, 2nd ed.; John Wiley & Sons: Hoboken, NJ, USA, 2007.

21. Medway, R.L.; Fulton, J. When More Gets You Less: A Meta-Analysis of the Effect of Concurrent Web Options on Mail Survey Response Rates. *Public Opin. Q.* **2012**, *76*, 733–746. [CrossRef]

22. Koo, M.; Skinner, H. Challenges of internet recruitment: A case study with disappointing results. *J. Med. Int. Res.* **2005**, *7*, e6. [CrossRef] [PubMed]

23. Jain, C.L.; Wyatt, C.M.; Burke, R.; Sepkowitz, K.; Begier, E.M. Knowledge of the Centers for Disease Control and Prevention's 2006 routine HIV testing recommendations among New York City internal medicine residents. *AIDS Patient Care STDS* **2009**, *23*, 167–176. [CrossRef] [PubMed]

24. Kramer, M.; Schmalenberg, C.; Brewer, B.B.; Verran, J.A.; Keller-Unger, J. Accurate assessment of clinical nurses' work environments: Response rate needed. *Res. Nurs. Health* **2009**, *32*, 229–240. [CrossRef] [PubMed]

25. Torghele, K.; Buyum, A.; Dubruiel, N.; Augustine, J.; Houlihan, C.; Alperin, M.; Miner, K.R. Logic Model Use in Developing a Survey Instrument for Program Evaluation: Emergency Preparedness Summits for Schools of Nursing in Georgia. *Public Health Nurs.* **2007**, *24*, 472–479. [CrossRef] [PubMed]

26. Petrovčič, A.; Petrič, G.; Lozar Manfreda, K. The effect of email invitation elements on response rate in a web survey within an online community. *Comput. Hum. Behav.* **2016**, *56*, 320–329. [CrossRef]

27. Zillmann, D.; Schmitz, A.; Skopek, J.; Blossfeld, H.-P. Survey topic and unit nonresponse. *Qual. Quant.* **2014**, *48*, 2069–2088. [CrossRef]

28. De Valck, K.D.; Langerak, F.; Verhoef, P.C.; Verlegh, P.W.J. Satisfaction with Virtual Communities of Interest: Effect on Members' Visit Frequency*. *Br. J. Manag.* **2007**, *18*, 241–256. [CrossRef]

29. Isenor, J.E.; Minard, L.V.; Stewart, S.A.; Curran, J.A.; Deal, H.; Rodrigues, G.; Sketris, I.S. Identification of the relationship between barriers and facilitators of pharmacist prescribing and self-reported prescribing activity using the theoretical domains framework. *Res. Soc. Adm. Pharm.* **2017**. [CrossRef] [PubMed]

30. Guirguis, L.M.; Hughes, C.A.; Makowsky, M.J.; Sadowski, C.A.; Schindel, T.J.; Yuksel, N.; Faruquee, C.F. Development and validation of a survey instrument to measure factors that influence pharmacist adoption of prescribing in Alberta, Canada. *Pharm. Pract.* **2018**, *16*, 1068. [CrossRef] [PubMed]

31. Tsuyuki, R.T.; Beahm, N.P.; Okada, H.; Al Hamarneh, Y.N. Pharmacists as accessible primary health care providers: Review of the evidence. *Can. Pharm. J.* **2018**, *151*, 4–5. [CrossRef] [PubMed]

32. Kosar, L.; Hu, N.; Lix, L.M.; Shevchuk, Y.; Teare, G.F.; Champagne, A.; Blackburn, D.F. Uptake of the Medication Assessment Program in Saskatchewan: Tracking claims during the first year. *Can. Pharm. J.* **2018**, *151*, 24–28. [CrossRef] [PubMed]

33. Weglicki, R.S.; Reynolds, J.; Rivers, P.H. Continuing professional development needs of nursing and allied health professionals with responsibility for prescribing. *Nurse Educ. Today* **2015**, *35*, 227–231. [CrossRef] [PubMed]

34. Rosenthal, M.M.; Holmes, E.R. The Professional Culture of Community Pharmacy and the Provision of MTM Services. *Pharmacy* **2018**, *6*. [CrossRef] [PubMed]

35. Henkel, P.J.; Marvanova, M. Maintaining Vitality: Pharmacists' Continuing Professional Education Decision-Making in the Upper Midwest. *Pharmacy* **2018**, *6*. [CrossRef] [PubMed]

18

Academic Career Progression of Chinese-Origin Pharmacy Faculty Members in Western Countries

Weixiang Zhang [†], Hao Zhong [†], Yitao Wang, Ging Chan, Yuanjia Hu, Hao Hu
and Defang Ouyang *

State Key Laboratory of Quality Research in Chinese Medicine, Institute of Chinese Medical Sciences (ICMS), University of Macau, Taipa, Macau, China; 13980967387@163.com (W.Z.); MB75822@umac.mo (H.Z.); YTWang@umac.mo (Y.W.); gchan@umac.mo (G.C.); YuanjiaHu@umac.mo (Y.H.); HaoHu@umac.mo (H.H.)
* Correspondence: defangouyang@umac.mo
† These authors contributed equally to this work.

Abstract: Background: The field of Pharmacy education is experiencing a paucity of underrepresented minorities (URMs) faculty worldwide. The aim of this study is to investigate the current professional status of Chinese-origin pharmacy faculty members, who are considered as a good model of URMs at pharmacy academia in western countries, and identify the influencing factors to their academic career progression in academic careers. **Methods:** An online questionnaire was sent to Chinese-origin academic staffs at pharmacy schools in US, UK, Canada, Australia, and New Zealand. The survey comprised demographic information, educational background, and the influencing factors to academic career progression. **Results:** The vast majority of Chinese faculty members who worked in US were male. Individuals with junior academic title comprised the largest proportion. Over 75% of Chinese-origin pharmacy academics were involved in scientific disciplines (e.g., pharmaceutics, pharmacology, and medicinal chemistry). Usually, Chinese-origin academic members spent 4 years obtaining their first academic jobs after finishing PhD degree, and need 5–6 years to get academic promotion. The contributing factors of academic promotion were high quality publications and external funding. **Conclusion:** Our research offers a deep insight into academic career progression for URMs and give some valuable advice for their pharmacy academic paths.

Keywords: underrepresented minorities; Chinese-origin faculty; academic career progression; academic; pharmacy

1. Introduction

With the development of globalization impacting education, western countries with English-speaking culture have attracted many scholars from non-English speaking countries [1]. One report by the National Center for Education Statistic (NCES) indicated that there was a total of 761,619 full-time faculty members at U.S degree-granting institutions in 2011. Among them, 79.3% of faculty members were White, while underrepresented minorities (NRMs) had reached to 20.7% (Black, Hispanic, Asian, Pacific Islander, and American Indian/Alaska Native). Asians showed the most obvious increase, which was from only 7.6% in 2007 to 8.8% in 2011 [2]. Academic institutions are challenged to increase the proportion of these NRMs faculty, which are more likely to suffer from injustice in faculty promotion [3], such as limited network opportunities, confronting bias and stereotypes, and lack of ethnic role models and mentors [4,5]. China has grown up the largest economy and population in the Asian and Chinese scholars working in the western counties are performing an obvious upward trend and becoming a non-neglectful group, so attention urgently needs to be taken for Chinese faculty members.

Pharmacy education in the US was experiencing challenges about the ratio of URM students [6]. A recent study showed that the composition of URM pharmacy faculty members (10% approximately) was much less than minority representation in the general American population, and there was very little growth in the number of URM pharmacy students and faculty members from 1989 to 2009 [7]. Nevertheless, the situation in UK pharmacy looked different from US pharmacy. A 2012 study investigated the ethnic composition of first-year pharmacy students at Aston pharmacy in the UK. The Aston pharmacy program has a history of over 100 years and among the ranks top 5 British pharmacy schools according to University Subject Table 2011 for pharmacy and pharmacology [8]. In this research, it was found that over 70% of first-year students at Aston pharmacy school originated from Asian counties, while white students were less than 10% [9]. American academic institutions should make effort to overcome these obstacles to make faculty workforce diverse.

At present, some researches about the academic career progression of URMs have been published. The aim of SE Kaplan et al.'s study [10] was to understand differences in productivity, advancement, retention, satisfaction, and compensation comparing underrepresented medical (URM) faculty with other faculty at multiple institutions. The result showed that no differences were identified in federal grant acquisition, senior leadership roles, career satisfaction, or compensation between URM and white faculty. Price EG et al. found racial differences led to disparities in qualifications for training programs and subsequent career path to faculty positions [5]. It revealed that some structural factors could hinder the recruitment and career advancements for URM faculty members. Other studies reported that major ethnic groups in pharmacy applicant pools were associated with higher grade point averages (GPAs) and pharmacy college admission test (PCATs) scores, and more likely to get into pharmacy colleges [11].

Currently, there is no quantitative study to investigate academic career progression of racial minority pharmacy faculty members. Chinese faculty, which constitute an important component of URM, can be considered as a good model of the minorities at pharmacy academia. Thus, the aim of this study was to investigate professional current status and the influencing factors of Chinese-origin pharmacy faculty members in western countries, and provide some advice for URMs.

2. Methodology

The British academic system is ranked from lecturer, senior lecturer, reader to professor, while the American system included assistant professor, associate professor, and professor. In this study, academic staff were identified, including lecturers/assistant professors, senior lecturers/associate professors, and readers/professors in the university. "Chinese-origin" referred to the ethnic Chinese who have received undergraduate education in China. "Chinese-origin" faculty members were investigated as URMs.

2.1. Research Instrument

An anonymous on-line questionnaire was used in the research that we carried out to investigate current academic career progression status of Chinese-origin faculty members. The questionnaire consisted of 20 questions and could be divided into three parts.

2.1.1. Demographic Information

In the first section of the questionnaire, a short introductory text about the intent of the questionnaire was presented followed by demographic information about Chinese-origin faculty: name, sex, age, country, institution, and academic discipline. Academic discipline contained pharmaceutics, pharmacology, medicinal chemistry, Clinic pharmacy (or pharmacy practice), pharmacy administration, and others.

2.1.2. Education Background

In the second section of the questionnaire, the contents mainly include two parts: the participants' major and professional degrees (bachelor, master, and PhD degree, respectively).

2.1.3. Career Development

In the third section of questionnaires, the aim was to obtain the information about the development of academic careers for participants, including academic ranks and influencing factors to the academic promotion. These influencing factors included high-quality publications, education background, research area, language skills, honors and awards, teaching, service, PhD supervision, recognition from peers, external fund supporting, and network. These questions were based on a 5-point Likert scale ("Very important", "Moderately important", "Slightly important", "Low important", "Not important"). The last question was an open-ended question about suggestions for Chinese pharmacy education.

2.2. Participants

At present, western countries are mainly of comprised the European Union member states, the United States, Canada, Australia, New Zealand, and parts of Latin America. After investigation of the status of pharmacy faculty members in these counties, it was found that most of Chinese-origin pharmacy faculty members were in pharmacy schools of five western countries: US, UK, Canada, Australia, and New Zealand. Thus, 331 participants were selected from the accredited pharmacy in these five countries. Contact E-mails of participants were obtained from the website of schools, as well as the biography, name and photograph of academic staffs. The project had been approved by University of Macau (UM) Ethic Committee.

2.3. Data Analysis

An online survey (Google Form) was sent to each faculty member separately. The responses information was collected by Google Form. Data statistics were analyzed using IBM SPSS Statistics version 19.0 (IBM, Chicago, IL, USA). The prior significance level was set at 0.05.

3. Results

3.1. Professional Status of Current Chinese-Origin Pharmacy Academics

Online surveys were sent to 331 Chinese-origin pharmacy faculty members and 59 effective responses were collected. The response rate was 18.8%. Figure 1 showed the country distribution and gender of Chinese-origin pharmacy faculty. The vast majority of Chinese faculty members (275) were in US, accounting for 83% of total workforce (N = 331). A total of 66% of Chinese-origin pharmacy faculty members were male, while female was only approximately one third.

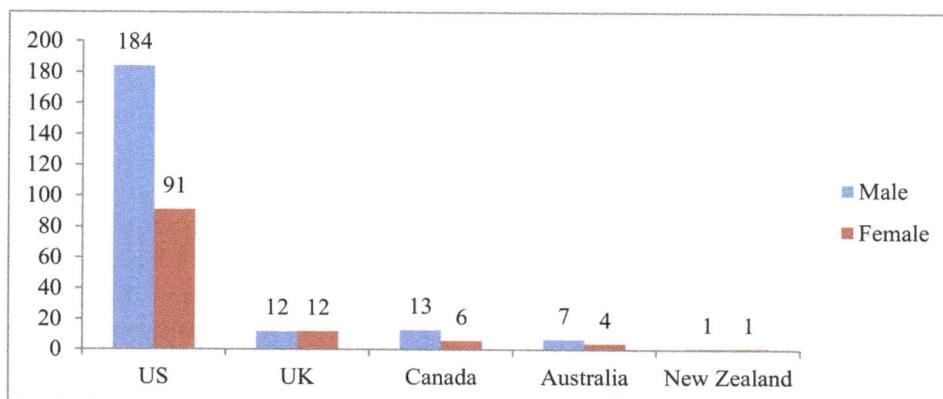

Figure 1. Distribution of Chinese-origin faculty members by the gender and country (N = 331).

Table 1 indicates the distribution of each academic rank among these five countries. It was clearly shown that junior faculty members (assistant professor in American system or lecturer in British system) comprised the largest proportion (40.5%), followed by middle-level academics with 32.3% (associate professor in American system or senior lecturer in British system), while only 27.2% were senior faculty members (such as reader and professor).

Table 1. Number of Chinese-origin faculty with different academic rank in each country (N = 331).

Academic Rank	No (%)
US	
Assistant Professor	114 (34.4)
Associate Professor	87 (26.3)
Professor	74 (22.4)
UK	
Lecturer	10 (3.0)
Senior Lecturer	12 (3.6)
Reader/Professor	2 (0.6)
Canada	
Assistant Professor	6 (1.8)
Associate Professor	5 (1.6)
Professor	8 (2.4)
Australia	
Lecturer	3 (0.9)
Senior Lecturer	2 (0.6)
Reader/Professor	6 (1.8)
New Zealand	
Lecturer	1 (0.3)
Senior Lecturer	1 (0.3)
Reader/Professor	0 (0)
Grand Total	
Assistant Professor/Lecturer	134 (40.5)
Associate Professor/Senior Lecturer	107 (32.3)
Professor/Reader	90 (27.2)

Table 2 clearly shows that the distribution of Chinese-origin faculty members by discipline and country. Most Chinese-origin faculty members were involved with the scientific disciplines, such as pharmaceutics (26.9%), pharmacology (30.5%), and medicinal chemistry (19.1%), while only 16.6% of them majored in clinical pharmacy and 6.9% in pharmacy administration.

Table 2. Status of Chinese-origin faculty by discipline and country (N = 331).

Discipline	Country (%)					Grand Total
	US	UK	Canada	Australia	New Zealand	
Clinical Pharmacy/pharmacy practice	49 (14.8)	1 (0.3)	1 (0.3)	4 (1.2)	0 (0)	55 (16.6)
Medicinal Chemistry	52 (15.6)	9 (2.7)	0 (0)	2 (0.6)	1 (0.3)	63 (19.1)
Pharmaceutics	68 (20.5)	11 (3.3)	6 (1.8)	3 (0.9)	1 (0.3)	89 (26.9)
Pharmacology	89 (26.9)	2 (0.6)	9 (2.7)	1 (0.3)	0 (0)	101 (30.5)
Pharmacy Administration	18 (5.4)	1 (0.3)	3 (0.9)	1 (0.3)	0 (0)	23 (6.9)
Grand total	275 (83.1)	24 (7.3)	19 (5.7)	11 (3.3)	2 (0.6)	331 (100)

3.2. Academic Career Progression in Pharmacy Academia of Chinese Faculty Members

Table 3 indicates the responded statistics ($n = 59$) for academic promotions of Chinese faculty members in their academic careers. Usually Chinese-origin academic members spent approximately 4 years to obtain their first academic jobs after finishing PhD degree. Moreover, it took them nearly 5–6 years to get academic promotion at each academic level.

Table 3. Academic promotion of Chinese faculty members ($n = 59$).

Promotion	Mean Years Spending	SD *
From PhD to first academic job	4.3	2.2
From assistant professor/lecturer to associate professor/senior lecturer	5.7	1.5
From associate professor/senior lecturer to professor	5.1	1.8

SD * = Standard Deviation.

Figure 2 indicates the importance ranking of the contributing factors to obtain the first academic jobs. The top three important factors were high quality publications, educational background, and research area. Language skills, strong reference, and grant were moderately important to getting academic jobs. In addition, several representative arguments were raised by some faculty members. For example, academic pedigree or work experiences in pharmaceutical industry was also important to getting the first academic jobs.

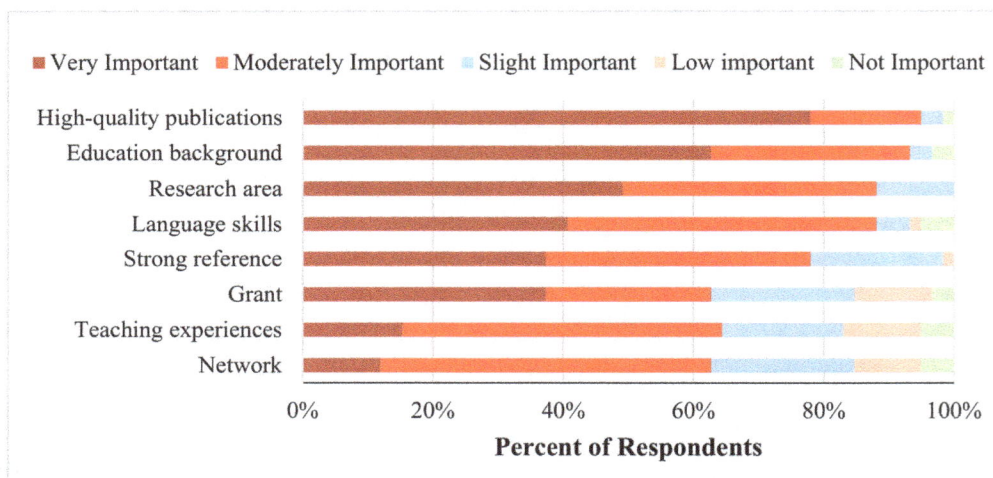

Figure 2. Ranking of contributing factors by importance in the first academic jobs for Chinese origin faculty ($n = 59$).

Figure 3 reveals the key factors to academic career progression for Chinese-origin pharmacy academics. It is not surprising that high quality publications and external fund support were two most important factors to their professional promotion. Recognition from international peers, honor/awards, teaching, and PhD supervision were also considered important to professional advancement. In addition, some respondents mentioned that generic skills, early occupation planning, and participation in school affairs and leadership were significant factors to academic career progression.

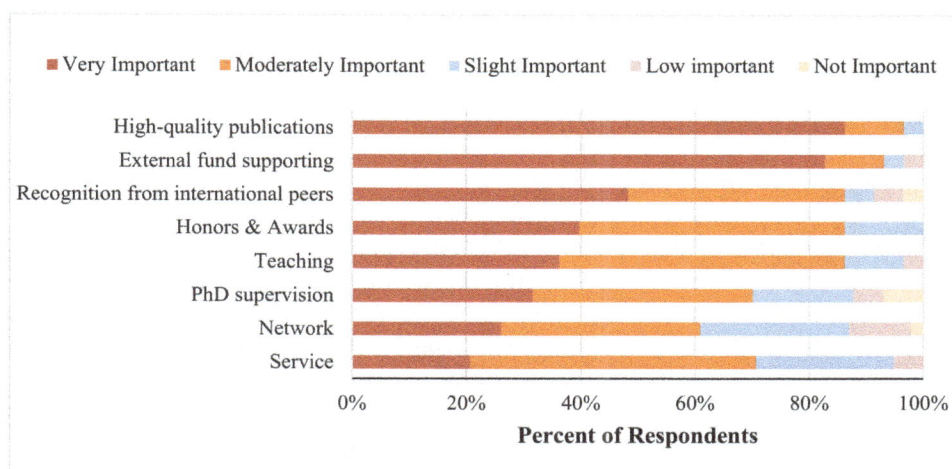

Figure 3. Ranking of contributing factors by importance to academic career progression for Chinese pharmacy faculty members ($n = 59$).

4. Discussion

The results showed that the number of Chinese-origin pharmacy faculty working in US comprised largest share, followed by UK, Canada, Australia, and New Zealand. One reason for this might be that the ranking is positively related to the number of accredited pharmacy schools (US: 134; UK: 26; Canada: 13; Australia: 18; New Zealand: 2). Another possible reason is that US is the first choice of higher education for Chinese students. One report showed that Chinese-origin students in 2016 had reached up to 550,000. About 60% of among these students applied to the US schools. The third explanation was that pharmacy education in US put more weight on faculty mentoring programs for future faculty development and academic achievement [12]. Over 70% of US pharmacy schools had faculty mentoring program as the significant component of faculty development and academic environment [13].

The majority of respondents majored in scientific disciplines (e.g., pharmaceutics, pharmacology and medicinal chemistry), while the number of members majoring in clinical pharmacy was less than 20%. This was quite different from the distribution of academic staff at pharmacy schools in western countries. Usually, the percentage of faculty members within clinical pharmacy accounted for over half of the whole pharmacy faculty workforce, which was significantly more than that of other science-based disciplines [14,15]. A possible reason for the big difference might be different mode of pharmacy education in China. In the past, the curriculum of Chinese pharmacy education focused mainly on chemistry courses, which was called "chemistry models". However, past pharmacy students in China were short of biomedical and clinical skills and practice experiences [16]. In general, clinical-related training courses took over 2 years at most pharmacy schools in western countries, but clinical training in Chinese system was less than a half-year [17]. This was consistent with the viewpoint from a respondent: "Chinese pharmacy schools do not train professional pharmacists. This is strange. They should train both pharmacists and researchers" (one participant from Australia).

The study also investigated influencing factors for academic career progression. High-quality publication still played the most important role in the process of getting their first academic jobs and professional advancements, which reflected the academic level and research area directly Academic performance is the most critical factor for getting the first academic job, such as educational background, research area, and language skills. With the further promotion of the academic career, external fund support and recognition from international peers become important. Chinese-origin faculty members usually spend 4 years getting the first job, but need 5–6 years to get academic promotion. The results are roughly consistent with previous studies. The impact factors mainly comprised academic performance, personal learning, and social change [18]. Currently, only few studies mention that fund supporting is key factor to career advancement.

5. Conclusions

The current research investigated academic career progression of Chinese-origin pharmacy faculty members in western countries from the multiple angles. Most Chinese-origin pharmacy faculty members worked in science-related subject due to different pharmacy training models between western countries and China. It would take more time to get the academic promotions for URMs. Publication still is the key factor to academic career progression for URMs, but the factors of assessment are relatively varied for academic career progression, such as external founding support and PHD supervision. So, scholars should make an effort to improve the educational background and release the high-quality publications at early states. After getting the jobs in academia, scholars need to broaden their views, not only focus on high-quality publications, but they also struggle for external funding support. Our research offers a deep insight into academic career progression for URMs and some valuable advice to Chinese pharmacy education. In the study, online survey was adopted, but only 59 effective responses were collected. The sample is so small that there may be deviation in the results. In addition, there is a lack of a comparative group in this study.

In further studies, researchers can investigate the mental status of Chinese-origin faculty who confront with the pressure of academic career progression. At the same time, the further studies can also compare Chinese-origin with other racial faculty to identify whether there exists any racial bias in career progression.

Author Contributions: Conceptualization, D.O., W.Z. and H.Z.; Methodology, W.Z., G.C. and Y.H.; Validation, H.Z. and H.H.; Formal Analysis, W.Z. and H.Z.; Investigation, W.Z. and Y.W.; Writing-Original Draft Preparation, W.Z. and H.Z.; Writing-review & Editing, G.C., H.H., Y.H. and Y.W.; Visualization, W.Z. and H.Z.; Supervision, D.O.; Project Administration, D.O.; Funding Acquisition, G.C.

Funding: This research was funded by the cooperative construction of a bid data platform for Chinese Medicine CP-001-2018 and The APC was funded by Zhuhai UM Science & Technology Research Institute.

Acknowledgments: We are grateful to all the study participants who generously gave their time and collaboration in the study.

References

1. Jöns, H.; Hoyler, M. Global geographies of higher education: The perspective of world university rankings. *Geoforum* **2013**, *46*, 45–59. [CrossRef]

2. Snyder, T.D.; Dillow, S.A. *Digest of Education Statistics 2012*; Nation Center For Education Statistics, Institue of Edcation Science, U.S. Department of Education: Washington, DC, USA, 2013.

3. Fang, D.; Moy, E.; Colburn, L.; Hurley, J. Racial and ethnic disparities in faculty promotion in academic medicine. *JAMA* **2000**, *284*, 1085–1092. [CrossRef] [PubMed]

4. Peterson, N.B.; Friedman, R.H.; Ash, A.S.; Franco, S.; Carr, P.L. Faculty self-reported experience with racial and ethnic discrimination in academic medicine. *J. Gen. Intern. Med.* **2004**, *19*, 259–265. [CrossRef] [PubMed]

5. Price, E.G.; Gozu, A.; Kern, D.E.; Powe, N.R.; Wand, G.S.; Golden, S.; Cooper, L.A. The role of cultural diversity climate in recruitment, promotion, and retention of faculty in academic medicine. *J. Gen. Intern. Med.* **2005**, *20*, 565–571. [CrossRef] [PubMed]

6. Hayes, B. Increasing the Representation of Underrepresented Minority Groups. *Am. J. Pharm. Educ.* **2008**, *72*, 14. [CrossRef] [PubMed]

7. Chisholm-Burns, M.A.; Spivey, C.A.; Billheimer, D.; Schlesselman, L.S.; Flowers, S.K.; Hammer, D.; Engle, J.P.; Nappi, J.M.; Pasko, M.T.; Ross, L.A.; et al. Multi-Institutional Study of Women and Underrepresented Minority Faculty. *Am. J. Pharm. Educ.* **2012**, *76*. [CrossRef]

8. Guide, T.C.U. University Subject Tables 2011: Pharmacology & Pharmacy. 2011. Available online: http://www.thecompleteuniversityguide.co.uk/league-tables/rankings?s=Pharmacology+%26+Pharmacy&y=2011 (accessed on 18 September 2018).

9. Ouyang, D. How to help first-year pharmacy students to gain the big picture. *J. Asian Assoc. Sch. Pharm.* **2012**, *1*, 194–202.

10. Kaplan, S.E.; Raj, A.; Carr, P.L.; Terrin, N.; Breeze, J.L.; Freund, K.M. Race/Ethnicity and Success in Academic Medicine: Findings From a Longitudinal Multi-Institutional Study. *Acad. Med.* **2018**, *93*, 616–622. [CrossRef] [PubMed]

11. Vongvanith, V.V.; Huntington, S.A.; Nkansah, N.T. Diversity Characteristics of the 2008–2009 Pharmacy College Application Service Applicant Pool. *Am. J. Pharm. Educ.* **2012**, *76*, 151. [CrossRef] [PubMed]

12. Zeind, C.S. Developing a Sustainable Faculty Mentoring Program. *Am. J. Pharm. Educ.* **2005**, *69*, 100. [CrossRef]

13. Wutoh, A.K.; Colebrook, M.N.; Holladay, J.W.; Scott, K.R.; Hogue, V.W.; Ayuk-Egbe, P.B.; Lombarbo, F.A. Faculty Mentoring Programs at Schools/Colleges of Pharmacy in the U.S. *J. Pharm. Teach.* **2000**, *8*, 61–72. [CrossRef]

14. Hagemeier, N.E.; Murawski, M.M.; Popovich, N.G. The Influence of Faculty Mentors on Junior Pharmacy Faculty Members' Career Decisions. *Am. J. Pharm. Educ.* **2013**, *77*, 51. [CrossRef] [PubMed]

15. MacKinnon, G.E. An Investigation of Pharmacy Faculty Attitudes Toward Faculty Development. *Am. J. Pharm. Educ.* **2003**, *67*, 11. [CrossRef]

16. Senlin, S.; Sanmin, H.; Xuefeng, X. To strengthen the Clinical pharmacy education and cultivatethe pharmaceutical care talents. *Pharm. Educ.* **2010**, *26*, 15–17.

17. Liang, H.; Zhang, X. Inspiration of Clinical Pharmacy Education Model Overseas to Chinese Pharmacy Education. *Med. Soc.* **2011**, *24*, 94–96.

18. Åkerlind, G.S. Academic growth and development-How do university academics experience it? *High. Educ.* **2005**, *50*, 1–32. [CrossRef]

19

A Qualitative Study Exploring the Role of Pharmacists in Medical Student Training for the Prescribing Safety Assessment

Fay Al-Kudhairi [1], Reem Kayyali [2,*], Vilius Savickas [2] 🆔 and Neel Sharma [3]

[1] Department of Pharmacy, University Hospital Lewisham, Lewisham High St, London SE13 6LH, UK; fay.al-kudhairi@nhs.net
[2] Department of Pharmacy, Faculty of Science, Engineering and Computing, Kingston University, Kingston-Upon-Thames KT1 2EE, UK; viliussavickas@gmail.com
[3] Division of Gastroenterology and Hepatology, National University Hospital Singapore, 5 Lower Kent Ridge Rd, Singapore 119074, Singapore; drneelsharma@outlook.com
* Correspondence: r.kayyali@kingston.ac.uk

Abstract: Five years after the introduction of the Prescribing Safety Assessment (PSA) in the UK, the role pharmacists play to help prepare medical students for this challenge is uncertain. Our study explored pharmacists' perceptions about their role in undergraduate medical training for the Prescribing Safety Assessment (PSA). One hundred and seventy-nine prospective participants from UK hospitals and education and training boards were emailed an interview schedule aimed at ascertaining their current involvement in undergraduate medical education, particularly the preparation for PSA. Responses received via email were thematically-analysed. A total of 27 hospital pharmacists and 3 pharmacists from local education and training boards participated in the interviews. Pharmacists were positive about their involvement in medical student training, recognising the added value they could provide in prescribing practice. However, respondents expressed concerns regarding resource availability and the need for formal educational practice mentoring. Despite a low response rate (17%), this research highlights the potential value of pharmacists' input into medical education and the need for a discussion on strategies to expand this role to maximise the benefits from having a pharmacist skill mix when teaching safe prescribing.

Keywords: inter-professional; education; pharmacist; medical; undergraduate; PSA

1. Introduction

An increasing amount of evidence suggests a positive reception of pharmacist-led inter-professional education (IPE) amongst medical undergraduates leading to an enhanced understanding of their roles within the multidisciplinary team and an ability to identify medication-related problems [1,2]. Similarly, pharmacist-led postgraduate training of doctors results in improved prescribing practice and medication safety [3,4]. Despite this, little is known about the extent of pharmacists' involvement in the education of their junior medical colleagues.

The need to explore the role of pharmacists in undergraduate medical education has intensified in recent years with increasing concerns over the prescribing competence of foundation doctors, in principle raised by the EQUIP study [5]. The development of the Prescribing Safety Assessment (PSA) [6] and the new undergraduate medical curricula [7], which aimed to address some of these concerns, created a further need to involve pharmacists in the preparation of the next generation of doctors.

A scoping questionnaire for former medical students revealed that 9 out of 10 respondents valued pharmacist-led training, which they felt would have supported their prescribing and preparedness for the PSA (data not shown). In turn, this study aimed to explore pharmacists' perceptions about their current involvement in the education and training of medical undergraduates in preparation for the PSA.

As the great majority of undergraduate clinical placements take place in the hospital environment [8], pharmacists working in secondary and/or tertiary care may be ideally placed to facilitate medical student education and preparedness for practice. Therefore, this qualitative study primarily targeted UK hospital pharmacists who might have the greatest amount of contact time with medical undergraduates.

2. Materials and Methods

A convenience and snowballing sampling strategy was used to recruit prospective participants. The contact details of prospective participants were obtained by one of the researchers via the Pharmalife website, which at the time facilitated the recruitment of pre-registration trainee pharmacists and contained the email addresses of the Lead Education and Training Pharmacists in each NHS Trust in England and Wales. The Education and Training Pharmacist in each Trust acted as a gatekeeper to snowball an email invitation to participate in an interview within their respective pharmacy department. The first author of the manuscript then approached individuals who expressed an interest to participate by email, providing them with a participant information sheet and an interview schedule. Participant's email response to questions in the interview schedule constituted an implied consent to take part.

A total of 176 pharmacists from National Health Service (NHS, UK) Trusts and three education and training pharmacists from local education and training boards (LETBs) across the UK were sent an email invitation to participate in semi-structured email interview. The choice of this interview method was preferred by interviewees over telephone or face-to-face alternatives due to increased flexibility and was expected to maximise the response rate [9].

The interview schedule consisted of 14 open questions designed to ascertain the perceived role of pharmacists in the education of medical undergraduates (Appendix A). Pharmacists were also asked about their knowledge related to the PSA and any impact this assessment might have had on their role in undergraduate medical education in order to support final-year medical students undertaking this assessment. The interview schedule was piloted with two pharmacists working within the academic institute who had education and training roles in NHS Trusts with minor changes. Thematic analysis of qualitative data was conducted using a 6-step method adapted from Braun and Clarke [10]. Analysis was carried out in a constant comparative manner until data saturation was reached. The stopping criterion for data saturation, which relates to the number of interviews conducted in the absence of any new data emerging, was six. Data saturation was reached after the 24th interview. One member of the research team transcribed the data, whilst two members were involved in the analysis including the coding and subsequent comparative analysis to identify any themes. The trial coding of the text involved assessing the accuracy and reliability of the coding procedure. As no disputes were found, the coding was maintained for the rest of the text, and conclusions were derived from the coded data.

3. Results

Twenty-seven pharmacists (all from different NHS Trusts) and all three pharmacists from LETBs took part in email interviews. The majority of respondents specialised in education and training of either or both other health care professionals (HCPs) and/or pre-registration trainee pharmacists ($n = 10/27$). Six respondents were either deputy chief, lead, highly specialist, or advanced pharmacists in their respective areas. The remainder of pharmacists specialised in other areas of clinical pharmacy, such as renal or critical care.

All pharmacist participants were asked to identify the advantages and limitations of pharmacists' involvement in the education and training of other HCPs (Table 1). The results derived from this question demonstrated that pharmacists believed their educational role had a positive impact on other HCPs, students, themselves, and patients. An emphasis was placed on pharmacists being experts in medicines who "can offer a unique perspective to teaching" and that, through regular interactions with other HCPs, pharmacists can "identify common errors to target future training." This in turn may lead to "improved basic knowledge [of prescribing], which improves patient safety." One participant felt that improved knowledge of medicines amongst junior doctors may also free up pharmacists' time traditionally used to answer medicines-related queries and would enable them to conduct "more specialised work and interventions", which would ultimately enhance patient care.

Table 1. A summary of themes relating to advantages and limitations of pharmacists' involvement in the training and education of other HCPs identified through the analysis of qualitative interview data ($n = 30$). Abbreviations: CPD—continuing professional development; IPE—inter-professional education; HCPs—healthcare professionals.

Advantages	Limitations
Pharmacists' specialist knowledge in medicines	Not all pharmacists are teachers by nature/no formal training
Pharmacists' perspective on patient, not disease, attention to detail	Teaching may have limited perspective and not be multi-disciplinary focused
Improved patient safety and care	Time taken from usual work commitments
Raises profile of pharmacists	Need dedicated teaching role in order to ensure compliance with sessions/appropriate follow up
Contributes to pharmacists' CPD	Pharmacists' lack of medical knowledge/medical experience
Encourages IPE between HCPs	Lack of awareness of pharmacists' knowledge and skills by other HCPs
Medical students benefit from practical knowledge of prescribing	Lack of funding and resources as support

Some pharmacists, however, did not feel supported enough to carry out training, either because "pharmacists do not routinely receive training on how to provide educational sessions" or due to a "lack of adequate resources and support from the organisation". Participants thought that such barriers may be overcome by "delivering educational sessions only where their expertise is called upon" and that certain sessions may be more appropriately delivered by experts from a different discipline.

All 27 hospital pharmacists indicated that either themselves or other pharmacists at their hospital were involved in the active education of other HCPs. However, in only 14 Trusts this involvement extended to medical undergraduate education. A range of pharmacist-led training sessions for medical students were listed by participants with safe prescribing as the most popular focus followed by controlled drugs, intravenous fluids, and calculations (Figure 1). Pharmacist participants anticipated that the training delivered to medical undergraduates "impacted on their practice and hopefully made them better prescribers in the future".

When asked if they had heard of the PSA, 23 said they had, with 12 either becoming more involved in teaching general therapeutics and prescribing to undergraduate medical students, or if already teaching medical students, tailoring their teaching to become more PSA-orientated as a result of the introduction of the assessment. When provided with an outline of the PSA and the associated competencies, all of the respondents agreed that pharmacists should be involved in educating medical students in preparation for the PSA. As "experts in medicines", pharmacists perceived themselves as "ideal HCPs" to teach medical undergraduates about the safety of prescribing. One pharmacist further added that "pharmacist-led teaching should not be focused only on the [prescribing safety] assessment, but rather the skills needed for future prescribing practice."

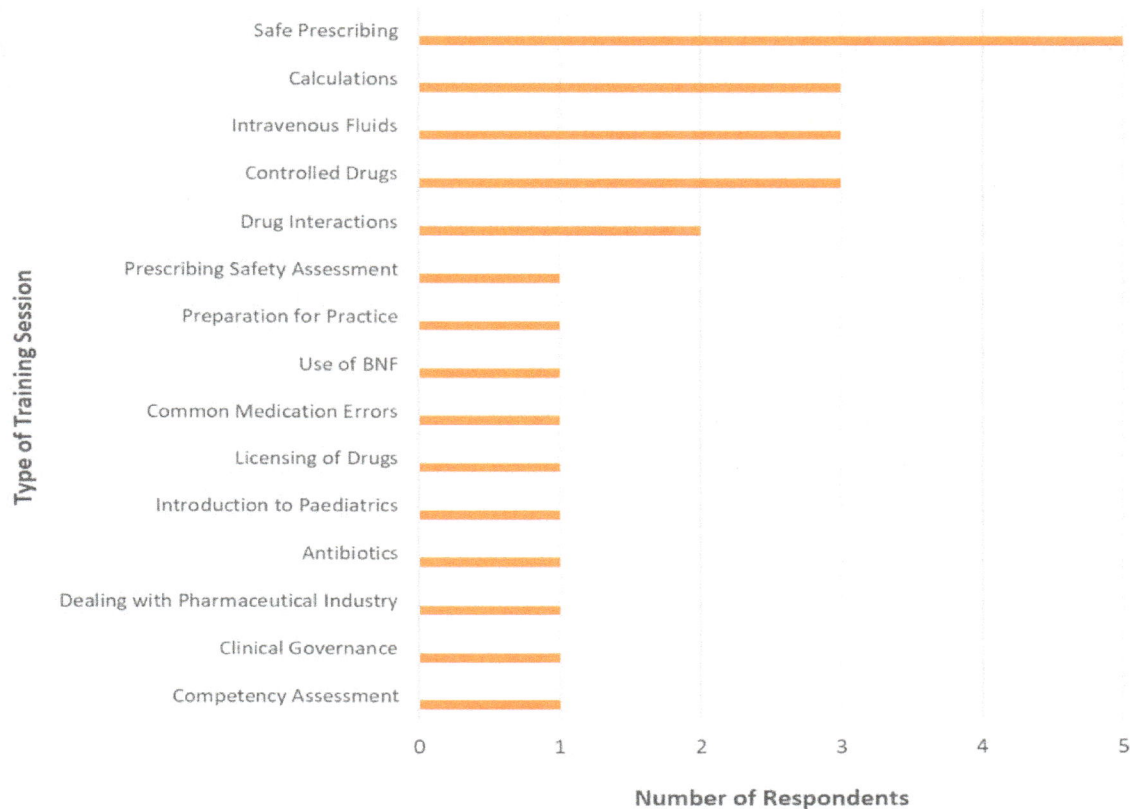

Figure 1. A range of training sessions delivered by pharmacists at the participating NHS Trusts ($n = 14/27$, excluding pharmacists from Local Education and Training Boards).

4. Discussion

This study aimed to highlight the role of pharmacists in enhancing the education of medical students in preparation for the PSA in the UK. Pharmacists expressed their beliefs about the benefits of their involvement. This focused predominantly on enhancing patient safety through appropriate prescribing knowledge delivery and the skillset they could transfer to medical students. Such perceptions about the significance of pharmacist's role were not unexpected considering the previous studies, which demonstrated an improvement in the quality of junior doctor prescribing following pharmacist-led educational interventions, thereby potentially leading to improved patient safety [3,4].

Concerns were raised, however, about the lack of resources available for pharmacists to assist fully with time and funding pressures being cited. Furthermore, pharmacists alluded to the fact that in order to teach effectively, formal understanding of educational practice is also necessary. While several courses have been made available to facilitate the development of pharmacist's educational skillset [11,12], it is clear that such courses may need to be made more widely available and flexible in order to accommodate the role of practicing pharmacists in undergraduate medical education, including the student preparation for the PSA.

At a time where health professional educators recognise the importance of IPE and the science of teaching, this study emphasised concerns that in reality there are notable factors that still need addressing. Some of these factors, for instance the lack of time and resources, may be partially addressed through better utilisation of nationally available e-learning courses for medical undergraduates and junior doctors (e.g., SCRIPT) [13]. The completion of such courses may be followed by discussion or feedback from the designated pharmacist facilitator—an educational model that is known to be effective in practice [4].

Our study findings are in contrast to existing data, which emphasised the existence of pharmacist-led teaching sessions on the wards, either one on one or in a group settings, as well as their involvement in clinical pharmacology and therapeutics [14,15].

5. Conclusions

Due to various barriers, few of the pharmacists in our study were actively involved in medical student education, yet respondents were generally positive about increasing their participation in prescribing-related training. Whilst we recognise the small sample size, we hope that our findings help to ensure that medical students' prescribing knowledge benefits from their pharmacist colleagues, and that they are supported adequately in their teaching endeavours.

Author Contributions: F.A. and R.K. contributed to study conceptualization, design of methodology, interview schedule validation, investigation, formal analysis, and writing—review & editing. R.K. also contributed to data curation, supervision, and project administration. V.S. contributed to formal analysis, data curation, writing—original draft preparation, and writing—review & editing. N.S. contributed to study conceptualization, design of methodology, writing—original draft preparation, and writing—review & editing. All authors read and approved the final version of the manuscript.

Funding: This research received no external funding.

Acknowledgments: All hospital pharmacists who agreed to participate in the interviews as part of the study.

References

1.   Vaughn, L.M.; Cross, B.; Bossaer, L.; Flores, E.K.; Moore, J.; Click, I. Analysis of an interprofessional home visit assignment: Student perceptions of team-based care, home visits, and medication-related problems. *Fam. Med.* **2014**, *46*, 522–526. [PubMed]

2.   Zorek, J.A.; MacLaughlin, E.J.; Fike, D.S.; MacLaughlin, A.A.; Samiuddin, M.; Young, R.B. Measuring changes in perception using the student perceptions of physician-pharmacist interprofessional clinical education (spice) instrument. *BMC Med. Educ.* **2014**, *14*, 101. [CrossRef] [PubMed]

3.   Simpson, J.H.; Lynch, R.; Grant, J.; Alroomi, L. Reducing medication errors in the neonatal intensive care unit. *Arch. Dis. Child. Fetal Neonatal Ed.* **2004**, *89*, F480–F482. [CrossRef] [PubMed]

4.   McLellan, L.; Dornan, T.; Newton, P.; Williams, S.D.; Lewis, P.; Steinke, D.; Tully, M.P. Pharmacist-led feedback workshops increase appropriate prescribing of antimicrobials. *J. Antimicrob. Chemother.* **2016**, *71*, 1415–1425. [CrossRef] [PubMed]

5.   Dornan, T.; Ashcroft, D.; Heathfield, H.; Lewis, P.; Miles, J.; Taylor, D.; Tully, M.; Wass, V. An in Depth Investigation into Causes of Prescribing Errors by Foundation Trainees in Relation to Their Medical Education. Equip Study. Available online: http://www.gmc-uk.org/FINAL_Report_prevalence_and_causes_of_prescribing_errors.pdf_28935150.pdf (accessed on 20 May 2018).

6.   Prescribing Safety Assessment. Available online: https://prescribingsafetyassessment.ac.uk/ (accessed on 20 May 2018).

7.   Outcomes for Graduates (Tomorrow's Doctors). Available online: https://www.gmc-uk.org/-/media/documents/outcomes-for-graduates-jul-15-1216_pdf-61408029.pdf (accessed on 20 May 2018).

8.   Harding, A.; Rosenthal, J.; Al-Seaidy, M.; Gray, D.P.; McKinley, R.K. Society for Academic Primary Care Heads of Teaching Group. Provision of medical student teaching in UK general practices: A cross-sectional questionnaire study. *Br. J. Gen. Pract.* **2015**, *65*, e409–e417. [CrossRef] [PubMed]

9.   Odeh, B.; Kayyali, R.; Nabhani-Gebara, S.; Philip, N. Implementing a telehealth service: Nurses' perceptions and experiences. *Br. J. Nurs.* **2014**, *23*, 1133–1137. [CrossRef] [PubMed]

10. Braun, V.; Clarke, V. Using thematic analysis in psychology. *Qual. Res. Psychol.* **2006**, *3*, 77–101. [CrossRef]

11. Health Education England. Practice Supervisor Training. Available online: https://www.lasepharmacy.hee.

12.   Health Education England. Training for Foundation Pharmacist Educational Supervisor. Available online: https://www.lasepharmacy.hee.nhs.uk/training-1/supervisor-training/foundation-pharmacist-educational-supervisor-training/ (accessed on 20 July 2018).

13.   University of Birmingham; Health Education England; Ocbmedia. Available online: https://www.safeprescriber.org/ (accessed on 20 July 2018).

14.   O'Shaughnessy, L.; Haq, I.; Maxwell, S.; Llewelyn, M. Teaching of clinical pharmacology and therapeutics in UK medical schools: Current status in 2009. *Br. J. Clin. Pharmacol.* **2010**, *70*, 143–148. [CrossRef] [PubMed]

15.   Kirkham, D.; Darbyshire, D.; Gordon, M.; Agius, S.; Baker, P. A solid grounding: Prescribing skills training. *Clin. Teach.* **2015**, *12*, 187–192. [CrossRef] [PubMed]

20

Eating Disorders in Relationship with Dietary Habits among Pharmacy Students

Magdalena Iorga [1] (iD)**, Isabela Manole** [2]**, Lavinia Pop** [3]**, Iulia-Diana Muraru** [1,*] **and Florin-Dumitru Petrariu** [4]

[1] Department of Behavioral Sciences, Faculty of Medicine, University of Medicine and Pharmacy "Grigore T. Popa" of Iasi, Iasi 700115, Romania; magdalena.iorga@umfiasi.ro

[2] Faculty of Pharmacy, University of Medicine and Pharmacy "Grigore T. Popa" of Iasi, Iasi 700115, Romania; isabella0290@gmail.com

[3] Nutrition and Dietetics, Faculty of Medicine, University of Medicine and Pharmacy "Grigore T. Popa" of Iasi, Iasi 700117, Romania; daianapopovici85@yahoo.com

[4] Department of Preventive Medicine and Interdisciplinarity, Faculty of Medicine, University of Medicine and Pharmacy "Grigore T. Popa" of Iasi, Iasi 700115, Romania; fpetrariu@mail.com

* Correspondence: iuliadianamuraru@gmail.com

Abstract: Changing dietary habits of university students is due to personal, social, educational or religious factors. The relationship between dietary habits and presence of eating disorders among university students is less known in Romania. **Material and Methods**: Ninety-one pharmacy students (91.21% women) were included in the research. Socio-demographic, anthropometric, medical, and psychological data were collected. Dietary self-declared habits were registered. The analysis of data was done using SPSS, v23. **Results**: A total of 69.2% of students had normal weight, 64.84% preferred to have lunch, and 23.08% eat during nights. The majority of subjects (95.6%), stated that they eat snacks daily. More than one-third of students keep diets to reduce their weight. Younger students tend to eat more main meals per week, snack more, and eat later after getting up in the morning. Subjects with high body dissatisfaction tended to have fewer main meals ($r = -0.265$, $p = 0.011$) and to skip breakfasts (-0.235, $p = 0.025$) and dinners ($r = -0.303$, $p < 0.001$). Pharmacy students that presented higher rate of emotional problems tend to sleep less and skip breakfast. **Conclusions**: Female pharmacy students had higher mean scores on all subscales than those found among Romanian women. A strong relationship between dietary habits and eating disorders was identified.

Keywords: pharmacy student; diet habits; eating disorders; anorexia; bulimia; BMI

1. Introduction

During their university studies, students change their dietary habits, and several factors were found to be responsible for it: changing location, living arrangements (skipping home-prepared food), respecting school schedule (leading to an increased number of snacks and skipping meals), having an easy access to fast-food (university campuses are providing fast-food for students), self-administrating palatable meals (students have the tendency to eat preferred meals), limitation by costs and easy to find food, etc. [1–5].

The persistence of dietary habits is not limited in time. These dietary habits were found to be stable over the years that is why developing a healthy nutritional behavior during academic years is important for both physical and mental health. Students were considered as a vulnerable group because they fail to meet dietary requirements for a long period of time. Lower scores for stress, bad eating behaviors, or poorer dietary habits were registered among students compared to general population. Studies revealed that medical students are practicing less healthy behaviors or eat more unhealthy food compared to non-medical students [6,7].

Unhealthy food is associated with high rates of chronicity, like obesity and cardiovascular disease, both identified in general population and among students. Some studies pointed that there was an increased rate of obesity among university students in the last twenty years; students start to gain weight since freshmen years and this process slows but still increases during the adult life [8–10]. Obesity and overweight rates registered among medical students were closely related to some dietary behaviors like: skipping breakfast, frequent fast food and low consumption of fruits and vegetables, or easy access to unhealthy food and carbohydrates from food machines or convenient fast-food stores [11–15].

Apart from these reasons, eating habits are also related to socio-cultural reasons. Western cultures are more prone to accept and promote thinness compared to eastern countries. Studies pointed out the influence of media on the ideal weight and how that ideal models influence to self-image of the body and also that the ideal weight of the body is closely related to the cultural ideal model. That is why, cultures where thinness is more agreed are more prone to registered high rates of eating disorders like anorexia and bulimia.

Acculturative stress is another aspect related to changing dietary habits for students who are studying abroad. One of the stressors is represented by the impossibility to find their favorite meals, their individual preferred food, or ingredients that they are used to using. Dietary acculturation is an extra distressful factor that may affect a student's life [16–18].

There is no other study in Romania investigating the relationship between eating disorders and dietary habits among pharmacy students. The aim of the study was to evaluate the presence of eating disorders among Romanian pharmacy students and their relationship with the patterns of dietary habits.

2. Materials and Methods

2.1. Study Design and Participants

A total of 91 students were included in the present research. All participants were enrolled, at the time of the investigation, in "University of Medicine and Pharmacy "Grigore T. Popa" of Iasi, Romania, Faculty of Pharmacy, from all five years of study. In total, the number of pharmacy students registered was 700, so the subjects investigated represented almost 10% of the targeted population.

The students voluntarily participated to the research. Participants were informed about the purpose of the study and they were informed from the beginning that they could withdraw from the study anytime they wanted to, with no penalties. The survey took approximately 25 min to complete.

A total of 120 questionnaires were distributed directly by the investigators. From the 115 returned documents (with a rate of response of 96%), 91 were taken into consideration for the research. Willingness to participate was considered as an inclusion criterion. The exclusion criteria were: documents were not fully filled-in, or were returned after the requested dead-line.

2.2. Questionnaires

A combined questionnaire including socio-demographic, medical, anthropometric, and psychological data was created.

2.2.1. Socio-Demographic Data

Because the present study is the first one focusing on eating habits and disease among pharmacy students in Romania, information like age, gender (male/female), environment (rural/urban), and year of study (one to five) were registered for this cross-sectional study.

2.2.2. Anthropometric and Medical Data

Information like weight, weight, body mass indices (BMI) and the existence of a chronic disease were also registered. Height and weight data were converted into Quetelet's BDI and the value was considered using *World Health Organization* (WHO) standards for European population: a BMI < 18.5 kg/m^2 was categorized as underweight, 18.5–24.9 kg/m^2 as the normal range, 25.0–29.9 kg/m^2 as pre-obese, 30–34.9 kg/m^2 as obese class I, 35.0–39.9 kg/m^2 as obese class II, and $\geq$40 kg/m^2 as obese Class III [10].

Also, an item was addressed in order to identify if students were satisfied with their weight, to declare if they used diets in order to reduce their weight. Information about having a chronic disease or being under medical treatment were also gathered.

2.2.3. Dietary Data

The study focused also on gathering information regarding the consumption of vegetables, fruits, snacks, or fast-food. The selection of dietary data was collected in order to respect also the religion and the restriction imposed by the practice of it.

2.2.4. Health-Related Behaviors

Special items were constructed in order to identify sleep-related problems (the number of hours of sleep), the number of weekly breakfasts, lunches, or dinners, preferred meal, serving snacks, the tendency to skip meals, eating during the night, and fasting.

2.2.5. Eating Disorders

Psychological problems referring to eating disorders were evaluated using *Eating Disorder Inventory (EDI)*. The original tool was designed by Gamer [19] for identifying eating disorders, and it is widely used both in research and in clinical practice to screen symptoms and psychological features related to eating disorder.

For the present study, EDI-3, Romanian Form [20] was used. The 91 items investigate the following aspects: three scales are related specific to eating disorders (drive for thinness—DT, bulimia—B, and body dissatisfaction—BD) and nine are general psychological scales in strong relationship with eating disorders (low self-esteem—LSE, personal alienation—PA, interpersonal insecurity—II, interpersonal alienation—IA, interoceptive deficits—ID, emotional dysregulation—ED, perfectionism—P, ascetism—AS, and maturity fears—MF).

A 6-point scale represents the response options for the items of EDI-3, ranging from *always* to *never*. The instrument has a number of 25 reversed items. In this case, we also reverse the coding. It is mandatory to choose a response for each item and individuals have to decide which one suits those best. The score for each subscale is obtained by summing up all scores for that scale.

EDI-3 is not an inventory designed for diagnosing eating disorders, but a tool to assess symptoms relevant to the development and maintaining of eating disorders. High scores on the first three scales are related to high risks of developing eating disorders. The other nine scales take into consideration important psychological aspects relevant to the evolution and persistence of eating disorders.

The adaptation and validation of EDI-3 on the Romanian population used individuals from the general population from six of the 41 counties in Romania and individuals with a diagnosis of eating disorders. For most of the subscale, there were no significant differences between male and female participants (in accordance with other studies), with two exceptions: drive for thinness and body dissatisfaction, with women scoring higher than men on these scales.

Test-retest reliability indicates a high stability in time for EDI-3, correlation coefficients varying between 0.613 and 0.844, with $p < 0.001$. The instrument also shows a good internal consistency on all scales as measured by alpha Cronbach coefficients ranged from 0.600 to 0.899. Correlations between the scores on the scales of EDI-3 and other eating disorders relevant instruments (Eating Attitudes

Test-26, Rosenberg self-esteem scale, Eysenck Personality Questionnaire, Beck Depression Inventory, Endler Multidimensional Anxiety Scales, etc.) indicate a good criterion validity. Intercorrelations between the scales of EDI-3 and factor analysis point to a good construct validity.

2.3. Statistical Analysis

The statistical analysis was done using SPSS IBM, version 23. (IBM, Tokio, Japan). Descriptive analysis used mean and standard deviations; Independent Samples t Tests were used in the case of one independent, categorical variable that has two levels/groups and one continuous dependent variable. The one-way analysis of variance (ANOVA) was also used to establish whether there are any statistically significant differences between the means of three or more independent (unrelated) groups. For Pearson correlations, interval measured variables were used. Differences were considered statistically significant at P value <0.05.

3. Results

3.1. Socio-Demographic, Anthropometric, and Medical Data

The majority of participants were females (N = 83, 91.21%), age range of 18–39 (M = 22.30 ± 2.71). The majority of female students is a common feature, the rate being specific to all rates registered by medical universities.

Socio-demographic (gender, age, environment), anthropometric (weight and BMI), and medical (having a chronic disease or being under medical treatment) data are described in Table 1.

Table 1. Socio-demographic, anthropometric, and medical data.

Variables	Results [1]
Gender	
female	83 (91.21%)
male	8 (8.79%)
Environment	
urban	54 (53.94%)
rural	37 (40.66%)
Religion	
Orthodox	70 (77.78%)
Catholic	10 (11%)
Others (Pentecostal, Adventist, etc.)	11 (11.21%)
Respecting religious fasts	29 (31.87%)
Weight (kg)	60.2 ± 10.56 (42 to 105)
Body mass index (BMI)	±
underweight	13 (14.3%)
normal weight	63 (69.2%)
pre-obese	12 (13.2%)
obese	0
Having a chronic disease	13 (14.29%)
Being under a medical treatment	15 (16.49%)

[1] Number (N) and percent (%), Mean (M) and standard deviation (st.dev).

3.2. Psychological Data—EDI-3

Results for EDI-3 subscales are presented in Table 2. The results obtained for both genders are presenting in Table 2, together with scores for men and women from general population in Romania. Comparing with women from general population, scores for female pharmacy students are higher for all subscales. For men, only five scores were registered to be higher than that of Romanian males: drive for thinness, body dissatisfaction, personal alienation, interoceptive deficits, and emotional dyssregulation.

Table 2. Comparative results for EDI-3 subscales for men and women.

EDI-3 Subscales	Pharmacy Students	Pharmacy Students	General Population	General Population
	Male	Female	Male	Female
Drive for thinness	3.37 ± 4.30	9.26 ± 7.65	2.66 ± 3.66	8.03 ± 7.54
Bulimia	1.12 ± 1.80	4.87 ± 5.97	2.04 ± 2.38	2.00 ± 3.18
Body dissatisfaction	7.25 ± 6.62	17.03 ± 10.62	5.18 ± 6.13	10.29 ± 9.28
Low self-esteem	2.75 ± 2.37	8.08 ± 5.98	3.28 ± 4.85	2.97 ± 3.19
Personal alienation	6.62 ± 1.40	10.40 ± 4.48	3.55 ± 4.12	4.48 ± 3.45
Interpersonal insecurity	6.35 ± 5.75	13.81 ± 7.75	7.07 ± 5.87	6.73 ± 4.95
Interpersonal alienation	5.03 ± 6.34	11.98 ± 9.62	7.04 ± 4.48	7.13 ± 4.06
Interoceptive deficits	7.82 ± 2.72	12.20 ± 3.50	4.79 ± 5.16	6.10 ± 4.34
Emotional dysregulation	6.24 ± 1.88	7.74 ± 2.12	5.36 ± 5.83	6.03 ± 4.60
Perfectionism	4.68 ± 7.84	10.96 ± 10.87	11.79 ± 5.34	10.42 ± 5.42
Ascetism	5.19 ± 3.29	7.77 ± 4.00	6.41 ± 3.66	6.81 ± 3.82
Maturity fears	6.65 ± 5.28	17.97 ± 10.37	10.62 ± 4.07	13.23 ± 5.81

[1] Means (M) and standard deviations (st.dev).

There is no association between age and BMI ($r = 0.059$, $p = 0.582$). Pearson correlations revealed negative significant associations between age and number of main meals per week ($r = -0.265$, $p = 0.012$) and the number of snacks per day ($r = -0.244$, $p = 0.021$). Also, there is a positive correlation between age and eating after getting up in the morning ($r = 0.337$, $p = 0.001$). More specifically, younger students tend to eat more main meals per week, snack more, and eat later after getting up in the morning.

Pearson correlations revealed that students with a high drive for thinness have higher body weights ($r = 0.282$, $p < 0.001$) and tend to skip dinners ($r = -0.344$, $p < 0.001$). As expected, a positive correlation was identified between weight and the subscales body dissatisfaction ($r = 0.342$, $p < 0.001$) and drive for thinness ($r = -0.285$, $p < 0.001$). Also, participants with high body dissatisfaction tend to have fewer main meals ($r = -0.265$, $p = 0.011$) and to skip breakfasts ($r = -0.235$, $p = 0.025$) and dinners ($r = -0.303$, $p < 0.001$).

Interpersonal alienation (reluctance to form close relationship) and maturity fears (the fear to face the demands specific to an adult life) had a negative correlation with number of lunches per week ($r = -0.295$, $p < 0.001$ and $r = -0.214$, $p = 0.042$, respectively), meaning that participants with high scores on this subscale tend to skip lunch.

For the subscale interoceptive deficits, it was identified a positive correlation with the number of eaten fruits ($r = 0.252$, $p = 0.021$). Interoceptive deficits scale measures the ability of an individual to discriminate between sensations (of hunger and satiety) and feelings.

A negative correlation was identified between emotional dysregulation and the number of hours of night sleep and number of breakfasts ($r = -0.222$, $p = 0.035$). So, pharmacy students that presented higher rate of emotional problems tend to sleep less and skip breakfast.

Also, a negative correlation was identified between ascetism and the number of main meals per week ($r = -0.265$, $p = 0.012$), meaning that students with high scores on ascetism tend to skip more main meals.

3.3. Diatery Habits and Health-Related Behaviors

3.3.1. Sleep-Related Data

Students were asked to estimate the number of nightsleep hours. The results revealed an $M = 7 \pm 1.02$ h of sleep every night and almost a quarter of them (24.12%) were having a nap after lunch almost every day.

The t test revealed significant differences between subjects who eat during nights ($M = 11.85$) and those who do not ($M = 9.54$) on personal alienation ($t(89) = 2.31$, $p = 0.035$). Personal alienation refers to low self-esteem. Results proved that students who used to eat during nights had higher scores on personal alienation.

3.3.2. Meals, Snacks, and Diets

Students were asked to mention which was their **preferred meal**: 64.84% of them usually prefer have lunch, 23.08% dinner, and 12.09% enjoy having breakfasts. A number of 21 subjects (23.08%) declared that they eat during nights. They had also to mentions how many times they succeed in serving breakfasts, lunches, and dinners. Results are presented in Table 3.

Table 3. Meals (breakfasts, lunches, dinners) per week.

How Many Times Per Week Do You Eat . . .	Never	1	2	3	4	5	6	Daily	M $\pm$ st.dev
breakfast	7.69%	5.49%	8.79%	16.48%	4.40%	14.29%	9.89%	32.97%	4.51 $\pm$ 2.34
lunch	1.10%	0%	2.20%	4.40%	12.09%	14.29%	6.59%	59.34%	5.92 $\pm$ 1.54
dinner	1.10%	0%	4.40%	9.89%	4.40%	13.19%	2.20%	64.84%	5.89 $\pm$ 1.72

[1] number of meals (%).

Students were also asked to report whether they eat snacks or not. The majority of them (95.6%), sustained that they eat snacks daily, with an $M = 2.33 \pm 1.25$.

More than one-third of students declared that they used to keep diets to reduce their weight ($N = 37, 40.7\%$). When comparing students who dieted for reducing weight to those who did not, the first group obtained statistically significant higher scores on each of the following six subscales: drive for thinness ($t(89) = 6.14$, $p < 0.001$), bulimia ($t(89) = 3.03$, $p = 0.004$), body dissatisfaction ($t(89) = 3.71$, $p < 0.001$), personal alienation ($t(89) = 2.01$, $p = 0.047$), emotional dysregulation ($t(89) = 2.02$, $p = 0.046$), and ascetism ($t(89) = 3.25$, $p = 0.002$).

3.3.3. Religious Fasts and Vegetable/Fruit Diet

The results of the Independent Samples t Test revealed that students who fast ($M = 9.24$) had lower scores than those who do not ($M = 12.96$) on interpersonal alienation ($t(89) = -3.21$, $p = 0.002$).

The answers to the items regarding the daily consumption of fruits and vegetables proved that 35.2% of students eat fruits daily and 57.1% of them declared they eat daily vegetables, with an $M = 2.02 \pm 1.41$ fruits and $M = 5.92 \pm 1.54$ vegetables per day.

One-Way ANOVA analyses showed significant differences between fruit consumption (1—daily, 2—two times a week, 3—three, four times a week, 4—not at all) and three of the subscales: drive for thinness ($F(3.87) = 4.57$, $p = 0.005$), emotional dysregulation ($F(3.87) = 3.24$, $p = 0.026$), and perfectionism ($F(3.87) = 3.86$, $p = 0.012$). The multiple comparisons analysis showed that students who ate fruits daily ($M = 11.53$) had a higher drive for thinness than those who eat fruits twice a week ($M = 5.23$); those who do not eat fruits ($M = 14.80$) had higher scores on emotional dysregulation than those who eat fruits three/four times a week ($M = 6.00$); and participants who do not eat fruits ($M = 16.60$) had higher scores on perfectionism than those who used to eat fruits two times ($M = 9.52$) or three/four times a week ($M = 9.97$).

3.3.4. Satisfaction with Personal Weight

A number of 53 (58.2%) students declared that they are content with their weight. The results of the Independent Samples t Tests showed significant differences between subjects who are content with their weight and those who are not on 9 of the 12 subscales of the EDI-3: drive for thinness ($t(89) = -5.40$, $p < 0.001$), bulimia ($t(89) = -4.42$, $p < 0.001$), body dissatisfaction ($t(89) = -8.31$, $p < 0.001$), low self-esteem ($t(89) = -3.08$, $p = 0.003$), personal alienation ($t(89) = -4.36$, $p < 0.001$), interpersonal alienation ($t(89) = -3.21$, $p = 0.002$), interoceptive deficits ($t(89) = -3.78$, $p < 0.001$), emotional dysregulation ($t(89) = -3.47$, $p = 0.001$), and ascetism ($t(89) = -4.85$, $p < 0.001$). More specifically, students who are content with their weight have a lower drive for thinness, lower scores on bulimia, higher self-esteem, lower scores on personal and interpersonal alienation, lower interoceptive deficits and emotional dysregulation, lower scores on ascetism, and are more satisfied with their bodies comparative with students dissatisfied with their weight.

3.3.5. Environment

Environment is closely link to several aspects of nutrition (more healthy food, private gardeners with fruits and vegetables) and more religious people. The analysis of data focused on the relationship between environment and the consumption of food (vegetables, fruits) or respecting religious fasts.

The chi square test revealed no statistical difference between students from rural areas and those from urban areas according to whether they respect religious fasts or not ($\chi^2(2) = 3.716$, $p = 0.054$) or whether they eat fruits ($\chi^2(3) = 1.173$, $p = 0.759$) or vegetables ($\chi2(1) = 0.004$, $p = 0.951$) on a daily basis.

Regarding EDI-3 analysis of data, the Independent Samples t Test, reveled a significant difference between students from **rural** areas ($M = 15.59$) and those from urban areas ($M = 11.70$) concerning the interpersonal insecurity (II) subscale of the EDI-3 ($t(89) = -2.91$, $p = 0.004$). More specifically, students from rural area score higher on interpersonal insecurity (II) than those from urban areas.

3.3.6. BMI

One-way ANOVA was used in order to identify the statistically significant differences between BMI categories. Significant differences were identified between underweight ($M = 3.92$), normal weight ($M = 8.74$), and pre-obese ($M = 13.71$) participants regarding the subscale DT ($F(2.85) = 5.43$, $p = 0.006$). Multiple comparisons using the Bonferroni method showed a significant difference between underweight and pre-obese students, the first group having a lower drive for thinness than the last group.

Significant statistical differences were also identified between underweight ($M = 11.38$), normal weight ($M = 15.11$), and pre-obese ($M = 25.08$) participants concerning the body dissatisfaction (BD) subscale ($F(2.85) = 6.98$, $p = 0.002$). Underweight students had lower scores on body dissatisfaction than pre-obese participants, the latter obtained higher scores than the former.

Positive correlations were identified between BMI and drive for thinness ($r = 0.291$, $p < 0.001$), bulimia, ($r = 0.391$, $p < 0.001$), body dissatisfaction ($r = 0.447$, $p < 0.001$), and ascetism ($r = 0.246$, $p = 0.019$).

4. Discussion

The present study identified a weight of $M = 60.2 \pm 10.56$ (ranged from 42 to 105 kg) and 69% of students are normal weight. No obese persons were identified among the questioned students. Because no other study was lead on pharmacy students' weight-related aspects, no comparative analysis could be done considering other results on Romanian pharmacy students. A previous study lead on Romanian students from many specialties, developed in 2012, registered a lower $M = 54.3 \pm 4.7$ for investigated Romanian student population. At that time, the score was lower in comparison with German students, with an $M = 60.3 \pm 9.3$ [21].

For female participants, our sample had higher mean score on all subscales than those found among Romanian women. For men, the majority of mean scores were higher than those reported among men from Romania, with the exception of low self-esteem, interpersonal insecurity, interpersonal alienation, ascetism, and maturity fears, where the means were lower [20].

A study lead on Hungarian medical and pharmacy students showed a low administration of milk, fruits, and vegetables [22]. Similar results were found by Allen et al. focusing on Canadian pharmacy students, identifying that students' dietary habits were far below Canadians' Food Guide recommendations [23]. Interesting results targeting students in Egypt showed that there is an important effect of nutrition awareness and knowledge on health habits and performance among Egyptian pharmacy students, meaning that knowledge is not sufficient to stimulate students from Pharmacy to practice healthy habits, this must be doubled by nutrition awareness [24]. Complementary results were presented by Tiralongo and Wallis, who showed that Australian pharmacy students must internalize first information prior respecting nutritional alternatives [25].

Sleep has consequences on both physical and psychological health. The results regarding the duration of night sleep showed that questioned students had an M = 7 ± 1.02 h of sleep every night. *American Academy of Sleep Medicine* recommended for this category of age 7–9 h for an optimal health [26].

The studies lead on pharmacist students in USA [27], Malaysia [28], and Poland [29] or focusing on working pharmacists [30] revealed that there is a high rate of consumption of vitamins, minerals, or other supplements and rates are even higher compared to other medical specialties or other science studies. It is natural to think that students or health professionals who are well-trained in drugs and their effect on health to consume with precociousness these medications [27]. One raison for high rate for the consumption of supplements could be related to the fact that these medical specialists are trained to be more aware about the importance of nutritional status and they are able to evaluate the fact that skipping meals or consuming unhealthy food lead to an unbalanced nutritional status with negative consequences on health. This self-evaluation of their dietary behaviors doubled by the knowledge in drug's component could be a reason for a self-administration of medicines. This habit was identified among medical students by a lot of researches focusing on this population [31,32] and among working pharmacists, with or without presenting a chronic disease [33,34]. The rates of self-administration of dietary supplements among pharmacy students balanced in different studies between 20% in Japan [35] and 47% in USA [27].

Our study identified that over 40% of the students admitted to dieting to lose weight, a higher rate than those observed in other studies [36]. Our results concerning the positive correlation between three scales of the EDI-3 (specifically the drive for thinness, bulimia, and body dissatisfaction) and weight and BMI are in accordance with those found in the Romanian population, with the exception of the relationship between bulimia and weight, where we found no associations [20].

The results pointed out that higher BMIs are associated with higher score on body dissatisfaction. Similar results found by Jaworowska and Bazylak [37]. The authors identified a relatively low percentage of pharmacy students satisfied with their body weights (34.4% for female and 37.1% for male participants), despite the fact that they were not overweight or obese. As-Sa'edi et al. [38] also found, a low percentage of female medical students satisfied with their bodies (26.40%), while the rest perceived themselves as either to thin or too heavy and expressed a desire to lose weight. In our study, only students with high BMIs tend to have a higher drive for thinness.

Female students desire a significantly thinner figure than men [39] and that their ideal figure is underweight [6]. In our study, a high desire to be thin is usually associated with high BMI. Albertson et al. [40] showed that a self-compassion meditation training spanning a period of 3 weeks improved body satisfaction for women.

Another finding in our sample is that students with high BMIs tend to score high on the bulimia scale of EDI-3, suggesting that this group of students are at a higher risk of developing symptoms for bulimia. Findings from other studies [41] point to the fact that weight suppression has an important effect on bulimic symptoms and this association could be maintained by the preoccupation with thinness.

When comparing college students and eating disorder patients, findings showed that the latter have lower mean levels of self-esteem [42] and that students with greater positive body image have higher levels of self-esteem [43]. Research suggest that, when comparing individuals with eating disorders with individuals without eating disorders, the first group has a tendency towards perfectionism in maladaptive ways [44]. Our results that students who do not eat fruits have higher scores on perfectionism than those who eat fruits two times or three, four times a week, suggesting that perfectionism could have significant implications for health and well-being.

Also, the results showed that that students with high scores on ascetism tend to skip more main meals. The results are in concordance with Gamer's results [19]. The ascetic motive for weight loss was common in early writings on anorexia nervosa and is still an important theme in some cases.

The present findings showed that students who fast had lower scores than those who do not fast on interpersonal alienation. The majority of subjects were Christians, representing also the major religion in Romania. Fasting is respected in general by the religious persons. Meaning that subjects are closed to religious rules, are used to going to church and fulfilling dietary restrictions during festal times. The result that students who fast are presenting less personal alienation is in congruency with the majority of studies, showing that the practice of religion has positive effects on personal, familial, social life, and on health [45–47]. Some recent study showed that a high prevalence of religious practice was associated with overweight/obesity, especially among Christian women [48].

Results proved that students who used to eat during nights obtained higher scores on personal alienation, so they had a low level of self-esteem. These findings are in congruence with previous researches on night-eaters. Individuals who used to eat during nights had higher scores on depression and lower self-esteem and usually eat later in the morning and present sleeping disturbance [49]. Further research would be interesting to focus on night-eating syndrome, in order to identify this psycho-pathological problem among students.

Strength and Limitations of the Study

The strong points of the research are due to the fact that no study was lead before in pharmacy students in Romania and there are not many international studies focusing on this population.

The first limitation is due to the fact that pharmacy students were recruited from one single university, so results cannot be generalized for all pharmacy student population in Romania. The university is gathering persons from the north-eastern part of the country. Because some studies on this population found differences considering the native region of the participants, further researches could focus on it. The second limitation refers to the small number of male respondents, so a comparative analysis must be considered with precociousness. The third limitation is related to the fact that no psychological comorbidity was taken into consideration, like the presence of depressive syndrome or any psychiatric diseases. These factors could influence dietary habits or health-related behaviors (preferences for specific foods, odd preferences, compulsory eating, self-rewarding eating behaviors, etc.). For example, insomnia was associated with higher severity of disordered eating and studies showed that both insomnia and disordered eating symptoms were related to depression [50].

5. Conclusions

The results of the present study showed that eating disorders were identified having higher rates among pharmacy students than in general population in Romania. Considering some key factors like age, environment, fasting, sleeping, respecting main meals, or encouraging the consumption of fruits and vegetables could help students and university policy makers to promote healthier eating behaviors among pharmacy students.

Author Contributions: Conceptualization, M.I.; Methodology, M.I.; Software, M.I., I.D.M., I.M.; Investigation, I.M., L.P.; Writing—Original Draft Preparation, M.I., I.D.M.; Writing—Review & Editing, M.I., I.D.M.

Funding: This research received no external funding.

References

1. El Ansari, W.; Maxwell, A.E.; Mikolajczyk, R.T.; Stock, C.; Naydenova, V.; Krämer, A. Promoting public health: Benefits and challenges of a Europeanwide research consortium on student health. *Cent. Eur. J. Public Health* **2007**, *15*, 58–65. [PubMed]

2. El Ansari, W.; Stock, C.; Mikolajczyk, R.T. Relationships between food consumption and living arrangements among university students in four European countries-a cross-sectional study. *Nutr. J.* **2012**, *11*, 28. [CrossRef] [PubMed]

3. García-Meseguer, M.J.; Burriel, F.C.; García, C.V.; Serrano-Urrea, R. Adherence to Mediterranean diet in a Spanish university population. *Appetite* **2014**, *78*, 156–164. [CrossRef] [PubMed]

4. Small, M.; Bailey-Davis, L.; Morgan, N.; Maggs, J. Changes in eating and physical activity behaviors across seven semesters of college: Living on or off campus matters. *Health Educ. Behav.* **2013**, *40*, 435–441. [CrossRef] [PubMed]

5. Ganasegeran, K.; Al-Dubai, S.A.; Qureshi, A.M.; Al-Abed, A.A.A.; Rizal, A.M.; Aljunid, S.M. Social and psychological factors affecting eating habits among university students in a Malaysian medical school: A cross-sectional study. *Nutr. J.* **2012**, *11*, 48. [CrossRef] [PubMed]

6. Yahia, N.; Wang, D.; Rapley, M.; Dey, R. Assessment of weight status, dietary habits and beliefs, physical activity, and nutritional knowledge among university students. *Perspect. Public Health* **2016**, *136*, 231–244. [CrossRef] [PubMed]

7. Lupi, S.; Bagordo, F.; Stefanati, A.; Grassi, T.; Piccinni, L.; Bergamini, M.; Donno, A.D. Assessment of lifestyle and eating habits among undergraduate students in northern Italy. *Annali Dell'istituto Superiore di Sanita* **2015**, *51*, 154–161. [PubMed]

8. World Health Organization. *Technical Report Series, No. 916. Diet, Nutrition and the Prevention of Chronic Diseases*; Report of a Joint FAO/WHO Expert Consultation; World Health Organization: Geneva, Switzerland, 2003.

9. Vella-Zarb, R.A.; Elgar, F.J. The "freshman 5": A meta-analysis of weight gain in the freshman year of college. *J. Am. Coll. Health* **2009**, *58*, 161–166. [CrossRef] [PubMed]

10. Gores, S.E. Addressing nutritional issues in the college-aged client: Strategies for the nurse practitioner. *J. Am. Acad. Nurse Pract.* **2008**, *20*, 5–10. [CrossRef] [PubMed]

11. Boeing, H.; Bechthold, A.; Bub, A.; Ellinger, S.; Haller, D.; Kroke, A. Critical review: Vegetables and fruit in the prevention of chronic diseases. *Eur. J. Nutr.* **2012**, *51*, 637–663. [CrossRef] [PubMed]

12. World Health Organization. Promoting fruit and vegetable consumption around the world. In *Global Strategy on Diet, Physical Activity and Health*; World Health Organization: Geneva, Switzerland, 2003.

13. World Health Organization. *Body Mass Index*; World Health Organization: Geneva, Switzerland, 2014.

14. Chourdakis, M.; Tzellos, T.; Papazisis, G.; Toulis, K.; Kouvelas, D. Eating habits, health attitudes and obesity indices among medical students in northern Greece. *Appetite* **2010**, *55*, 722–725. [CrossRef] [PubMed]

15. Shah, T.; Purohit, G.; Nair, S.P.; Patel, B.; Rawal, Y.; Shah, R.M. Assessment of obesity, overweight and its association with the fast food consumption in medical students. *J. Clin. Diagn. Res JCDR* **2014**, *8*, CC05. [CrossRef] [PubMed]

16. Socolov, S.; Munteanu, C.; Alwan, S.; Soponaru, C.; Iorga, M. Socio-demographic characteristics, educational motivation and geo-cultural comfortability related to the process of adaptation of freshman international students in a Romanian university. *Med. Surg. J.* **2017**, *121*, 787–793.

17. Perez-Cueto, F.; Verbeke, W.; Lachat, C.; Remaut-De Winter, A.M. Changes in dietary habits following temporal migration. The case of international students in Belgium. *Appetite* **2009**, *52*, 83–88. [CrossRef] [PubMed]

18. Edwards, J.S.A.; Hartwell, H.L.; Brown, L. Changes in food neophobia and dietary habits of international students. *J. Hum. Nutr. Diet.* **2010**, *23*, 301–311. [CrossRef] [PubMed]

19. Garner, D.M.; Olmstead, M.P.; Polivy, J. Development and validation of a multidimensional eating disorder inventory for anorexia nervosa and bulimia. *Intern J. Eat. Dis.* **1983**, *2*, 15–34. [CrossRef]

20. Miclea, S.; Joja, O.; Albu, M. Studiul de adaptare şi standardizare a Inventarului tulburărilor de comportament alimentar (EDI-3) pe populaţia din România. In *Garner DM Manualul Inventarului Tulburărilor de Comportament Alimentar EDI-3*; SC Cognitrom SRL: Cluj-Napoca, România, 2011.

21. Joja, O.; Von Wietersheim, J. A cross-cultural comparison between EDI results of Romanian and German students. *Procedia Soc. Behav. Sci.* **2012**, *33*, 1037–1041. [CrossRef]

22. Biró, L.; Rabin, B.; Regöly-Mérei, A.; Nagy, K.; Pintér, B.; Beretvás, E.; Antal, M. Dietary habits of medical and pharmacy students at Semmelweis University, Budapest. *Acta Aliment.* **2005**, *34*, 463–471. [CrossRef]

23. Allen, J.P.; Taylor, J.G.; Rozwadowski, M.M.; Boyko, J.A.; Blackburn, D.F. Adherence to Canada's Food Guide among pharmacy students. *Can. Pharm. J. Rev. Pharm. Can.* **2011**, *144*, 79–84. [CrossRef]

24. El-Ahmady, S.; El-Wakeel, L. The Effects of Nutrition Awareness and Knowledge on Health Habits and Performance among Pharmacy Students in Egypt. *J. Community Health* **2017**, *42*, 213–220. [CrossRef] [PubMed]

25. Tiralongo, E.; Wallis, M. Attitudes and perceptions of Australian pharmacy students towards Complementary and Alternative Medicine—A pilot study. *BMC Complement. Altern. Med.* **2008**, *8*, 2. [CrossRef] [PubMed]

26. Paruthi, S.; Brooks, L.J.; D'Ambrosio, C.; Hall, W.A.; Kotagal, S.; Lloyd, R.M.; Malow, B.A.; Maski, K.; Nichols, C.; Quan, S.F.; et al. Consensus Statement of the American Academy of Sleep Medicine on the Recommended Amount of Sleep for Healthy Children: Methodology and Discussion. *J. Clin. Sleep Med.* **2016**, *12*, 1549–1561. [CrossRef] [PubMed]

27. Rabinowitz, J.; Heppard, D., Jr.; Pearen, B.N. Use of vitamin and mineral supplements by pharmacy students. *Am. J. Hosp. Pharm.* **1993**, *50*, 674–678.

28. Al-Naggar, R.A.; Chen, R. Prevalence of vitamin-mineral supplements use and associated factors among young Malaysians. *Asian Pac. J. Cancer Prev.* **2011**, *12*, 1023–1029. [PubMed]

29. Jaworowska, A.; Bazylak, G. Residental factors affecting nutrient intake and nutritional status of female pharmacy students in Bydgoszcz. *Roczniki Panstwowego Zakladu Higieny* **2007**, *58*, 245–251. [PubMed]

30. Gardiner, P.; Woods, C.; Kemper, K.J. Dietary supplement use among health care professionals enrolled in an online curriculum on herbs and dietary supplements. *BMC Complement. Altern. Med.* **2006**, *6*, 21. [CrossRef] [PubMed]

31. Iorga, M.; Soponaru, C.; Ciuhodaru, T. The Influence of Medical Knowledge on Self-Medication among Nursing Students. In Proceedings of the Edulearn16 8th International Conference on Education and New Learning Technologies, Barcelona, Spain, 4–6 July 2016; pp. 3713–3720.

32. Gavrilescu, I.M.; Dondas, C.; Munteanu, C.; Socolov, S.; Pantilimonescu, T.; Iorga, M. Psychological Profile of Freshman Pharmacy Students. *Med. Surg. J.* **2017**, *121*, 770–778.

33. Iorga, M.; Dondaş, C.; Soponaru, C.; Antofie, I. Determinants of Hospital Pharmacists' Job Satisfaction in Romanian Hospitals. *Pharmacy* **2017**, *5*, 66. [CrossRef] [PubMed]

34. Iorga, M.; Dondas, C.; Sztankovszky, L.Z.; Antofie, I. Burnout Syndrome among Hospital Pharmacists in Romania. *Farmacia* **2018**, *66*, 181–188.

35. Shimizu, R.; Sakamoto, Y.; Nishizawa, T.; Iguchi, S.; Yamaoka, Y. Survey of current conditions regarding awareness of the nutritional role of supplements for pharmacy students. *Yakugaku Zasshi J. Pharm. Soc. Jpn.* **2007**, *127*, 1461–1471. [CrossRef]

36. Tavolacci, M.P.; Grigioni, S.; Richard, L.; Meyrignac, G.; Déchelotte, P.; Ladner, J. Eating Disorders and Associated Health Risks Among University Students. *J. Nutr. Educ. Behav.* **2015**, *47*, 412–420. [CrossRef] [PubMed]

37. Jaworowska, A.; Bazylak, G. An outbreak of body weight dissatisfaction associated with self-perceived BMI and dieting among female pharmacy students. *Biomed. Pharmacother.* **2009**, *63*, 679–692. [CrossRef] [PubMed]

38. As-Sa'edi, E.; Sheerah, S.; Al-Ayoubi, R.; Al-Jehani, A.; Tajaddin, W.; Hanan Habeeb, H. Body image dissatisfaction: Prevalence and relation to body mass index among female medical students in Taibah University. *J. Taibah Univ. Med. Sci.* **2013**, *8*, 126–133.

39. Zaccagni, L.; Masotti, S.; Donati, R.; Mazzoni, G.; Gualdi-Russo, E. Body image and weight perceptions in relation to actual measurements by means of a new index and level of physical activity in Italian university students. *J. Transl. Med.* **2014**, *12*, 42. [CrossRef] [PubMed]

40. Albertson, A.M.; Reicks, M.l.; Joshi, N.; Gugger, C.K. Whole grain consumption trends and associations with body weight measures in the United States: Results from the cross sectional National Health and Nutrition Examination Survey 2001–2012. *Nutr. J.* **2015**, *15*, 8. [CrossRef] [PubMed]

41. Bodell, L.P.; Brown, T.A.; Keel, P.K. Weight suppression predicts bulimic symptoms at 20-year follow-up: The mediating role of drive for thinness. *J. Abnorm. Psychol.* **2017**, *126*, 32–37. [CrossRef] [PubMed]

42. Kelly, A.C.; Vimalakanthan, K.; Carter, J.C. Understanding the roles of self-esteem, self-compassion, and fear of self-compassion in eating disorder pathology: An examination of female students and eating disorder patients. *Eat. Behav.* **2014**, *15*, 388–391. [CrossRef] [PubMed]

43. Gillen, M.M. Associations between positive body image and indicators of men's and women's mental and physical health. *Body Image* **2015**, *13*, 67–74. [CrossRef] [PubMed]

44. Ashby, J.S.; Kottman, T.; Schoen, E. Perfectionism and eating disorders reconsidered. *J. Ment. Health Couns.* **1998**, *20*, 261–271.

45. Alcorta, C. Religion, social signaling, and health: A psychoneuroimmunological approach. *Relig. Brain Behav.* **2017**, *7*, 243–246. [CrossRef]

46. Lucchetti, G.; Lucchetti, A.L.G. Spirituality, religion, and health: Over the last 15 years of field research (1999–2013). *Intern. J. Psychol. Med.* **2014**, *48*, 199–215. [CrossRef] [PubMed]

47. Scott, R. Religion benefits health. *Br. J. Gen. Pract.* **2014**, *64*, 353. [CrossRef] [PubMed]

48. Peltzer, K.; Pengpid, S.; Samuels, T.; Özcan, N.K.; Mantilla, C.; Rahamefy, O.H.; Gasparishvili, A. Prevalence of overweight/obesity and its associated factors among university students from 22 countries. *Int. J. Environ. Res. Public Health* **2014**, *11*, 7425–7441. [CrossRef] [PubMed]

49. Gluck, M.E.; Geliebter, A.; Satov, T. Night eating syndrome is associated with depression, low self-esteem, reduced daytime hunger, and less weight loss in obese outpatients. *Obes. Res.* **2001**, *9*, 264–267. [CrossRef] [PubMed]

50. Lombardo, C.; Battagliese, G.; Baglioni, C.; David, M.; Violani, C.; Riemann, D. Severity of insomnia, disordered eating symptoms, and depression in female university students. *Clin. Psychol.* **2014**, *18*, 108–115. [CrossRef]

Permissions

All chapters in this book were first published in PHARMACY, by MDPI; hereby published with permission under the Creative Commons Attribution License or equivalent. Every chapter published in this book has been scrutinized by our experts. Their significance has been extensively debated. The topics covered herein carry significant findings which will fuel the growth of the discipline. They may even be implemented as practical applications or may be referred to as a beginning point for another development.

The contributors of this book come from diverse backgrounds, making this book a truly international effort. This book will bring forth new frontiers with its revolutionizing research information and detailed analysis of the nascent developments around the world.

We would like to thank all the contributing authors for lending their expertise to make the book truly unique.

They have played a crucial role in the development of this book. Without their invaluable contributions this book wouldn't have been possible. They have made vital efforts to compile up to date information on the varied aspects of this subject to make this book a valuable addition to the collection of many professionals and students.

This book was conceptualized with the vision of imparting up-to-date information and advanced data in this field. To ensure the same, a matchless editorial board was set up. Every individual on the board went through rigorous rounds of assessment to prove their worth. After which they invested a large part of their time researching and compiling the most relevant data for our readers.

The editorial board has been involved in producing this book since its inception. They have spent rigorous hours researching and exploring the diverse topics which have resulted in the successful publishing of this book. They have passed on their knowledge of decades through this book. To expedite this challenging task, the publisher supported the team at every step. A small team of assistant editors was also appointed to further simplify the editing procedure and attain best results for the readers.

Apart from the editorial board, the designing team has also invested a significant amount of their time in understanding the subject and creating the most relevant covers. They scrutinized every image to scout for the most suitable representation of the subject and create an appropriate cover for the book.

The publishing team has been an ardent support to the editorial, designing and production team. Their endless efforts to recruit the best for this project, has resulted in the accomplishment of this book. They are a veteran in the field of academics and their pool of knowledge is as vast as their experience in printing. Their expertise and guidance has proved useful at every step. Their uncompromising quality standards have made this book an exceptional effort. Their encouragement from time to time has been an inspiration for everyone.

The publisher and the editorial board hope that this book will prove to be a valuable piece of knowledge for researchers, students, practitioners and scholars across the globe.

List of Contributors

Andries Koster
Department of Pharmaceutical Sciences, Utrecht University, The Netherlands and European Association of Faculties of Pharmacy (EAFP), Utrecht 3508 TB, The Netherlands

Tom Schalekamp
Department of Pharmaceutical Sciences, Utrecht University, Utrecht 3508 TB, The Netherlands

Irma Meijerman
Department of Pharmaceutical Sciences, The Netherlands and Centre for Teaching and Learning, Utrecht University, Utrecht 3508 TB, The Netherlands

Marie Barnard, Donna West-Strum, Yi Yang and Erin Holmes
Department of Pharmacy Administration, School of Pharmacy, University of Mississippi, 223 Faser Hall, University, MS 38677, USA

Maria Gustafsson and Sofia Mattsson
Department of Pharmacology and Clinical Neuroscience, Umeå University, SE-90187 Umeå, Sweden

Gisselle Gallego
School of Medicine, The University of Notre Dame, New South Wales 2010, Australia

Roland N. Dickerson, G. Christopher Wood, Joseph M. Swanson and Rex O. Brown
Department of Clinical Pharmacy and Translational Science, University of Tennessee College of Pharmacy, 881 Madison Ave., Memphis, TN 38163, USA

Lakhan Kanji, Sensen Xu and Afonso Cavaco
Department of Social Pharmacy, Faculty of Pharmacy, University of Lisbon, Av. Prof. Gama Pinto, 1649-003 Lisboa, Portugal

Melissa S. Medina
College of Pharmacy, The University of Oklahoma, 1110 N Stonewall Ave, Oklahoma City, OK 73117, USA

Shamima Khan
CRE Services, Inc., 1560 Broadway, Suite 812, New York, NY 10036, USA

Joshua J. Spooner
College of Pharmacy and Health Sciences, Western New England University, 1215Wilbraham Road, Springfield, MA 01119, USA

Harlan E. Spotts
College of Business, Western New England University, 1215 Wilbraham Road, Springfield, MA 01119, USA

Marita Barrett, Anna Keating and Deirdre Lynch
Pharmacy Department, Cork University Hospital, Cork T12 DC4A, Ireland

Geraldine Scanlon, Mary Kigathi and Fidelma Corcoran
Adult Mental Health Unit, Cork University Hospital, Cork T12 DC4A, Ireland

Laura J. Sahm
School of Pharmacy, University College Cork, Cork T12 YN60, Ireland
Pharmacy Department, Mercy University Hospital, Cork T12 WE28, Ireland

Lee Baker
Amayeza Info Services, Johannesburg 1709, South Africa

Jordan R. Covvey, Anthony J. Guarascio, Lauren A. O'Donnell and Kevin J. Tidgewell
Duquesne University School of Pharmacy, 600 Forbes Ave, Pittsburgh, PA 15282, USA

Sasikala Chinnappan
Department of Life Sciences, International Medical University, Kuala Lumpur 57000, Malaysia

Palanisamy Sivanandy
Department of Pharmacy Practice, International Medical University, Kuala Lumpur 57000, Malaysia

Rajenthina Sagaran
School of Pharmacy, La Trobe University, Bendigo 3552, Australia

Nagashekhara Molugulu
Department of Pharmaceutical Technology, International Medical University, Kuala Lumpur 57000, Malaysia

Cheryl D. Cropp and Jennifer Beall
McWhorter School of Pharmacy, Samford University, 800 Lakeshore Drive, Birmingham, AL 35229, USA

Ellen Buckner and Amanda Barron
Ida Moffett School of Nursing, Samford University, 800 Lakeshore Drive, Birmingham, AL 35229, USA

Frankie Wallis
University of Alabama at Birmingham Hospital, NP1333, 1802 6th Avenue South, Birmingham, AL 35249-7010, USA

Akshaya Srikanth Bhagavathula and Yonas Getaye Tefera
Department of Clinical Pharmacy, University of Gondar-College of Medicine and Health Sciences, School of Pharmacy, Gondar 196, Ethiopia

Deepak Kumar Bandari
Department of Clinical Pharmacy, Vaagdevi College of Pharmacy, Warangal 506001, Telangana, India

Shazia Qasim Jamshed
Department of Pharmacy Practice, Kulliyyah of Pharmacy, International Islamic University Malaysia, Kuantan 25200, Pahang, Malaysia

Asim Ahmed Elnour
Faculty of Pharmacy, Fathima College of Health Sciences, Al Ain Campus, Al Ain 24162, UAE

Abdulla Shehab
Department of Internal Medicine, College of Medicine and Health Sciences, UAE University, Al Ain 17666, UAE

Tanja Gmeiner, Nejc Horvat, Mitja Kos, Aleš Obreza, Tomaž Vovk, Iztok Grabnar and Borut Božič
Faculty of Pharmacy, University of Ljubljana, Askerčeva 7, 1000 Ljubljana, Slovenia

Michelle Bones
Department of Veterans Affairs, Voluntary Service, 1601 Kirkwood Highway, Wilmington, DE 19805 USA

Martin Nunlee
Department of Business Administration, College of Business, Delaware State University, 1200 North Dupont Highway, Dover, DE 19901-2277, USA

Saima Mahmood Malhi, Hassan Raza, Kiran Ajmal, Sumbul Shamim, Saniya Ata, Salman Farooq, Syed Muhammad Sharib and Sidrat-ul Muntaha
Faculty of Pharmaceutical Sciences, Dow College of Pharmacy, Dow University of Health Sciences, OJHA Campus, Karachi 74200, Pakistan

Brenna Shearer
College of Pharmacy, Faculty of Health Sciences, University of Manitoba, Winnipeg, MB R3E 0T5, Canada
Independent Researcher Pharmacists Manitoba, Winnipeg, MB R3C 4H1, Canada

Sheila Ng, Drena Dunford and I fan Kuo
College of Pharmacy, Faculty of Health Sciences, University of Manitoba, Winnipeg, MB R3E 0T5, Canada

Weixiang Zhang, Hao Zhong, Yitao Wang, Ging Chan, Yuanjia Hu, Hao Hu and Defang Ouyang
State Key Laboratory of Quality Research in Chinese Medicine, Institute of Chinese Medical Sciences (ICMS), University of Macau, Taipa, Macau, China

Fay Al-Kudhairi
Department of Pharmacy, University Hospital Lewisham, Lewisham High St, London SE13 6LH, UK

Reem Kayyali and Vilius Savickas
Department of Pharmacy, Faculty of Science, Engineering and Computing, Kingston University, Kingston-Upon-Thames KT1 2EE, UK

Neel Sharma
Division of Gastroenterology and Hepatology, National University Hospital Singapore, 5 Lower Kent Ridge Rd, Singapore 119074, Singapore

Magdalena Iorga and Iulia-Diana Muraru
Department of Behavioral Sciences, Faculty of Medicine, University of Medicine and Pharmacy "Grigore T. Popa" of Iasi, Iasi 700115, Romania

Isabela Manole
Faculty of Pharmacy, University of Medicine and Pharmacy "Grigore T. Popa" of Iasi, Iasi 700115, Romania

Lavinia Pop
Nutrition and Dietetics, Faculty of Medicine, University of Medicine and Pharmacy "Grigore T. Popa" of Iasi, Iasi 700117, Romania

Florin-Dumitru Petrariu
Department of Preventive Medicine and Interdisciplinarity, Faculty of Medicine, University of Medicine and Pharmacy "Grigore T. Popa" of Iasi, Iasi 700115, Romania

Index